Obstetric Intervention

Obstetric Interventions

Edited by

P. Joep Dörr
Formerly of HMC Haaglanden Medical Centre, Westeinde, The Hague, the Netherlands

Vincent M. Khouw
VMK Designs, Utrecht, the Netherlands

Frank A. Chervenak
Department of Obstetrics and Gynecology, Weill Cornell Medical Center, New York, USA

Amos Grunebaum
Department of Obstetrics and Gynecology, Weill Cornell Medical Center, New York, USA

Yves Jacquemyn
Department of Obstetrics and Gynecology, Antwerp University Hospital, Edegem, Belgium

Jan G. Nijhuis
Department of Obstetrics and Gynecology, Maastricht University Medical Centre, Maastricht, the Netherlands

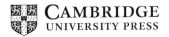
CAMBRIDGE
UNIVERSITY PRESS

CAMBRIDGE
UNIVERSITY PRESS

University Printing House, Cambridge CB2 8BS, United Kingdom

Cambridge University Press is part of the University of Cambridge.

It furthers the University's mission by disseminating knowledge in the pursuit of education, learning, and research at the highest international levels of excellence.

www.cambridge.org
Information on this title: www.cambridge.org/9781316632567

© Cambridge University Press 2017

First published 2017

Printed in the United Kingdom by Clays, St Ives plc

A catalogue record for this publication is available from the British Library

Library of Congress Cataloguing in Publication data
Dorr, P.J. (P. Joep), –2014, editor.
Obstetric interventions / edited by P.J. Dorr, V.M. Khouw, F.A. Chervenak, A. Grunebaum, Y. Jacquemyn, J.G. Nijhuis.
Obstetrische interventies. English
Cambridge, United Kingdom ; New York : Cambridge University Press, 2017. | Translation of the Obstetrische interventies / redactie P. Joep Dörr, Vincent M. Khouw, Yves Jacquemyn, Frank A. Chervenak, Jan G. Nijhuis ; tekeningen: Vincent M. Khouw. Derde druk. 2014. Translated by Robert Croese. | Includes bibliographical references and index.
LCCN 2016057369 | ISBN 9781316632567 (alk. paper)
| MESH: Obstetric Labor Complications – surgery | Obstetric Surgical Procedures
LCC RG701 | NLM WQ 330 | DDC 618.5–dc23
LC record available at https://lccn.loc.gov/2016057369

ISBN 978-1-316-63256-7 Mixed Media
ISBN 978-1-316-63258-1 Paperback
ISBN 978-1-316-85028-2 Cambridge Core

Additional resources for this publication at www.cambridge.org/9781316632567

....

Contents

Animations

Animations will appear in the online version of this title on Cambridge Core.

Contributors

H.J. van Beekhuizen, MD, PhD
Department of Obstetrics and Gynecology, Erasmus University Medical Centre, Rotterdam, the Netherlands

P.P. van den Berg, MD, PhD
Department of Obstetrics and Gynecology, Groningen University Medical Centre, Groningen, the Netherlands

H.W. Bruinse, MD, PhD
Former Professor of Clinical Obstetrics, Department of Obstetrics and Gynecology, Utrecht University Medical Centre, Utrecht, the Netherlands

F.A. Chervenak, MD
Department of Obstetrics and Gynecology, Weill Cornell Medical Center, New York, USA

J.B. Derks, MD, PhD
Department of Obstetrics and Gynecology, Utrecht University Medical Centre, Utrecht, the Netherlands

J. van Dillen, MD, PhD
Department of Obstetrics and Gynecology, Radboud University Nijmegen Medical Centre, Nijmegen, the Netherlands

M. van Dillen-Putman, midwife
Department of Obstetrics and Gynecology, Radboud University Nijmegen Medical Centre, Nijmegen, the Netherlands

P.J. Dörr, MD, PhD
Gynaecologist, formerly of HMC Haaglanden Medical Centre, The Hague, the Netherlands; Professor, formerly of Department of Education and Teaching, Leiden University Medical Centre, Leiden, the Netherlands

F.M. van Dunné, MD, PhD
Department of Obstetrics and Gynecology, Medical Centre Haaglanden, The Hague, the Netherlands

J.J. Duvekot, MD, PhD
Department of Obstetrics and Gynecology, Erasmus University Medical Centre, Rotterdam, the Netherlands

G.G.M. Essed, MD, PhD
Former Gynaecologist, Department of Obstetrics and Gynecology, Maastricht University Medical Centre, Maastricht, the Netherlands; Anton de Kom University of Suriname, Paramaribo, Suriname

A. Grunebaum, MD
Department of Obstetrics and Gynecology, Weill Cornell Medical Center, New York, USA

W.J.A. Gyselaers, MD, PhD
Department of Obstetrics and Gynecology, East Limburg Hospital, Genk, Belgium

M. Hanssens, MD, PhD
Department of Obstetrics and Gynecology, University Hospital, Leuven, Belgium

K.M. Heetkamp, MSc
The School of Midwifery at the Rotterdam University of Applied Sciences, Rotterdam, the Netherlands

Y. Jacquemyn, MD, PhD
Department of Obstetrics and Gynecology, Antwerp University Hospital, Edegem, Belgium

S. Keizer, midwife
Midwifery Practice Mundo Midwives, The Hague, the Netherlands

V.M. Khouw, MSc
VMK Designs, Utrecht, the Netherlands

M. Kok, MD, PhD
Department of Obstetrics and Gynecology, Academic Medical Centre, Amsterdam, the Netherlands

M. Laubach, MD
Department of Obstetrics, University Hospital Brussels, Brussels, Belgium

J.P. de Leeuw, MD, PhD
Former Gynaecologist, Alrijne Hospital, Leiderdorp, the Netherlands

F.K. Lotgering, MD, PhD
Department of Obstetrics and Gynecology, Utrecht University Medical Centre, Utrecht, the Netherlands

L.B. McCullough, PhD
Center for Medical Ethics and Health Policy, Baylor College of Medicine, Houston, USA

W. Mingelen, MD
Department of Obstetrics and Gynecology, HMC Haaglanden Medical Centre, The Hague, the Netherlands

J.G. Nijhuis, MD, PhD
Department of Obstetrics and Gynecology, Maastricht University Medical Centre, Maastricht, the Netherlands

S.G. Oei, MD, PhD
Department of Obstetrics and Gynecology, Maxima Medical Centre, Veldhoven; Eindhoven University of Technology, Eindhoven, the Netherlands

E. Roets, MD
Department of Obstetrics and Gynecology, University Hospital Ghent, Ghent, Belgium

J. van Roosmalen, MD, PhD
Department of Obstetrics and Gynecology, Leiden University Medical Centre, Leiden, the Netherlands

M.C. de Ruiter, MD, PhD
Department of Obstetrics and Gynecology, Leiden University Medical Centre, Leiden, the Netherlands

J.H. Schagen van Leeuwen, MD, PhD
Department of Obstetrics and Gynecology, St. Antonius Hospital, Nieuwegein, the Netherlands

H.C.J. Scheepers, MD, PhD
Department of Obstetrics and Gynecology, Maastricht University Medical Centre, Maastricht, the Netherlands

S.A. Scherjon, MD, PhD
Department of Obstetrics and Gynecology, Groningen University Medical Centre, Groningen, the Netherlands

A.J. Schneider, MD, PhD
Department of Obstetrics and Gynecology, Erasmus University Medical Centre, Rotterdam, the Netherlands

H.W. Torij, MSc
Rotterdam University of Applied Sciences, Rotterdam, the Netherlands

A.T.M. Verhoeven, MD, PhD
Former Gynaecologist, Rijnstate Hospital, Arnhem, the Netherlands

M.E. Vierhout, MD, PhD
Department of Obstetrics and Gynecology, Radboud University Nijmegen Medical Centre, Nijmegen, the Netherlands

M. Weemhoff, MD, PhD
Department of Obstetrics and Gynecology, Zuyderland Medical Centre, Heerlen, the Netherlands

B. Wibbens, MD
Department of Obstetrics and Gynecology, Amstelland Hospital, Amstelveen, the Netherlands

C. Willekes, MD, PhD
Department of Obstetrics and Gynecology, Maastricht University Medical Centre, Maastricht, the Netherlands

Preface

This past century has seen significant changes in obstetrics due to dramatic technological advances. More often than not these changes have led to positive improvements in antepartum and intrapartum care. Nonetheless, a timeless challenge for all providers continues to be how to best take care of a pregnant woman and her soon to be born child on labor and delivery.

The purpose of this book is to merge traditional obstetrics with what we have learned through technology and evidence-based medicine illustrated by state of the art 3D illustrations and animations.

Too often tradition and local customs have determined our approach to labor and delivery management and training. It is essential today that management and training are based on the best available evidence so that optimal care can be given to pregnant women and soon to be born children. Each chapter in our text is referenced by a comprehensive literature review seeking the best available international evidence.

The anatomy chapter lays the foundation for the book, by explicating the passage of the child through the birth canal during normal and pathological childbirth. Animations are used to further clarify the different birth mechanisms. Throughout the book we provide insight into the mechanisms of normal childbirth and the choices of obstetric interventions in the delivery room and operating room using text, 3D drawings, and animations. This combination gives our book a unique perspective. We also discuss the important topic of ethical dimensions of the birth process including the crucial aspect of informed consent.

Furthermore, by using the code that comes with the book, one can open the 3D animations, which are even more powerful than the static pictures alone.

The first two editions of this book were based on a Dutch initiative and therefore written in Dutch. However, because obstetrics in the twenty-first century has truly become a global enterprise, we decided to have international collaboration as maternal and perinatal morbidity and mortality are a global problem. We hope that this book will facilitate education and help all those who care for pregnant women and their children throughout the world to improve their basic understanding of the birth process and understand and prevent potential complications that can arise.

It is very sad that the initiator of this project, Joep Dörr, died in 2014, just before the book was completely ready. We have honored him by keeping his name as first author on this edition.

P. Joep Dörr
Vincent M. Khouw
Frank A. Chervenak
Amos Grunebaum
Yves Jacquemyn
Jan G. Nijhuis

Classification of Evidence Levels

LE A1: Systematic reviews covering at least some A2-level studies, in which the results of the individual studies are consistent

LE A2: Randomized comparative clinical studies of good quality, sufficient size, and consistency

LE B: Randomized clinical trials of moderate quality or insufficient size, or other comparative studies (non-randomized, comparative cohort study, patient–control study)

LE C: Non-comparative study

LE D: Expert opinion

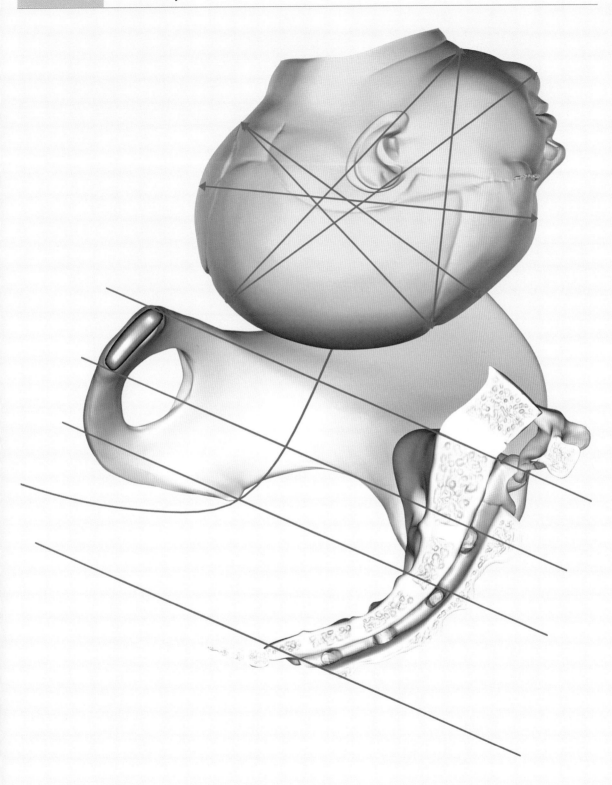

Anatomy

P.J. Dörr, S. Keizer, M. Weemhoff, M.C. de Ruiter, and V.M. Khouw

Introduction

Knowledge of the anatomy, the fetal skull, and the bony and soft-tissue birth canal is required to understand the passage of the infant through the birth canal in either normal or pathological birth.

To produce the graphic figures depicting the fetal skull and the birth canal, the authors used many atlases and textbooks. The most important publications are listed in the bibliography.[1-3]

Fetal Skull

The five skull bones (the two frontal bones, the two parietal bones, and the one occipital bone) of the fetus are not joined together yet, but separated from each other by sutures and fontanels (Figure 1.1).

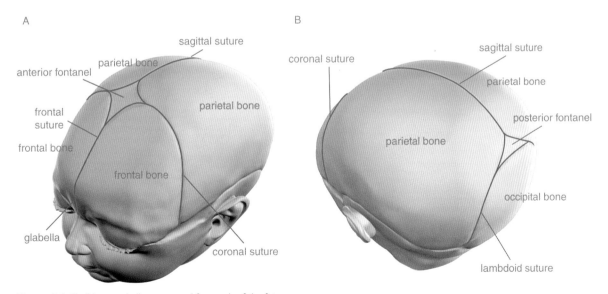

Figure 1.1 Skull bones, skull sutures, and fontanels of the fetus.

Obstetric Interventions, ed. P. Joep Dörr, Vincent M. Khouw, Frank A. Chervenak, Amos Grunebaum, Yves Jacquemyn, and Jan G. Nijhuis. Published by Cambridge University Press. © Cambridge University Press 2017.

The fetal skull is malleable since the parietal bones can slide over the frontal bones and the occipital bone: this is called molding (or moulage). Molding allows the skull to adapt to the birth canal.

The sutures and fontanels can be determined through internal examination for the orientation (attitude and position) of the head in the true pelvis. The posterior fontanel (triangular), the sagittal suture, and the anterior fontanel (diamond-shaped) are crucial orientation points in this examination (Figure 1.2).

The most important skull dimensions are shown in Table 1.1 and Figure 1.3.

Table 1.1 Skull dimensions

Distance (d.) and circumference (c.)	cm	From – to	Presentation
d. suboccipitobregmatic	9.5–10	Neck – middle anterior fontanel	Occiput presentation with maximum flexion
c. suboccipitobregmatic	32–33		
d. suboccipitofrontal	10	Neck – forehead	Normal occiput presentation
c. suboccipitofrontal	34		
d. fronto-occipital	12	Glabella – back of head	Sinciput presentation
c. fronto-occipital	34–35		
d. mento-occipital	13.5–14	Chin – back of head	Brow presentation
c. mento-occipital	35		
d. submentobregmatic	9.5	Lower jaw – middle anterior fontanel	Facial presentation
c. submentobregmatic	34		
d. biparietal	9.5	Greatest transverse diameter	
d. bitemporal	8–8.5	Smallest transverse diameter	

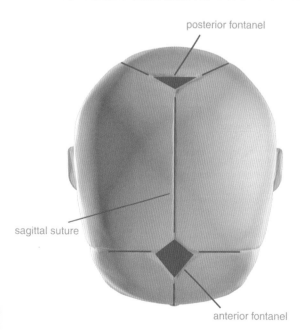

posterior fontanel

sagittal suture

anterior fontanel

Figure 1.2 Fontanels and sagittal suture.

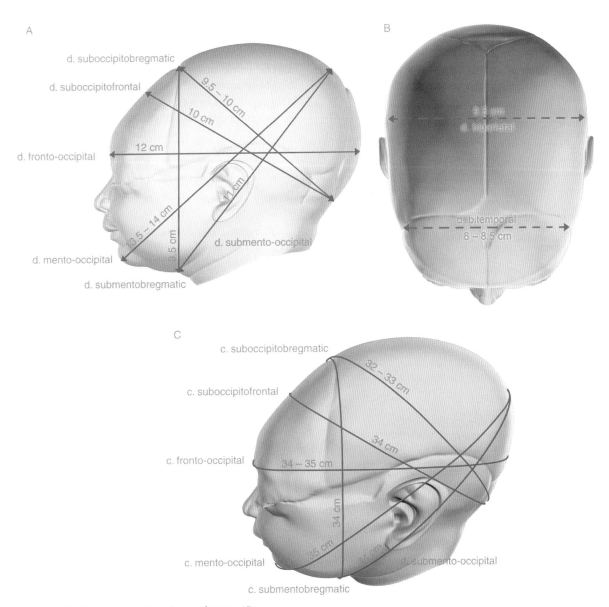

A

d. suboccipitobregmatic

d. suboccipitofrontal

9.5 – 10 cm

10 cm

12 cm

d. fronto-occipital

11 cm

9.5 – 14 cm

9.5 cm

d. mento-occipital

d. submento-occipital

d. submentobregmatic

B

9.5 cm
d. biparietal

d. bitemporal
8 – 8.5 cm

C

c. suboccipitobregmatic

32 – 33 cm

c. suboccipitofrontal

34 cm

c. fronto-occipital

34 – 35 cm

34 cm

35 cm

c. mento-occipital

c. submento-occipital

c. submentobregmatic

Figure 1.3A–C Distances (A, B) and circumferences (C).

Birth Canal

The birth canal consists of:

- *the bony birth canal:* the true pelvis;
- *the soft-tissue birth canal:* the lower uterine segment, the cervix, the vagina, the vulva, and the pelvic floor musculature.

The Bony Birth Canal

The bony pelvis consists of the two innominate or hip bones, the sacrum, and the coccyx. The innominate bones consist of the ilium, the ischium, and the pubic bone. Anteriorly, the pubic bones are conjoined by the pubic symphysis. Posteriorly, the ilium bones are conjoined to the sacrum by means of the sacroiliac joints. The sacrum is connected to the coccyx by means of the sacrococcygeal joint. During pregnancy, a slight and individually varying relaxation occurs to the connective tissue of the pubic symphysis and the sacroiliac joints. Because of this relaxation, more room is created in the pelvis (Figure 1.4).

The boundary between the false and the – obstetrically more important – true pelvis is formed by the plane of the (true) pelvic inlet. The true

5

pelvis has different dimensions at different points. The plane of the midpelvis, with the ischial spines as reference points, has the smallest diameter. The plane of the pelvic inlet has a transverse oval

shape. The plane of the pelvic outlet has an oval shape in anteroposterior direction (Table 1.2, Figures 1.5 and 1.6).

The pelvic axis passes through the midpoints of the above-mentioned planes. This central axis of the birth canal runs in a straight line from the pelvic inlet to the midpelvis and then bends at an angle of approximately 90° around the pubic symphysis to the pelvic outlet (Figure 1.7).

Table 1.2 Pelvic planes

Plane	Boundaries: F(ront), L(ateral), B(ack)	Dimensions (cm): F(ront), B(ack), Tr(ansverse)
Pelvic inlet	F: upper edge of pubic symphysis L: innominate line B: promontory	FB: 10.5–11.5 Tr: 13
Maximum pelvic breadth	F: middle posterior plane of pubic symphysis L: obturator foramen B: third sacral vertebra	FB: 12–13 Tr: 12–13
Midpelvis	F: lower edge of pubic symphysis L: ischial spine B: boundary of fourth/fifth sacral vertebra	FB: 11–12 Tr: 10.5–11.5
Pelvic outlet Two triangles	Anterior triangle: F: lower edge of pubic symphysis L: ischial tuberosity Posterior triangle: L: ischial tuberosity B: sacrococcygeal joint	FB: 9.5–12 Tr: 11–12

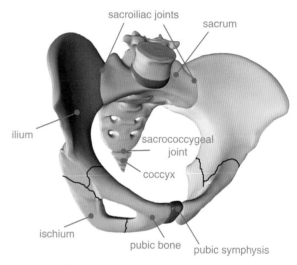

Figure 1.4 Pelvis.

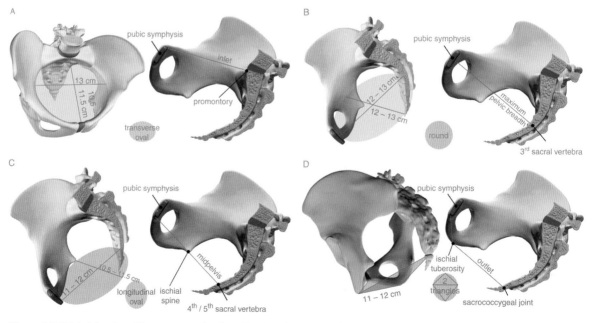

Figure 1.5 Pelvic inlet plane (A), maximum pelvic breadth (B), midpelvis (C), pelvic outlet (D).

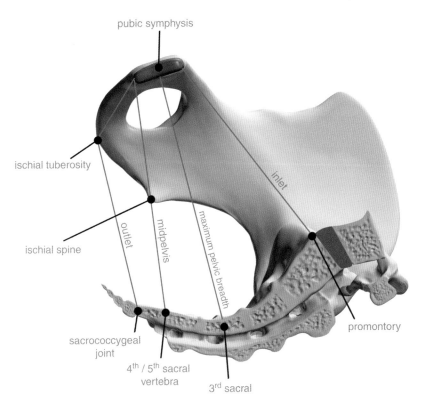

pubic symphysis

ischial tuberosity

ischial spine

inlet

maximum pelvic breadth

midpelvis

outlet

promontory

sacrococcygeal joint

4th / 5th sacral vertebra

3rd sacral

Figure 1.6 Pelvic planes.

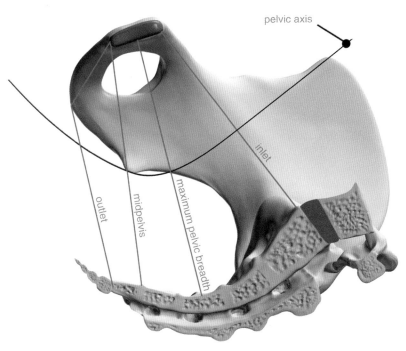

pelvic axis

inlet

maximum pelvic breadth

midpelvis

outlet

Figure 1.7 Pelvic axis.

Engagement of the presenting part is determined by the lower-most engaged presenting (bony) part of the infant (the head in a cephalic presentation) relative to the true pelvis. For this purpose, the true pelvis is divided into four parallel planes: the planes of Hodge (Table 1.3 and Figure 1.8).

In the English-language literature, the engagement of the presenting part is described relative to the ischial spines. The level of the interspinal line (Hodge 3) is referred to as the "zero (0) station." The indication of

Table 1.3 Planes of Hodge classification

Plane of Hodge	Position in the true pelvis
Hodge 1	Plane of the pelvic inlet
Hodge 2	Plane parallel to H1, through the lower edge of the pubic symphysis
Hodge 3	Plane parallel to H1 and H2, through the ischial spines
Hodge 4	Plane parallel to H1, H2, and H3, through the sacrococcygeal joint

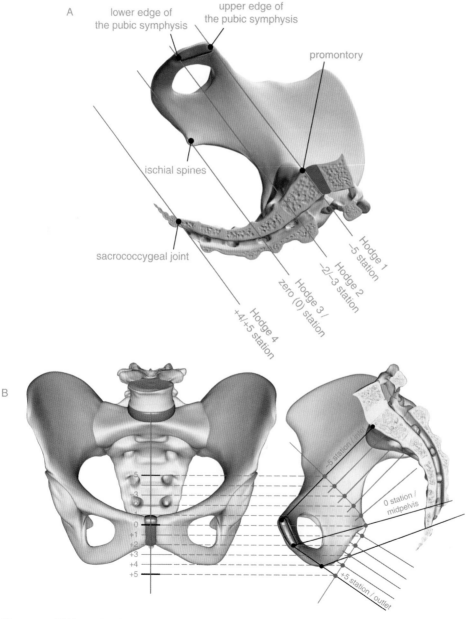

Figure 1.8 (A) Planes of Hodge. (B) The indication of the engagement of the presenting part on passage from the pelvic inlet to the pelvic floor.

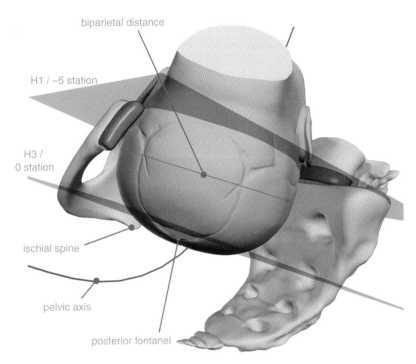

biparietal distance

H1 / −5 station

H3 / 0 station

ischial spine

pelvic axis

posterior fontanel

Figure 1.9 Head is engaged past the H3/0 station.

the engagement of the presenting part on passage from the pelvic inlet to the interspinal line is −5 through −1 (cm) and from the interspinal line to the pelvic floor is +1 through +5 (cm) (Figure 1.8B). "Station +5" means that the presenting part is positioned on the pelvic floor. If the head (in an occiput presentation) is engaged past the third plane of Hodge ("0 station"), the largest diameter of the head (the biparietal distance) has essentially passed the pelvic inlet and the child can in principle be born vaginally (Figure 1.9).

In firm molding of the fetal head, with the lowermost engaged part at or past the third plane of Hodge, the largest diameter of the head may not have passed the pelvic inlet yet (Figure 1.10).

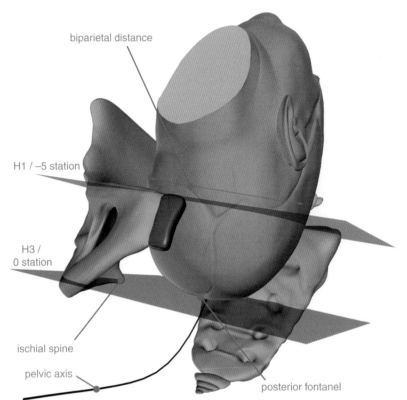

biparietal distance

H1 / −5 station

H3 / 0 station

ischial spine

pelvic axis

posterior fontanel

Figure 1.10 Firmly molded head is engaged up to the H3/0 station.

Pelvic Shapes

The classification of Caldwell and Moloy (1933, 1934) is based on the shape of the pelvis. Knowledge of this classification provides an understanding of the mechanism of childbirth with different pelvic shapes (Figure 1.11).

- *The gynecoid pelvis:* has a transverse oval pelvic entry, the pubic arch is wide, the true pelvis is cylinder-shaped, the ischial spines are not prominent, and the sacrum is biconcave.

- *The android or male-like pelvis:* has a "triangular" pelvic inlet, the pubic arch is narrow, the true pelvis is funnel-shaped, the sacrum is less concave, and the ischial spines are prominent.
- *The anthropoid pelvis:* the pelvic inlet is oval-shaped in an anteroposterior direction; the other characteristics are the same as the android pelvis.
- *The platypelloid pelvis:* has a pelvic inlet with a short anteroposterior dimension and further characteristics as in the gynecoid pelvis.

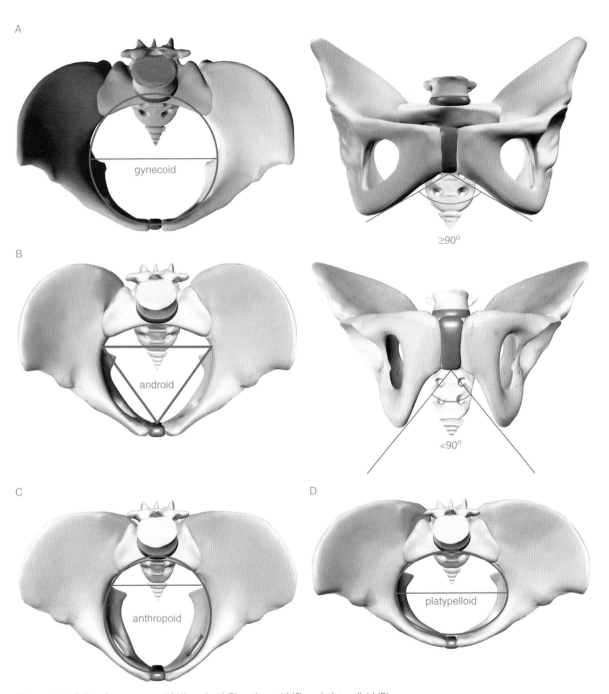

Figure 1.11 Pelvic shapes: gynecoid (A), android (B), anthropoid (C), and platypelloid (D).

Internal Pelvic Examination

The internal pelvic examination can give an indication of the pelvic dimensions. The orientation points are at the following anatomical structures:

- *The promontory:* can usually not be reached with the examination fingers (Figure 1.12). If,

however, the promontory is reached, the *diagonal conjugate* – the distance from the lower edge of the pubic symphysis to the promontory (normal 12–13 cm) – can be "measured." The *true conjugate* (the distance from the upper edge of the pubic symphysis to the promontory) is the

11

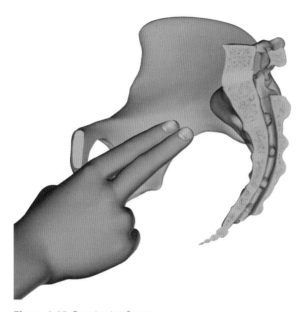

Figure 1.12 Examination fingers.

anteroposterior diameter of the pelvic inlet and is 1.5 cm shorter than the diagonal conjugate, and therefore 10.5–11.5 cm (Figures 1.13 and 1.14).

- *The innominate line:* in a normal pelvis, the lateral and the posterior part of the innominate line cannot be reached.
- *The rear of the pubic symphysis:* is normally smooth. Be aware of exostoses.
- *The sacrum:* is normally hollow in two directions (biconcave). Be aware of ridges.
- *The coccyx:* is normally located at the end of the sacrum and points to the front.
- *The ischial spines:* are not normally prominent.
- *The distance between the ischial tuberosity:* the transverse distance of the pelvic outlet is determined by placing the knuckles (bend of the fingers at the margin of the middle and distal phalanges) from the second to the fourth fingers between the ischial tuberosity. There is normally room for four knuckles.

Figure 1.13 Diagonal conjugate and true conjugate.

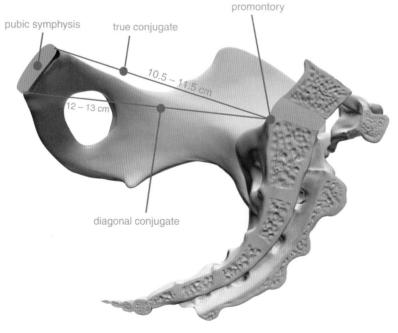

pubic symphysis

true conjugate

promontory

10.5 – 11.5 cm

12 – 13 cm

diagonal conjugate

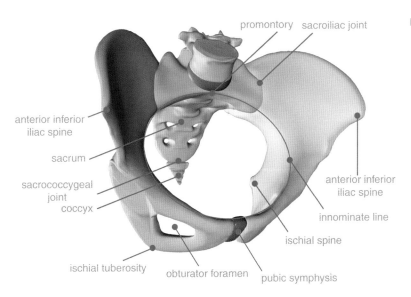

Figure 1.14 Pelvic orientation points.

promontory sacroiliac joint

anterior inferior
iliac spine

sacrum

sacrococcygeal
joint
coccyx

anterior inferior
iliac spine

innominate line

ischial spine

ischial tuberosity obturator foramen pubic symphysis

Abnormal pelves can develop due to poor diet in the past, vitamin D shortage (rickets), and traumas. An internal pelvic examination is frequently painful and has limited value. Additionally, the reproducibility of the examination is poor. The only justification for an internal pelvic examination in pregnant women is a baby in breech position. If on internal pelvic examination abnormalities are encountered, a decision will be made to perform a cesarean section.

The added value of pelvic examinations with the use of X-rays, CT scans, or magnetic resonance imaging (MRI) has not been demonstrated.[4,5]

The Soft-Tissue Birth Canal

The soft-tissue birth canal is made up of the lower uterine segment, the completely effaced and opened cervix, the vagina, the vulva, and the pelvic floor musculature (Figure 1.15).

During the final phase of the expulsion the birth canal is elongated due to the diastasis of the pelvic floor musculature.

Pelvic Floor

The perineum can be divided into an anterior urogenital triangle and a posterior anal triangle. The anterior urogenital triangle is divided by the perineal membrane into a superficial and a deep perineal space. The perineal membrane is situated in a horizontal position. Anteriorly the perineal membrane is continuous with the insertion of the tendinous arch to the pubic bone. Posteriorly the membrane is connected to the membranous perineal body.

The erectile tissue and the clitoris are located in the superficial perineal space and fused into the perineal membrane. The erectile tissue is covered by the ischiocavernosus and the bulbospongiosus muscles. The superficial transverse perineal muscle divides the perineum into the urogenital and anal triangles. Together with the urethrovaginal muscle, the axons of the bulbospongiosus muscle, and the external anal sphincter, this muscle forms the perineal body between the vagina and the anus (Figure 1.16).

The perineal membrane consists of an anterior and a posterior part. The posterior part consists of a bilateral transverse fibrous layer that connects the lateral vaginal walls and the perineal body to the inferior rami of the pubic bone and the rami of the ischium. The anterior part of the perineal membrane covers three muscles situated in the deep perineal space. Alongside the circular external urethral sphincter there is the compressor urethra muscle of the inferior pubic ramus in front of the urethra to the contralateral side, to unite there with this muscle from the other side. Next to that, there is a sling-shaped muscle – the urethrovaginal muscle – that runs from the inferior pubic ramus and fuses behind the vagina in the perineal body (Figure 1.17).[6]

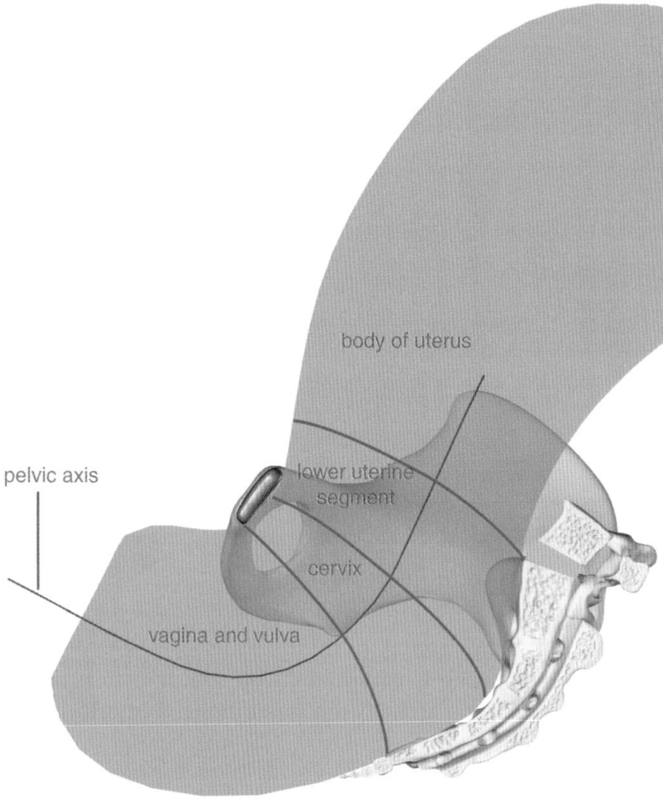

Figure 1.15 Soft-tissue birth canal.

body of uterus

pelvic axis

lower uterine segment

cervix

vagina and vulva

Figure 1.16 Superficial perineal space.

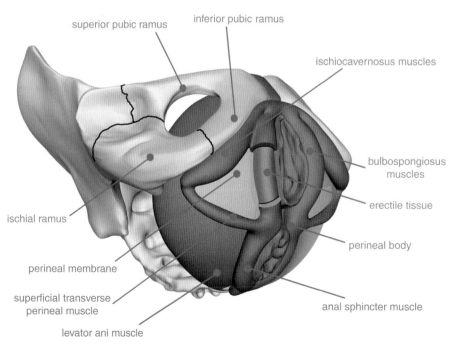

superior pubic ramus

inferior pubic ramus

ischiocavernosus muscles

bulbospongiosus muscles

erectile tissue

perineal body

ischial ramus

perineal membrane

superficial transverse perineal muscle

levator ani muscle

anal sphincter muscle

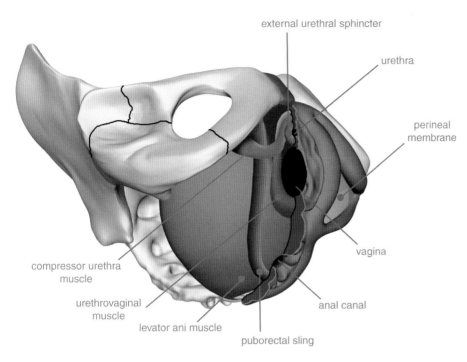

external urethral sphincter

urethra

perineal membrane

vagina

anal canal

puborectal sling

levator ani muscle

urethrovaginal muscle

compressor urethra muscle

Figure 1.17 Deep perineal space.

The anal triangle contains the anal canal, the anal sphincters, and laterally the ischioanal fossae. The boundary of the bottom of the anal triangle is formed by the levator ani muscle, of which the puborectal muscle, the medial part of the levator, forms a sling-shaped loop around the anal canal and attaches ventrally to the pubic bone.

References

1 Dudenhausen JW. Praktische Geburtshilfe mit geburtshilflichen Operationen. Berlin-New York: Walter de Gruyter, 2011.

2 Cunningham F, Leveno K, Bloom S, et al. Williams Obstetrics. New York: McGraw-Hill, 2009

3 Putz R, Pabst R. Sobotta, Atlas van de menselijke anatomie. Houten: Bohn Stafleu van Loghum, 2006.

4 Rozenburg P. Is there a role for X-ray pelvimetry in the twenty-first century. Gynecol Obstet Fertil. 2007;**35**:6–12.

5 Spörri S, Gyr T, Schollerer A, et al. Methods, techniques and assessment criteria in obstetric pelvimetry. Z Geburtshilfe Perinatol. 1994;**198**:37–46.

6 Stoker J, Wallner C. The anatomy of the pelvic floor and sphincters. In: Stoker J, Taylor S, DeLancey JOL (eds). Imaging pelvic floor disorders. New York: Springer Verlag, 2008.

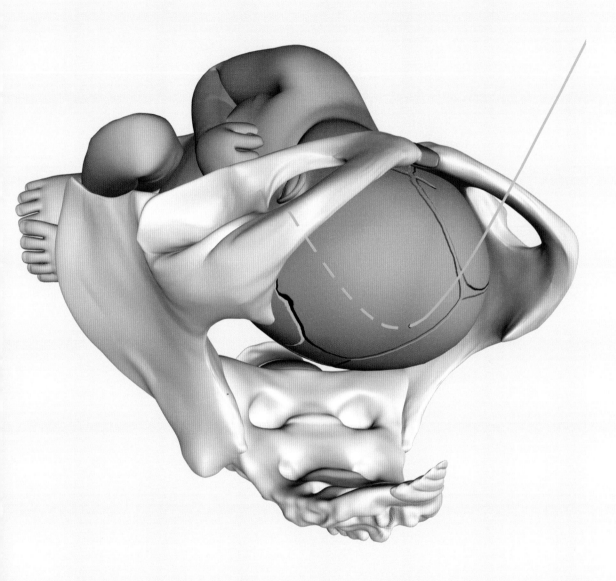

Chapter

2

Normal Labor and Delivery

H.W. Torij, K.M. Heetkamp, A. Grunebaum, M. van Dillen-Putman, and J. van Dillen

Introduction

In this chapter the mechanisms of labor and delivery with various cephalic presentations will be explained as insightfully as possible through the use of text, graphics, and animations. To describe the mechanisms of labor and delivery a variety of existing manuals and reference books have been used.[1-14]

The so-called "planes of Hodge" and the stations – representing the different levels of descending through the birth canal – will be described and used to explain, illustrate, and animate labor and delivery mechanisms. This provides good insight into the different and changing attitudes and positions of the fetal head as it descends through the birth channel in the various cephalic presentations.

Definitions

In order to comprehend the passage of the fetus through the birth canal, an understanding of the mechanisms of normal labor and delivery is required. To describe these mechanisms, the following definitions will be used in this chapter.

Orientation of the Fetus

The orientation of the fetus in the uterus is determined by lie, presenting part, attitude, and position.

- *Lie:* This refers to the relationship between the long axis of the fetus and that of the woman. Longitudinal lies differentiate between cephalic presentations (96%) and breech presentations (3–4%). Additionally, transverse and divergent presentations are differentiated (<0.5%) (Figure 2.1). The percentages refer to term pregnancies.
- *Presenting part:* This refers to the part of the fetus that lies deepest in the birth canal and that therefore is the closest to the outlet of the birth canal. Thus, in the case of a vertex presentation, the occiput is the presenting part and in a transverse presentation, the shoulder, the trunk, or the hip are the presenting parts (Figure 2.1).
- *Attitude:* Attitude refers to the position of the head relative to the trunk (Figure 2.2).

The following are differentiated:

- *flexion presentations (most common):* in which the chin of the fetus is pointed toward the chest; these include the occiput and the sinciput presentations;
- *extension presentations:* in which the occiput of the fetus points toward the dorsum; these include the brow and face presentations.

- *Position:* This refers to the orientation of the presenting part of the fetus relative to the pelvis (Figure 2.3).

Position is determined by the *determining point:*

- in a flexion presentation, the determining point is the occiput (*occiput presentation*);
- in an extension presentation, the determining point is the chin (*mental presentation*);
- in a breech presentation, the determining point is the sacrum (*sacral presentation*).

Obstetric Interventions, ed. P. Joep Dörr, Vincent M. Khouw, Frank A. Chervenak, Amos Grunebaum, Yves Jacquemyn, and Jan G. Nijhuis. Published by Cambridge University Press. © Cambridge University Press 2017.

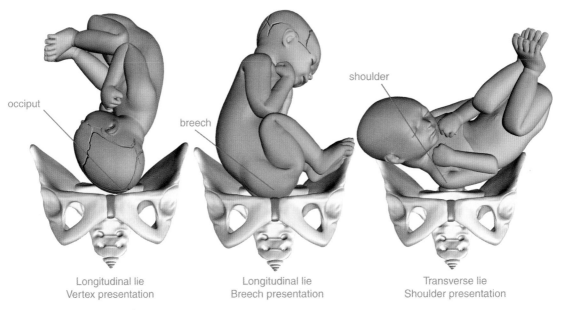

Longitudinal lie
Vertex presentation

Longitudinal lie
Breech presentation

Transverse lie
Shoulder presentation

Figure 2.1 Presentations and presenting parts.

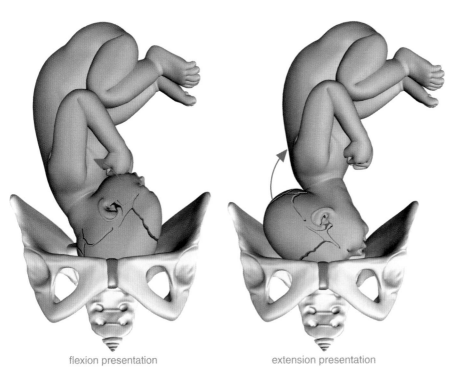

Figure 2.2 Flexion and extension presentations.

flexion presentation

extension presentation

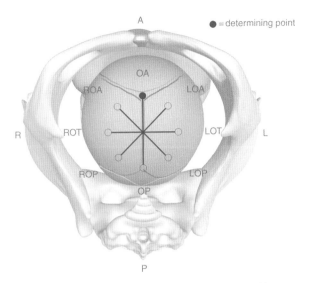

Figure 2.3 Positions of the head in occiput presentation (the determining point is the occiput).

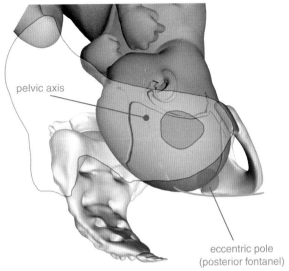

Figure 2.4 Eccentric pole.

Notation of the Fetal Presentation Attitude and Position

Presentation and attitude are indicated with capital letters.

Presentation/attitude	Determining point
Occiput presentation	Occiput (O)
Sinciput presentation	Occiput (O)
Brow presentation	Mentum (M)
Face presentation	Mentum (M)
Breech presentation	Sacrum (S)

Example

In an occiput presentation, the determining point is the occiput (O). The occiput can have the following positions relative to the pelvis:

A = anterior	P = posterior
LOA = left anterior	LOP = left posterior
ROA = right anterior	ROP = right posterior
LOT = left transverse	ROT = right transverse

Thus, LOA stands for a left occiput anterior presentation.

Eccentric Pole

The eccentric pole is the deepest point of the presenting part lying outside the pelvic axis (Figure 2.4).

Rotation

While descending into the pelvis and during expulsion the head rotates (simultaneously) around the frontal, sagittal, and vertical axes.

- *Rotation around the frontal axis* (Figure 2.5): On engagement, the head usually flexes, thereby allowing the smallest circumference to pass through the pelvic cavity.
- *Rotation around the sagittal axis* (Figure 2.6): The following are differentiated (Figure 2.7):
  - synclitism: the sagittal suture transverses the pelvic axis;
  - anterior asynclitism: the sagittal suture lies behind the pelvic axis;
  - posterior asynclitism: the sagittal suture lies in front of the pelvic axis.
- *Rotation around the longitudinal axis (lengthwise rotation)* (Figure 2.8): The following are differentiated:
  - *internal rotation:* rotation of the infant's head around the longitudinal axis, whereby the eccentric pole usually turns to the front;

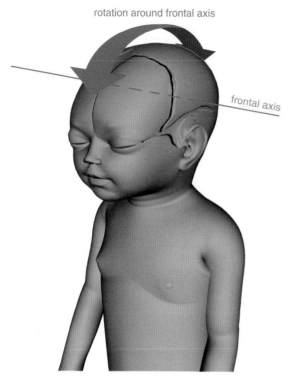

Figure 2.5 Rotation around the frontal axis.

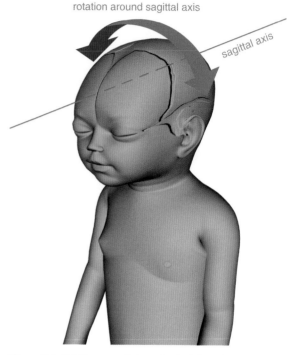

Figure 2.6 Rotation around the sagittal axis in occiput presentation.

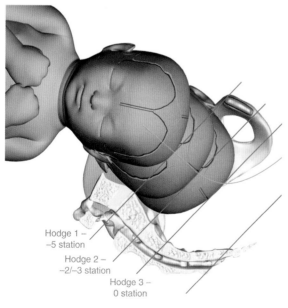

Figure 2.7 Synclitism.

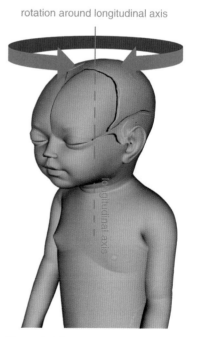

Figure 2.8 Rotation around the longitudinal axis.

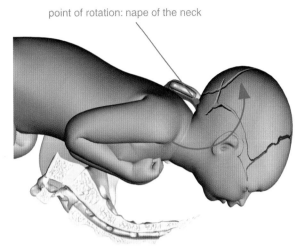

point of rotation: nape of the neck

Figure 2.9 Point of rotation in occiput presentation.

–   *external rotation:* rotation of the infant's head around the longitudinal axis following delivery of the head, in which the occiput turns to the right or the left toward the infant's dorsum.

Point of Rotation (Hypomochlion)

The point of rotation is that part of the fetal head that passes over the symphysis pubis during delivery (Figure 2.9).

In this chapter we describe the passage of the fetus in cephalic presentation through the pelvis with different attitudes and positions of the fetal head. It is important to realize that – besides attitude and position – there are many other factors that influence the passage through the birth canal. The duration of labor, determining whether a woman is in labor at the right moment (not too early and not too late), the strength of contractions, and of course the size of the fetal head in relation to the size of the pelvis influence the passage through the birth canal.

Owing to the focus of this chapter on mechanisms of labor and delivery, other characteristics of the first and second stage of labor will not be described.

Mechanisms of Labor and Delivery in Occiput Presentation, Occiput Anterior

Labor in vertex presentation with the occiput to the front is the most efficient way for a normally proportioned infant to pass through a gynecoid pelvis and be born.

Characteristics

In an occiput presentation:

- the lie is: cephalic presentation;
- the presenting part is: the occiput;
- the attitude is: flexion presentation;
- the determining point is: the occiput;
- the eccentric pole is: the occiput;
- the diameters of the head descending through the pelvis are: the suboccipitofrontal (10 cm) diameter and the biparietal (9.5 cm) diameter;
- the point of rotation is: the posterior hairline.

Incidence

Occiput presentation births occur in 85–88% of all deliveries.[15] Most often it is an occiput presentation with the occiput anterior.

Notation

Occiput presentation: determining point (O) anterior (A), thus: OA.

Diagnosis

- External examination: cephalic presentation.
- Vaginal examination: posterior fontanel in or near the pelvic axis.

Mechanism of Labor from Hodge 1, −5 Station Through Birth

See Animations 2.1 and 2.2.

In the majority of nulliparous women with pregnancy duration of 36 weeks, the head is already engaged, whereas in the majority of multiparous women the head is just barely or not yet engaged at the start of the delivery process.

Hodge 1, −5 Station

- At term, the dorsum of approximately 70% of infants is left anterior, 25% right posterior, and 5% right anterior or left posterior. Therefore, most infants start the descent into the pelvis with the occiput left anterior (LOA). Owing to the transverse-oval shape of the pelvic inlet, the head descends in a transverse or oblique orientation (usually LOT) (Figure 2.10).
- Since the head has to pass over the promontory (rotation around the sagittal axis), the skull at Hodge 1 is in asynclitic position (Figure 2.10). The sagittal suture is anterior to the pelvic axis, making this a posterior asynclitism.

23

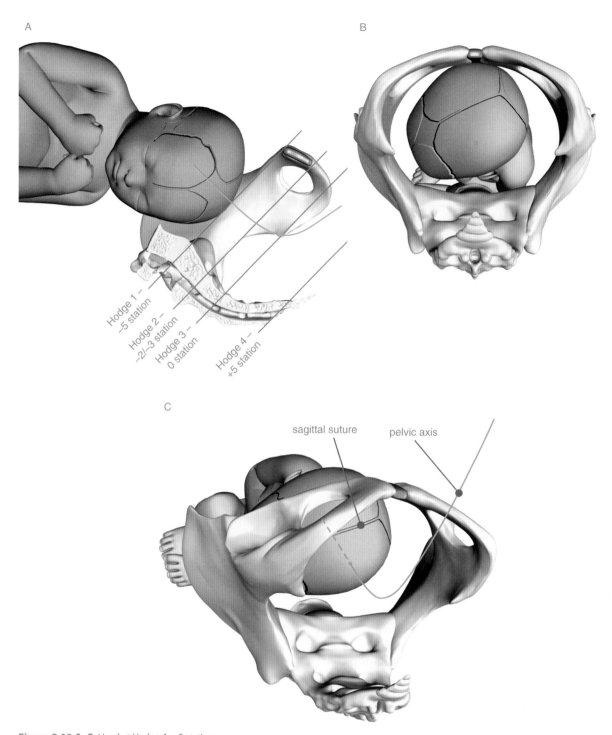

A

B

C

sagittal suture   pelvic axis

Hodge 1 –
–5 station

Hodge 2 –
–2/–3 station

Hodge 3 –
0 station

Hodge 4 –
+5 station

Figure 2.10 A–C Head at Hodge 1, –5 station.

Hodge 2, −2/−3 Station

- In this plane, the head has descended about one-third of the way.
- Flexion increases (rotation around the frontal axis), causing the posterior fontanel to be positioned closer to the pelvic axis.

- The head passes a little more over the sacral promontory at this point. The sagittal suture is now almost positioned in the pelvic axis. Synclitism is reached between Hodge 2, −2/−3 station and Hodge 3, 0 station (Figure 2.11).

A

B

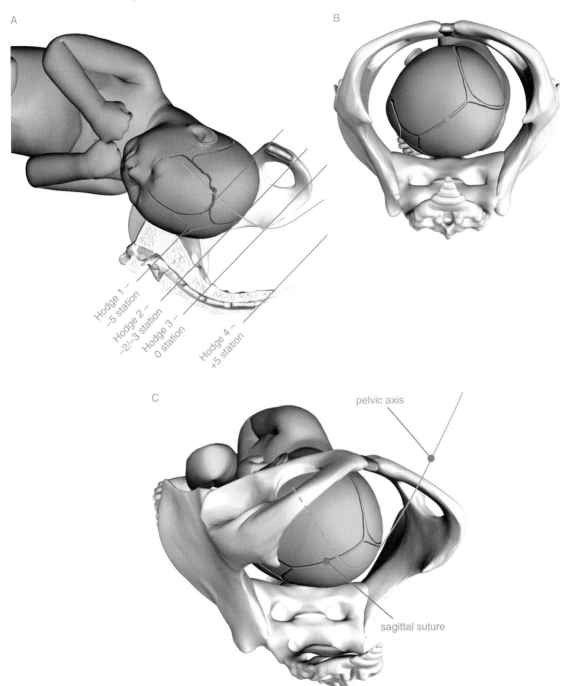

C

pelvic axis

sagittal suture

Hodge 1 – −5 station
Hodge 2 – −2/−3 station
Hodge 3 – 0 station
Hodge 4 – +5 station

Figure 2.11A–C Head at Hodge 2, −2/−3 station.

Hodge 3, 0 Station

- At this point the head has descended about half way. The largest diameter of the head (the biparietal diameter) has passed the pelvic inlet. In principle, the infant can now be born vaginally.

- The head has now pivoted completely around the sacral promontory. The sagittal suture is positioned behind the pelvic axis (anterior asynclitism) (Figure 2.12).

- The flexion of the head increases some more. The posterior fontanel gets closer to the pelvic axis and an eccentric pole develops (Figure 2.13).

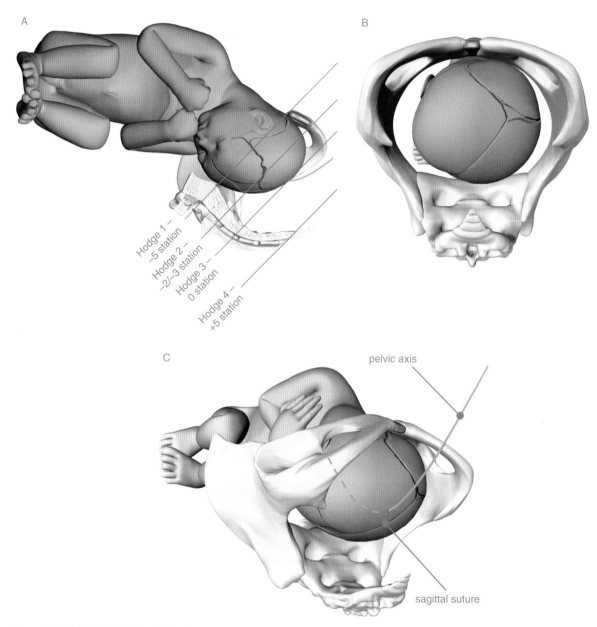

Figure 2.12A–C Head at Hodge 3, 0 station.

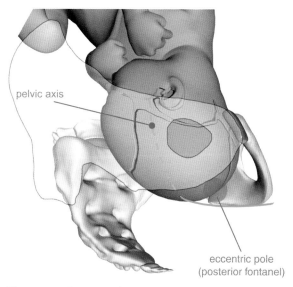

Figure 2.13 Eccentric pole.

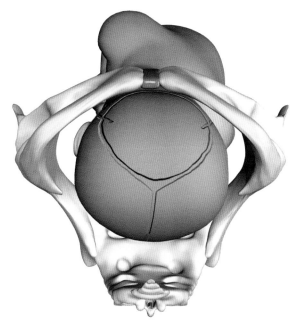

Figure 2.14 Rotated head on pelvic floor.

Internal Rotation

Through this maneuver, the occiput rotates to the front. This is a rotation around the long axis. This internal rotation is necessary to be able to pass the pelvic outlet, whose anteroposterior dimension is greater than the transverse dimension (Figure 2.14). In most women the internal rotation is complete when the head reaches the pelvic floor.

Internal rotation occurs due to:

- the shape of the birth canal: from Hodge 3, 0 station, the birth canal curves 90° toward the front (Figure 2.15);
- the flexibility of the head relative to the trunk: in a flexion attitude, the head will flex further while descending (and extends further in an extension attitude);
- the eccentric pole: due to the contractions, the eccentric pole rotates to the front on passing the bend in the birth canal.

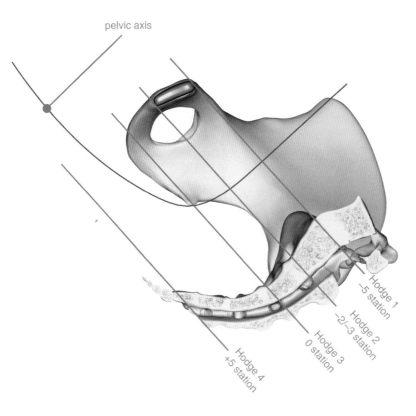

pelvic axis

Figure 2.15 Pelvic axis.

Hodge 1
−5 station

Hodge 2
−2/−3 station

Hodge 3
0 station

Hodge 4
+5 station

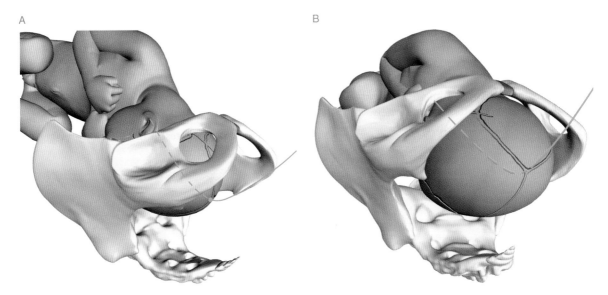

A

B

Figure 2.16A–B Persistent mechanism.

Persistent Mechanism

Sometimes, in an occiput presentation, the head is situated in a persistent mechanism. This means that the head is flexed at maximum and the posterior fontanel (the deepest point) is positioned in the pelvic axis (Figure 2.16). In that position there is no eccentric pole, which sometimes causes the rotation to take place later. An occiput presentation with persistent mechanism can occur when there is a discrepancy between the head and the pelvis.

Hodge 4, +5 Station

- The head is now at the level of the pelvic outlet. The internal rotation is usually complete. The position is OA (Figure 2.17).

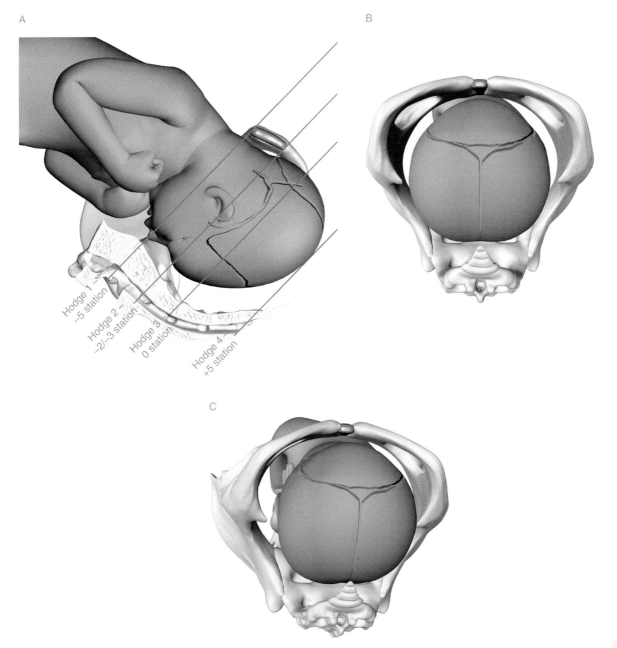

Figure 2.17A–C Head at Hodge 4, +5 station.

Birth of the Head

Crowning of the Head

When the head is rotated, flexion decreases due to the forward-bending curve in the birth canal. With each contraction the skull pushes against the pelvic floor. The perineum becomes increasingly more curved due to the pressure from the pushing skull. With each contraction the anus is open and the vulva becomes wider. The back of the head finally becomes visible

in the vulva during a contraction and will retract again between contractions. This is called *crowning* (Figure 2.18).

Extension of the Head

The head becomes more visible as it descends. When the neck groove is under the symphysis (brow under the posterior edge of the vulva), the head no longer retracts during a pause in the contractions: the head is extended (Figure 2.19).

A   B

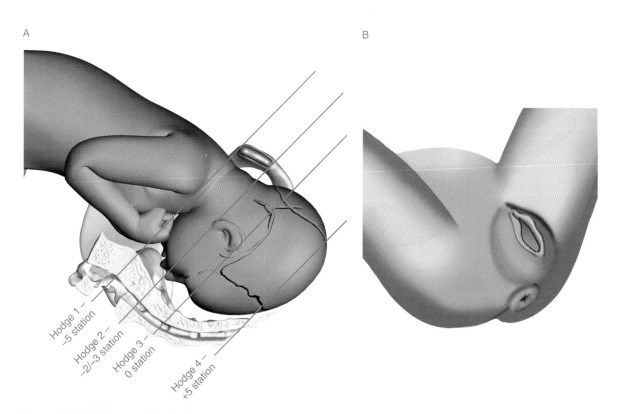

Figure 2.18A–B Crowning of the head.

A

B

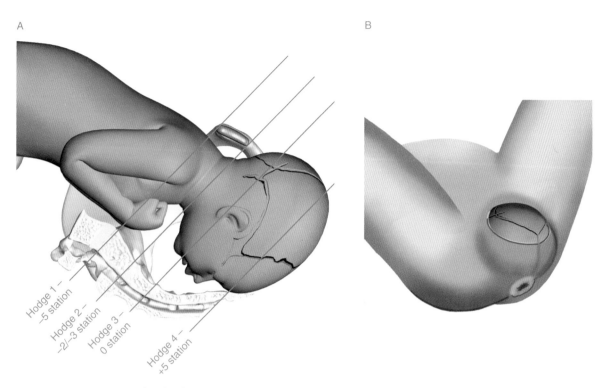

Hodge 1 –
–5 station

Hodge 2 –
–2/–3 station

Hodge 3 –
0 station

Hodge 4 –
+5 station

Figure 2.19A–B Extension of the head.

Delivery of the Head

During one of the following contractions the head extends and is born by rotation around the symphysis. The pivot point is the nape of the neck (Figure 2.20). When the largest dimension of the head is expelled, it is referred to as the delivery of the head.

During delivery of the head, a choice can be made between two methods: *hands on* or *hands off.*

Hands On –– In the hands-on method the perineum is supported by holding one hand on the perineum. The other hand is placed on the head of the infant during the extension of the head and pressure may be exerted on the head to promote deflection of the head (Figure 2.21). Warm compresses reduce the chance of third- and fourth-degree perineal tears (relative risk [RR] 0.48; 95% CI 0.28–0.84)[16] (Figure 2.21).

Hands Off –– In the hands-off method, the hands are not on the head or on the perineum.

Research outcomes are not unequivocal concerning the hands-on versus the hands-off method related to the effect on perineal tears. The hands-on versus hands-off method shows no effect on the incidence of an intact perineum or on third- or fourth-degree tears [LE A1].[16] An episiotomy has been seen significantly more often when the hands on method is performed (RR 0.69; 95% CI 0.50–0.96).[15] A training program (hands-on method, correct performing of episiotomy) focusing on protection of the perineum may result in a reduction of anal sphincter injuries.[17]

Engagement of the Shoulders

The shoulders follow the shape of the birth canal: the scapular arch passes the pelvic inlet in a transverse direction and the plane of the pelvic outlet in the anteroposterior direction.

A

B

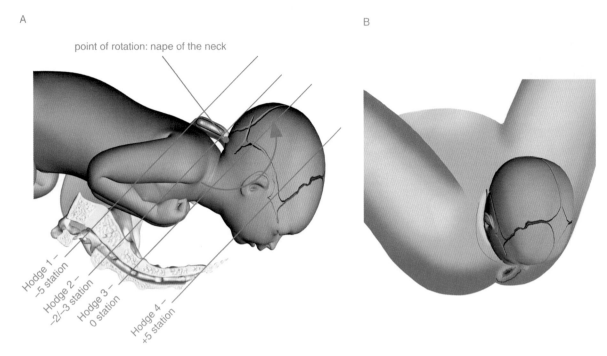

point of rotation: nape of the neck

Hodge 1 –
–5 station

Hodge 2 –
–2/–3 station

Hodge 3 –
0 station

Hodge 4 –
+5 station

Figure 2.20A–B Delivery of the head.

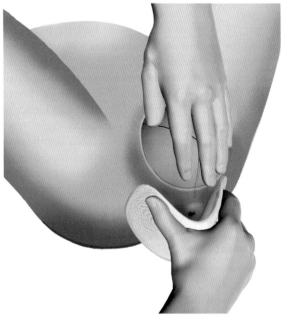

Figure 2.21 Hands on.

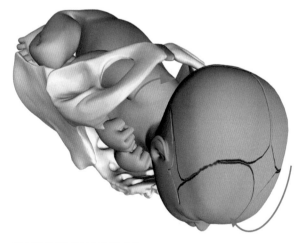

Figure 2.22 External rotation.

External Rotation

The external rotation is a rotation of the infant's head around the long axis after delivery of the head, in which the occiput turns to the left or to the right (depending on the location of the dorsum) (Figure 2.22).

Delivery of the Shoulders

After the external rotation the head is grasped biparietally and mildly bent toward the sacrum, causing the

A

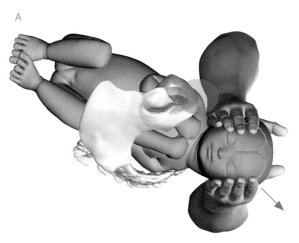

B

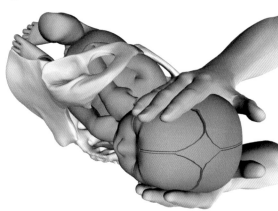

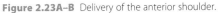

Figure 2.23A–B Delivery of the anterior shoulder.

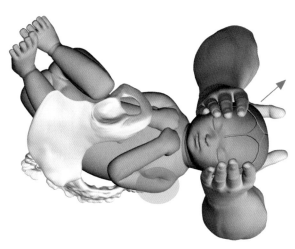

Figure 2.24 Delivery of the posterior shoulder.

anterior shoulder to be delivered first from below the pubic arch (Figure 2.23).

Next, the head is moved toward the symphysis, whereupon the posterior shoulder is delivered over the perineum (Figure 2.24).

During delivery of the posterior shoulder close attention must be paid to the perineum, making sure that it does not rupture. In a vertical delivery, in which the woman leans forward, or in an 'all-fours' position (on hands and knees), the posterior shoulder is sometimes delivered first.

Delivery of the Trunk
After delivery of the shoulders and the axillary folds are visible, the axillas are hooked with the pinkies. Then the trunk, the buttocks, and the extremities are delivered in the direction of the birth canal (Figure 2.25).

A

B

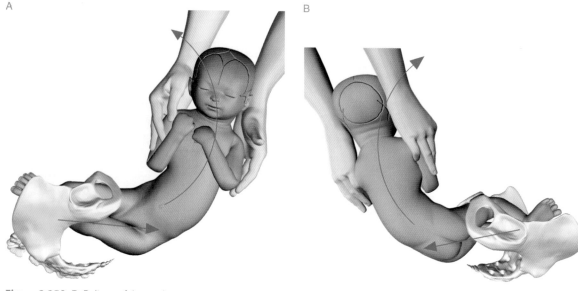

Figure 2.25A–B Delivery of the trunk.

Mechanisms of Labor and Delivery in Sinciput Presentation

Characteristics

In a sinciput presentation:

- the lie is: cephalic presentation;
- the presenting part is: the part of the head that lies at or near the anterior fontanel;
- the attitude is: a position between a flexion and an extended presentation;
- the determining point is: the occiput;
- there is no eccentric pole;
- the dimensions of the head that pass through the pelvis are: the fronto-occipital diameter (12 cm); the transverse distance is the bitemporal diameter (8–8.5 cm);
- the point of rotation is: the glabella.

Notation

Sinciput presentation, with the occiput (determining point) posterior: sinciput OP.

Causes

Normally, the reasons for a sinciput presentation will not be known.

The causes for sinciput presentation could be:

- fetal disorders:

  - congenital disorders, such as a neck tumor (struma, hygroma colli);
  - round shape of the head (no eccentric pole);
  - dead fetus;

- minimal resistance between the head and the birth canal (small head, wide birth canal);
- entwinement (often multiple);
- a platypelloid pelvis (short anteroposterior dimension): in sinciput presentations the head engages with the bitemporal diameter (which is smaller than the biparietal diameter in an occipital presentation) and adapts itself thereby to the platypelloid pelvis;
- weak contractions.

Diagnosis

- External examination: cephalic presentation.
- Vaginal examination: anterior fontanel in or near the pelvic axis: in complete dilation – depending on the engagement – the posterior fontanel and the orbital ridges can sometimes also be felt.

Table 2.1 Differences between sinciput presentation and occiput presentation with the occiput posterior

Sinciput posterior	Occiput posterior
Absence of flexion	Flexion
Greatest circumference of the head has passed the pelvic inlet past H3, 0 station	Greatest circumference of the head has passed the pelvic inlet at H3, 0 station
On crowning of the head, the anterior fontanel lies in the pelvic axis (at the level of the posterior commissure)	On crowning of the head, the anterior fontanel lies closely beneath the symphysis; this is sometimes difficult to feel because of the flexion
The posterior fontanel cannot be reached on the pelvic floor; higher in the pelvis the posterior fontanel should be palpable toward the back and the orbital margins further to the front	The posterior fontanel can be reached without difficulty in the pelvic floor, although it is usually masked by a large caput succedaneum
The point of rotation is the glabella	The point of rotation is the anterior hairline
On delivery, the frontal bone appears in the vulva	On delivery, the anterior fontanel appears in the vulva
Caput succedaneum near the anterior fontanel	Caput succedaneum near the posterior fontanel

Comment

A sinciput presentation with the occiput posterior (OP) is sometimes difficult to differentiate from an occiput presentation with the OP (Table 2.1). Both are presentations with the back in posterior position, in which the infant is born face forward. In both presentations the dilation and expulsion duration may be prolonged. Sometimes the posterior fontanel is equally distant from the pelvic axis as the anterior fontanel. This is a medial position between sinciput posterior and occiput posterior and is called the *military attitude*.

Labor Mechanism in Sinciput Presentation from Hodge 1 through Birth

See Animations 2.3 and 2.4.

Hodge 1, −5 Station

The sinciput descends with the sagittal suture in oblique or transverse direction. The head then descends with the bitemporal diameter (8–8.5 cm), which is smaller than the biparietal diameter (9.5 cm) (Figure 2.26).

To be able to pass the promontory the head lies in asynclitism. The sagittal suture lies in front of the pelvic axis, thus there is a posterior asynclitism.

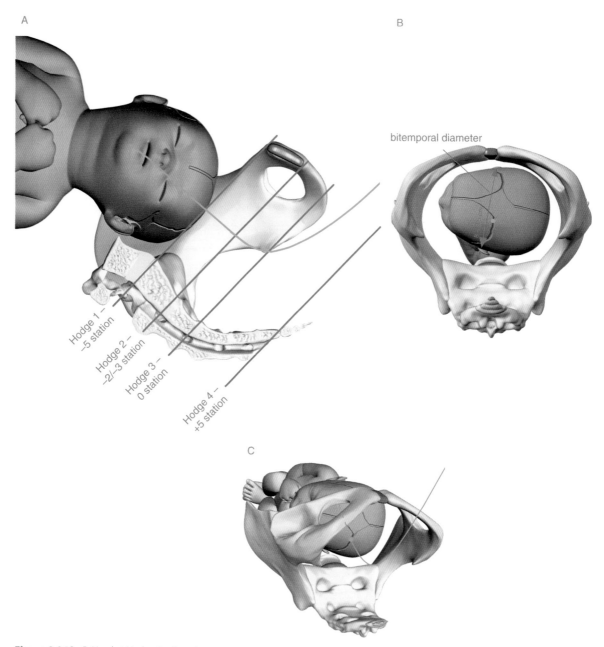

A

B

bitemporal diameter

Hodge 1 –
−5 station

Hodge 2 –
−2/−3 station

Hodge 3 –
0 station

Hodge 4 –
+5 station

C

Figure 2.26A–C Head at Hodge 1, −5 station.

Hodge 2, −2/−3 Station

If the sinciput presentation persists, the head will descend deeper, but engagement will be slower due to the larger dimensions of the penetration plane (fronto-occipital circumference, 34–35 cm).

The head tilts (rotation around the sagittal axis) over the sacral promontory and goes toward synclitism (Figure 2.27).

Hodge 3, 0 Station

At this point the head has descended a little less than half way because the head is less flexed compared to a head in occiput anterior (OA) presentation. When the head has descended past H3, the largest diameter of the head (the biparietal diameter) has passed the pelvic inlet. It can then be assumed that when a fetus in sinciput presentation

A

B

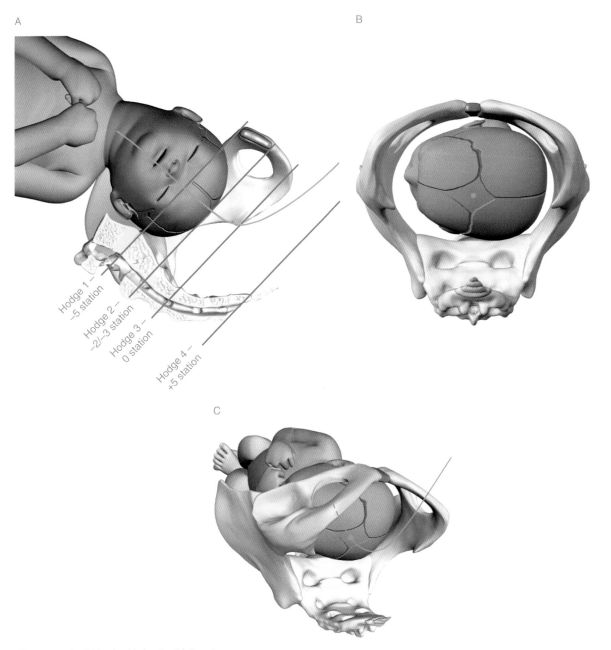

Hodge 1 –
–5 station

Hodge 2 –
–2/–3 station

Hodge 3 –
0 station

Hodge 4 –
+5 station

C

Figure 2.27A–C Head at Hodge 2, –2/–3 station.

has descended past the H3 plane, the infant can be delivered vaginally.

The moment at which the head has completely rotated around the promontory and lies in anterior asynclitism occurs later than in an OA presentation (Figure 2.28).

Rotation

If flexion does not occur during the descent, the sinciput presentation persists. Rotation does not take place because the rotation factors are lacking.

In a sinciput LOP or ROP a rotation of the head occurs at H3, 0 station in which the sagittal suture lies

A

B

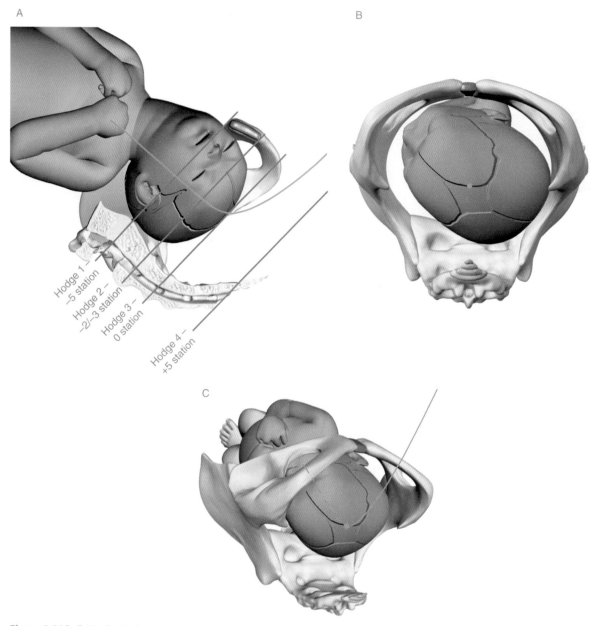

C

Figure 2.28A–C Head at Hodge 3.

in the anteroposterior diameter of the pelvis. In this rotation the posterior fontanel will turn to the rear.

In case of a sinciput presentation in the LOA or ROA position at H3, 0 station, the sinciput presentation will in most cases evolve into an occiput presentation. In these positions flexion occurs quite easily (greater resistance in back

than in front past the curve of the pelvic axis), giving rise to an eccentric pole. The occiput rotates to the front and the delivery takes place as in an OA delivery.

A sinciput OP does not evolve easily into an occiput OP, as the head at this pelvic location is no longer able to inflect from this position.

A

B

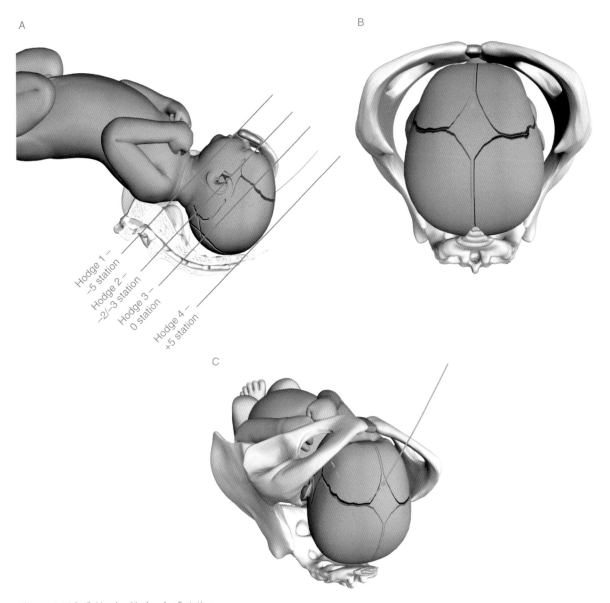

Hodge 1 –
–5 station
Hodge 2 –
–2/–3 station
Hodge 3 –
0 station
Hodge 4 –
+5 station

C

Figure 2.29A–C Head at Hodge 4, +5 station.

Hodge 4, +5 Station

In a sinciput presentation the anterior fontanel lies in the pelvic axis. This means that at the plane of the pelvic outlet the anterior fontanel lies at the level of the posterior commissure (Figure 2.29).

Birth of the Head

The brow and the anterior fontanel are the first to penetrate the vulva (Figure 2.30). In a sinciput OP birth, the glabella (point of rotation) is located under the symphysis pubis (Figure 2.31). Flexion causes the occiput to be born first over the perineum, after which the face is born through extension.

During the crowning, extension, and delivery process there is an increased chance of perineal laceration in both sinciput and occiput posterior positions compared to OA position, since:

- the head passes the pelvic outlet with the fronto-occipital diameter (12 cm). In an OA delivery the suboccipitofrontal diameter (10 cm) passes through;

- the head descends straight down to the glabella, before rotation around the symphysis pubis takes place;
- the occiput is wider than the forehead;
- the shape of the forehead fits less perfectly under the pubic arch than the neck.

After the head is born, the delivery continues as in occiput OA.

Possible Interventions in Sinciput Presentations

- In the event of an engaged head in the presence of a normal pelvis, the mother may be asked to lie in a side position on the side of the fetal back (Figure 2.32). This is done to promote flexion and attempt a transition from a sinciput to a normal occiput presentation. Through flexion an eccentric pole develops again.
- By changing position or by moving around. This may also help to improve flexion.

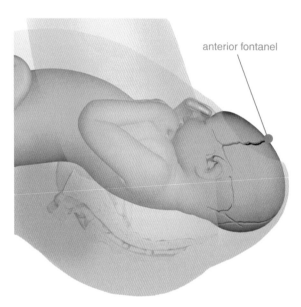

anterior fontanel

Figure 2.30 Crowning of the head.

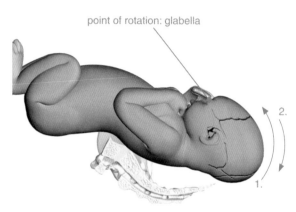

point of rotation: glabella

2.

1.

Figure 2.31 Point of rotation: glabella.

A

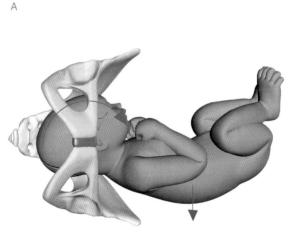

B

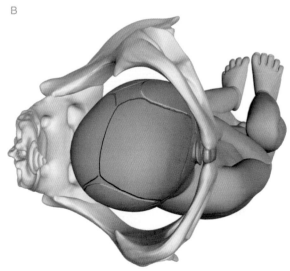

Figure 2.32A–B Stimulation of flexion.

Mechanism of Labor and Delivery in Occiput Presentation, Occiput Posterior

Characteristics

In an occiput presentation with the occiput in posterior position:

- the lie is: cephalic presentation;
- the presenting part is: the head;
- the attitude is: flexion position;
- the determining point is: the occiput;
- the eccentric pole is: the posterior fontanel;
- the dimensions of the head that pass through the pelvis are: the suboccipitofrontal diameter (10 cm) and the biparietal diameter (9.5 cm);
- the point of rotation is: the anterior hairline.

Incidence

Occiput presentation births with the occiput in posterior position occur in 5.5% of all deliveries.[18]

Notation

Occiput presentation with the occiput (determining point: O) posterior: OP.

Causes

Usually, the reason for an occiput posterior presentation is not known.

The causes for an occiput presentation with the occiput posterior could be:

- small infant;
- dead infant;
- incongruency between head and pelvis.

Diagnosis

- External examination: cephalic presentation.
- Vaginal examination: the posterior fontanel is situated (left or right) posterior; the anterior fontanel (left or right) is located anterior.

Comment

For an explanation of the difference between an occiput presentation with the occiput posterior and a sinciput presentation with the occiput posterior, see Section: Mechanisms of Labor and Delivery in Sinciput Presentation.

Labor Mechanism with Occiput Presentation with Occiput Posterior from Hodge 1 through Birth

See Animations 2.5 and 2.6.

Hodge 1, −5 Station

In 25–30% of the infants, descent into the pelvis starts with the dorsum in posterior position. The head engages with the occiput left or right transverse or left or right posterior (LOT, ROT, LOP, or ROP) (Figure 2.33).

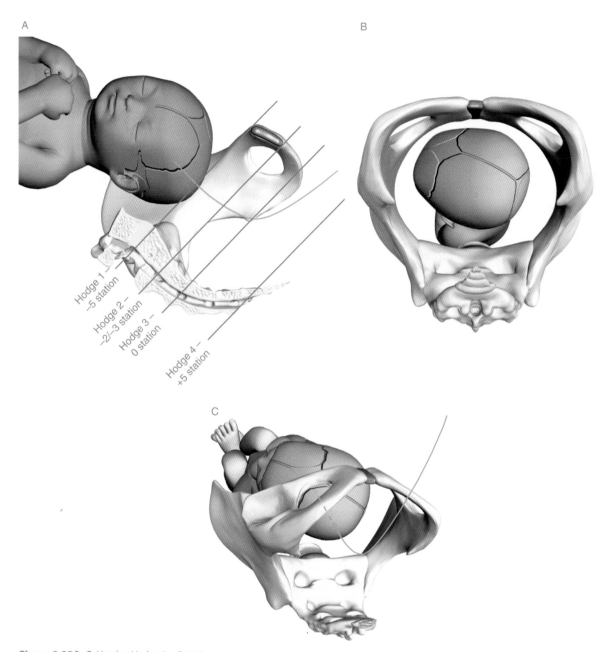

A

B

C

Hodge 1 –
–5 station

Hodge 2 –
–2/–3 station

Hodge 3 –
0 station

Hodge 4 –
+5 station

Figure 2.33A–C Head at Hodge 1, –5 station.

Hodge 2, −2/−3 Station

At this plane the head is coming a little deeper and inflects (rotation around the frontal axis). The posterior fontanel comes situated a little closer to the pelvic axis (Figure 2.34).

At this level the head passes over the promontory and moves toward synclitism. Synclitism is reached between Hodge 2, −2/−3 station and Hodge 3, 0 station (rotation around the sagittal axis).

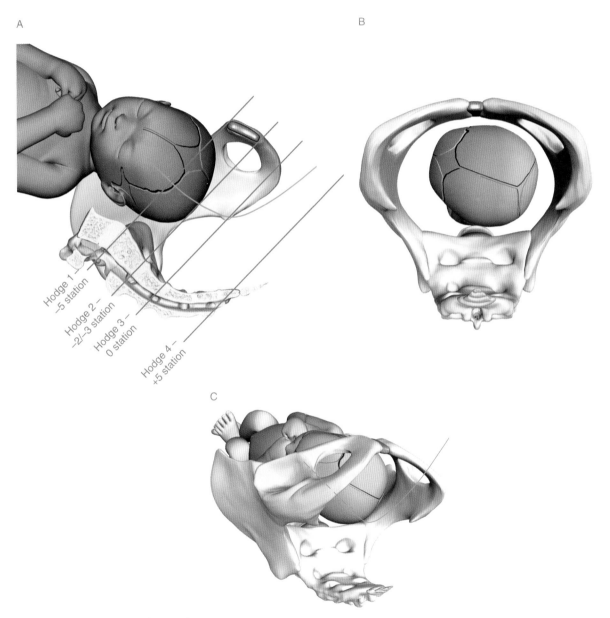

Figure 2.34A–C Head at Hodge 2, −2/−3 station.

Hodge 3, 0 Station

At this point the head has descended about half way. The largest diameter of the head (the biparietal diameter) has passed the pelvic inlet.

The head has now rotated completely around the sacral promontory and the sagittal suture is positioned behind the pelvic axis. There is now anterior asynclitism (Figure 2.35).

Rotation

If the head presents at H3, 0 station in ROP or LOP, there are two possibilities:

- The occiput rotates 135° forward to an OA and the labor will proceed as in an occiput OA delivery.
- The occiput rotates 45° to the back, to an occiput OP.

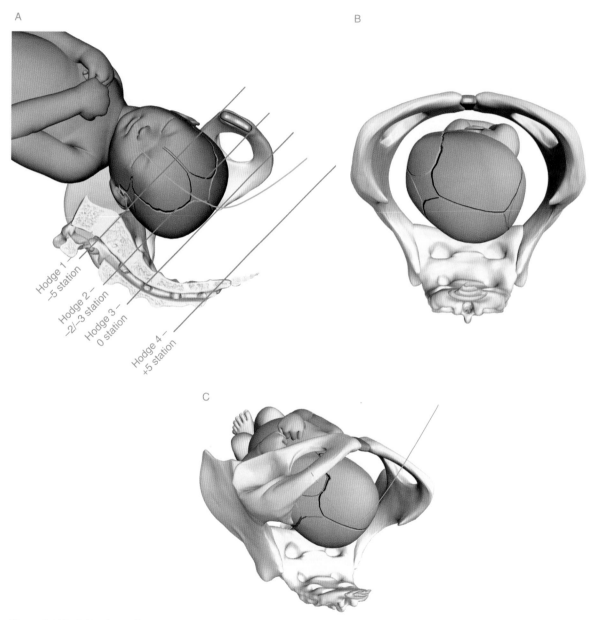

A

B

Hodge 1 – –5 station
Hodge 2 – –2/–3 station
Hodge 3 – 0 station
Hodge 4 – +5 station

C

Figure 2.35A–C Head at Hodge 3, 0 station.

A
B

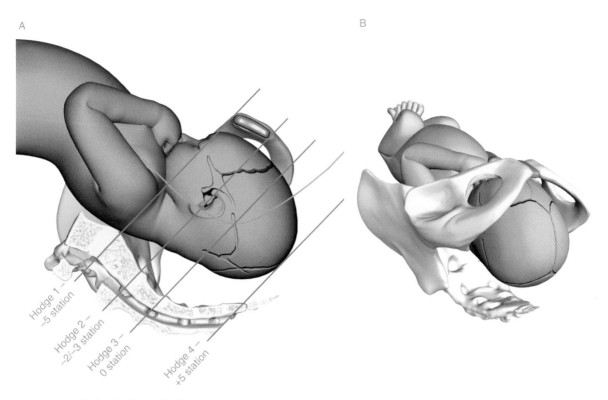

Hodge 1 –
–5 station

Hodge 2 –
–2/–3 station

Hodge 3 –
0 station

Hodge 4 –
+5 station

Figure 2.36A–B Head at Hodge 4, +5 station.

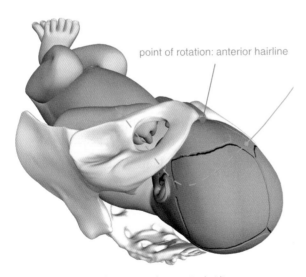

point of rotation: anterior hairline

Figure 2.37 Point of rotation is the anterior hairline.

Hodge 4, +5 Station

At Hodge 4, +5 station, the head lies at the level of the pelvic outlet in OP position (Figure 2.36).

Birth of the Head

After maximum flexion of the head, the occiput is born up to the neck groove (the point of rotation is the anterior hairline, the area of the anterior fontanel) (Figure 2.37). Then the head becomes extended, whereby the sinciput, the brow, and the face are expelled under the symphysis (Figure 2.38).

In an occiput posterior birth, the tension on the perineum is even greater than in a sinciput presentation birth, since the head engages "straight down" until after the birth of the occiput.

From the moment the head is born, labor proceeds as in occiput OA.

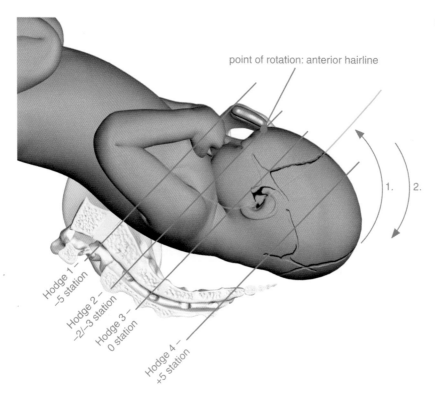

Figure 2.38 Birth of the head.

point of rotation: anterior hairline

1. 2.

Hodge 1 –
−5 station

Hodge 2 –
−2/−3 station

Hodge 3 –
0 station

Hodge 4 –
+5 station

Mechanism of Labor and Delivery in Brow Presentation

Characteristics

In a brow presentation:

- the lie is: cephalic presentation;
- the presenting part is: the brow of the head;
- the attitude is: a (moderate) extension presentation;
- the determining point is: the chin (mentum);
- the eccentric pole is: the chin (mentum);
- the diameter that has to pass the pelvis: the mento-occipital diameter (13.5–14 cm);
- the point of rotation is: the fossae caninae (cheekbones).

Incidence

The incidence of brow presentation is 0.01–0.05%.

Notation

Brow presentation with the chin (determining point: mentum) anterior: MA.

Causes

As in a face presentation, the reasons for brow presentation are circumstances that produce extension instead of flexion of the head. These circumstances could be:

- disorders in the infant, for instance:
  - anencephaly;
  - neck tumor (struma, hygroma colli);
- entwinement;
- weak abdominal wall (multipara);
- incongruency between head and pelvis.

For most brow presentations the causes will not be known.

Diagnosis

- External examination: cephalic presentation, in which:
  - the most amount of resistance can be felt on the side of the small extremities;
  - the (back of the) head remains palpable for a long time above the pelvic inlet;
  - the heart tones of the infant can be heard best on the side of the small extremities.

- Vaginal examination, in which:
  - the anterior fontanel and the orbital ridges are palpable on both sides of the pelvic axis;
  - the bridge of the nose, the frontal suture, the glabella, and sometimes the mouth are also palpable, but the chin can never be felt (in contrast with the face presentation, in which the chin is always palpable and the anterior fontanel is never palpable).

Comment

In an incomplete dilation it is possible that only the anterior fontanel will be palpable and that the orbital ridges are not palpable yet. This could cause confusion with the sinciput presentation. But in the brow position the anterior fontanel does not lie in the pelvic axis, such as is the case in a sinciput presentation.

Labor Mechanism with Brow Presentation from Hodge 1, −5 Station through Birth

See Animations 2.7 and 2.8.

Usually, when a brow presentation occurs a cesarean section is indicated. The greatest diameter in a brow presentation, the mento-occipital diameter (13.5–14 cm), is larger than the transverse diameter of the pelvic inlet (13 cm). Often the head cannot descend further than the second plane of Hodge, −2/−3 station. Therefore, a spontaneous birth is only possible in the case of a small fetus and/or a large pelvis. In this case, a face presentation will present due to increased extension or a sinciput presentation as a result of flexion (see sinciput presentation and face presentation).

Hodge 1, −5 Station

In a brow presentation the head usually descends with the chin left or right anterior (Figure 2.39).

Hodge 2, −2/−3 Station and Hodge 3, 0 Station

Usually the head cannot descend further. If, however, this is the case, the head descends further with the chin left or right anterior (Figures 2.40 and 2.41).

Internal Rotation

The rotation takes place when the brow is on the pelvic floor, since only at that point the occiput has passed the promontory. The eccentric pole is the chin. The chin turns to the front with the cheekbones under the symphysis.

Hodge 4, +5 Station

The rotation takes place at Hodge 4, +5 station. The chin turns to the front with the fossae caninae (cheekbones) under the symphysis (Figure 2.42).

Birth of the Head

The head rotates around the symphysis with the fossae caninae (cheekbones) as the point of rotation, whereby the occiput is born first through flexion. After that the face is born under the symphysis through extension.

The head is often born with the sagittal suture in the oblique diameter of the pelvic outlet, since adaptation of one of the cheekbones under the symphysis creates more room (Figure 2.43).

After the head has been born in a brow presentation, the labor proceeds from that point onward as in an occiput OP delivery.

Possible Interventions in a Brow Presentation

- Choose a side-lying position: on the side of the abdomen of the fetus to promote extension (face presentation).
- Choose a side-lying position: on the side of the back of the infant to promote flexion (sinciput presentation).

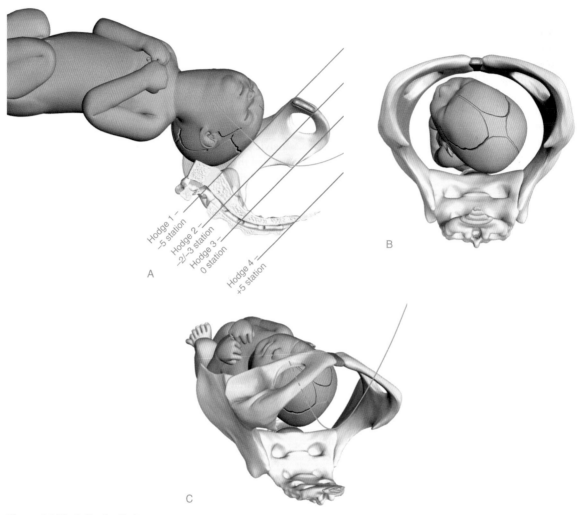

Hodge 1 —
−5 station
Hodge 2 —
−2/−3 station
Hodge 3 —
0 station
Hodge 4 —
+5 station

A

B

C

Figure 2.39A–C Head at Hodge 1, −5 station.

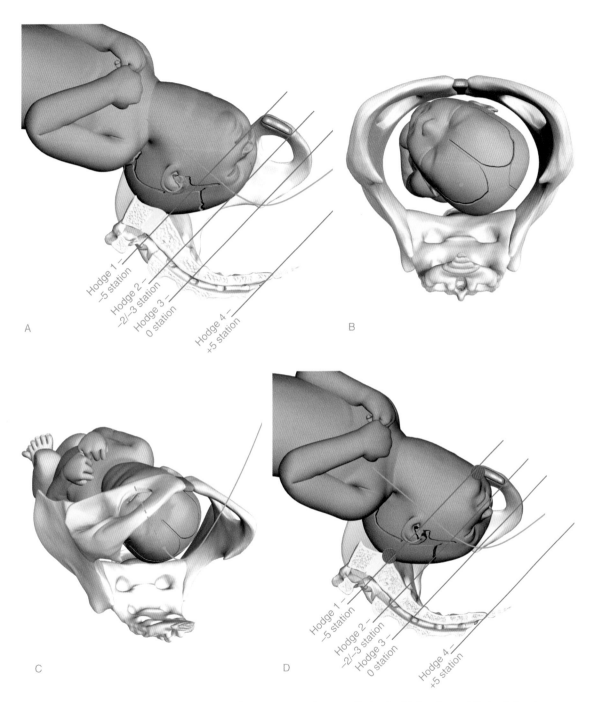

A

Hodge 1 —
−5 station

Hodge 2 —
−2/−3 station

Hodge 3 —
0 station

Hodge 4 —
+5 station

B

C

D

Hodge 1 —
−5 station

Hodge 2 —
−2/−3 station

Hodge 3 —
0 station

Hodge 4 —
+5 station

Figure 2.40A–D Head at Hodge 2, −2/−3 station: descent stagnates between Hodge 2, −2/−3 station and Hodge 3, 0 station.

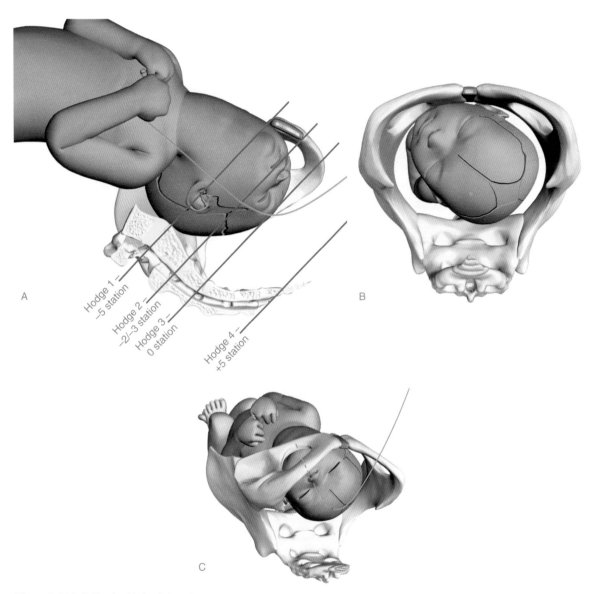

A

Hodge 1 –
–5 station

Hodge 2 –
–2/–3 station

Hodge 3 –
0 station

Hodge 4 –
+5 station

B

C

Figure 2.41A–C Head at Hodge 3, 0 station.

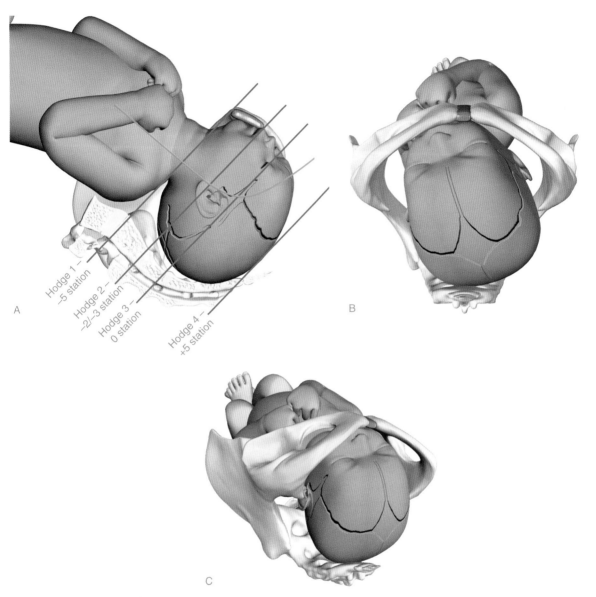

A

Hodge 1 –
–5 station

Hodge 2 –
–2/–3 station

Hodge 3 –
0 station

Hodge 4 –
+5 station

B

C

Figure 2.42A–C Head at Hodge 4, +5 station.

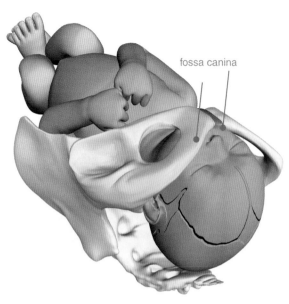

fossa canina

Figure 2.43 Point of rotation.

Mechanism of Labor and Delivery in Face Presentation

Characteristics

In a face presentation:

- the lie is: a cephalic presentation;
- the presenting part is: the face of the head;
- the attitude is: hyperextended presentation;
- the determining point is: the chin (mentum);
- the eccentric pole is: the chin (mentum);
- the dimension of the head that passes the pelvis: the submentobregmatic diameter (9.5 cm);
- the point of rotation: the larynx.

Incidence

Face presentation births occur in 0.05–0.5% of all deliveries.

Notation

Face presentation with chin (determining point: mentum) anterior: MA.

Causes

Causes for face presentations are circumstances in which extension of the head occurs rather than flexion. These circumstances could be:

- disorders in the infant, such as:
  - anencephaly;
  - neck tumor (struma, hygroma colli);
- entwinement;
- weak abdominal wall (multipara);
- incongruency between head and pelvis.

For most face presentations the causes will not be known.

Diagnosis

- External examination: cephalic presentation, in which:
  - the most amount of resistance can be felt on the side of the small extremities;
  - the (back of the) head remains palpable for a long time above the pelvic inlet;
  - the heart tones of the infant can be heard best on the side of the small extremities.

- Vaginal examination, in which:
  - the orbital ridges and the chin with the mouth are palpable on both sides of the pelvic axis;
  - the caput succedaneum develops in the face; the eyelids, nose, and lips may be acutely swollen, making it sometimes difficult to determine a face presentation.

Comment

Upon internal examination it is sometimes difficult to differentiate between a face presentation and a breech presentation. A mistake is possible if the anus is mistaken for the mouth. A distinction can be made by remembering that the anus lies central in an imaginary line that connects the two (palpable) ischial tuberosities, while these bony identification points cannot be felt on both sides of the mouth.

Labor Mechanism in a Face Presentation from H1 through Birth

There is usually no face presentation at the onset of the descent, but a brow presentation. When descending into the pelvis, the head will extend further and thereby become a face presentation (see Animations 2.9 and 2.10).

Hodge 1, −5 Station

If the head is in face presentation at the start of the descent, this will usually be with the chin at LA/LT or RA/RT. As in an occiput presentation, the head will have to rotate around the sagittal axis to be able to pass the promontory in a face presentation (Figure 2.44).

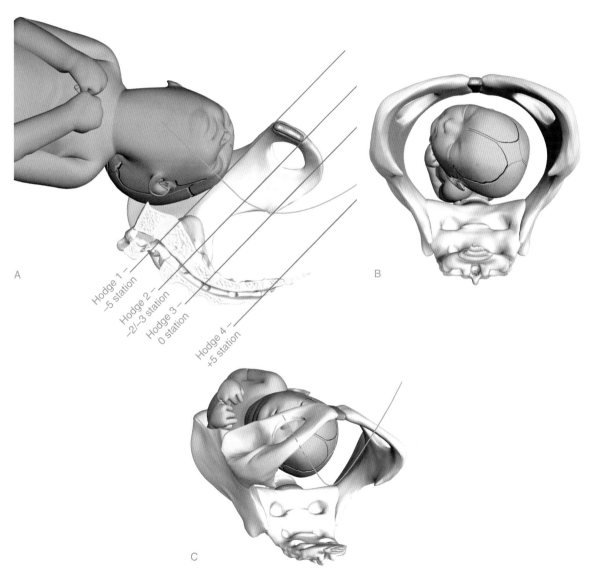

A

Hodge 1 −
−5 station

Hodge 2 −
−2/−3 station

Hodge 3 −
0 station

Hodge 4 −
+5 station

B

C

Figure 2.44A–C Head at Hodge 1, −5 station.

Hodge 2, −2/−3 Station

The head descends deeper in the same position as at Hodge 1. The descent is slower, on the one hand because of the irregularly shaped presenting part and on the other hand because the head crowns with the submento-occipital diameter (13.5–14 cm) compared to the suboccipitofrontal diameter (10 cm) in an occipital presentation (Figure 2.45).

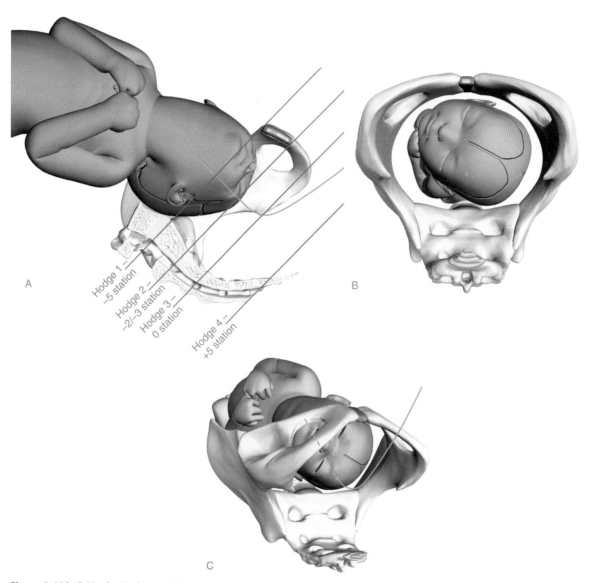

Figure 2.45A–C Head at Hodge 2, −2/−3 station.

Hodge 3, 0 Station

The head descends deeper in the same position as at Hodge 1 and will extend further (rotation around the frontal axis) (Figure 2.46).

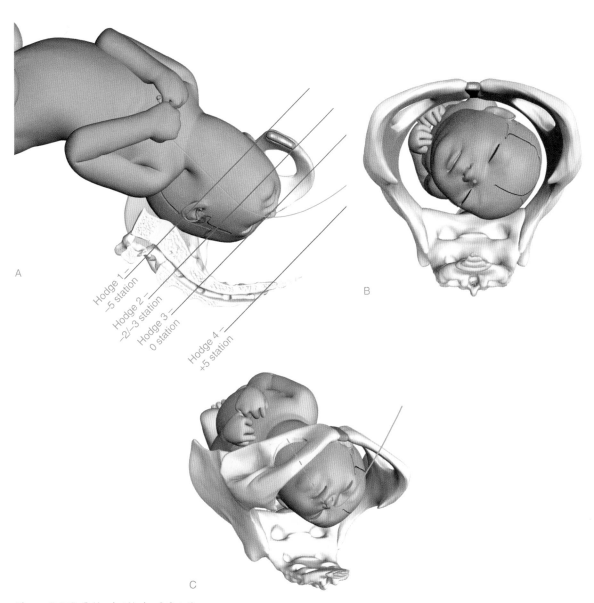

Figure 2.46A–C Head at Hodge 3, 0 station.

Internal rotation

Internal rotation ultimately takes place at Hodge 4, +5 station. The largest dimension of the head has finally passed the pelvic inlet when the face is on the pelvic floor (Hodge 4, +5 station). The chin is the eccentric pole and when going deeper it is the first part to reach the bend of the birth canal (Figure 2.47).

If in the rotation the chin turns to the back, a spontaneous birth is not possible (the head is hyperextended and cannot descend further) (Figure 2.48).

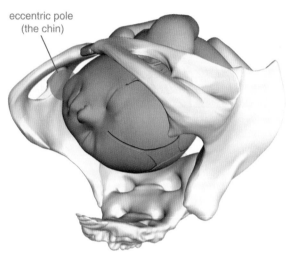

Figure 2.47 Eccentric pole.

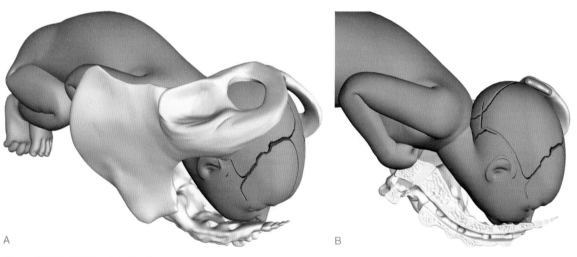

Figure 2.48A–B Chin rotated to the back.

Hodge 4, +5 Station

Rotation takes place at Hodge 4 (Figure 2.49).

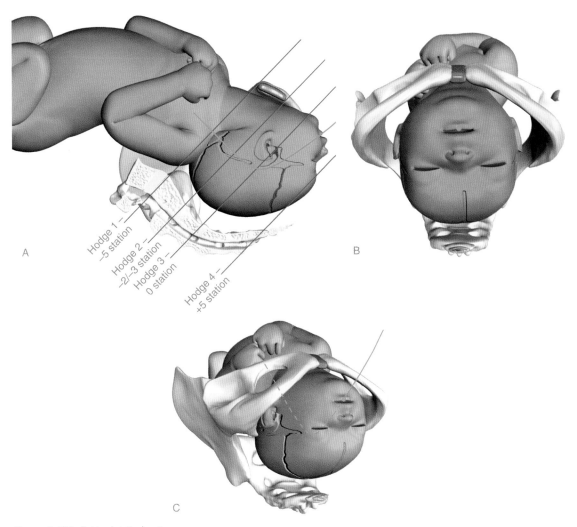

A

Hodge 1 –
–5 station

Hodge 2 –
–2/–3 station

Hodge 3 –
0 station

Hodge 4 –
+5 station

B

C

Figure 2.49A–C Head at Hodge 4.

Birth of the Head

The initial part that is visible in the vulva is the mouth, after which the nose, the eyes, and the forehead are born (Figure 2.50). Then flexion occurs with the larynx as the point of rotation (Figure 2.51), causing the stretched occiput to be born.

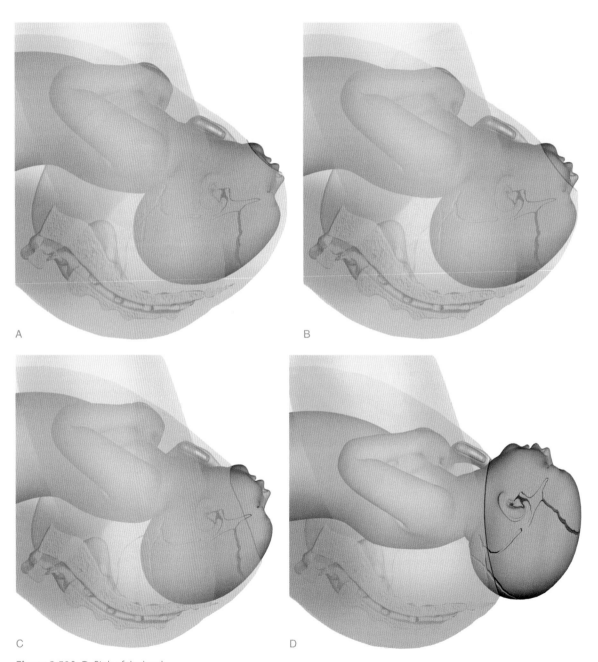

A

B

C

D

Figure 2.50A–D Birth of the head.

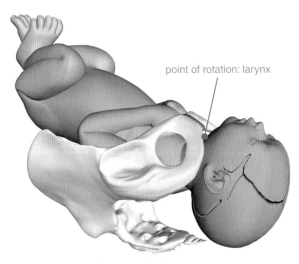

Figure 2.51 Point of rotation: the larynx.

point of rotation: larynx

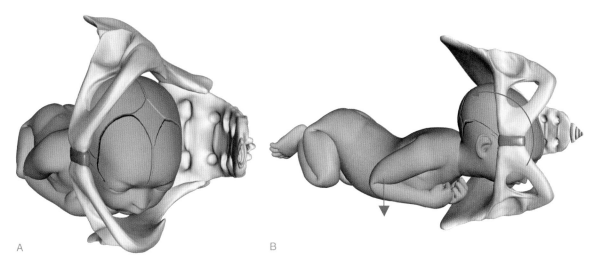

A

B

Figure 2.52A–B Stimulation of extension.

During crowning, extension, and delivery there is a greater chance of perineal laceration than with delivery in an OA position.

- The head crowns and extends with the submento-bregmatic diameter (9.5 cm).
- Through flexion, the head delivers with the submento-occipital diameter (11.5 cm).

After the birth of the head the delivery proceeds in the same manner as in an occiput OP delivery.

Comment

- To reach optimal extension, the mother may be asked to move into a side-lying position on the side of the abdomen of the infant (Figure 2.52).
- Edema of the larynx may occur due to prolonged hyperextension of the neck. This may cause stridor after birth. The presence of a pediatrician or a neonatologist is therefore recommended.

Mechanism of Labor in Persistent Occiput Anterior or Posterior Position

There are two forms of persistent occiput position:

- the persistent occiput anterior position (occipito-pubic position);
- the persistent occiput posterior position (occipito-sacral position).

Characteristics

In a persistent occiput position:

- the lie is: cephalic presentation;
- the presenting part is: the head;
- the sagittal suture lies nearly or completely in the anteroposterior diameter (true conjugate) before the largest circumference of the head has passed the pelvic inlet;
- there usually is an occiput presentation;
- the attitude is: flexion position;
- the determining point is: the occiput;
- the dimensions of the head that pass through the pelvis are: the suboccipitofrontal diameter (10 cm) and the biparietal diameter (9.5 cm).

Incidence

Of all vertex presentations, 0.7–1.6% are persistent occiput anterior or posterior presentations.

Notation

In a persistent occiput position with the occiput anterior or posterior, respectively, the notations are:

- OA – occipitopubic position;
- OP – occipitosacral position.

Causes

The reasons for a persistent occipital position are not clear.

Diagnosis

- External examination:
  - cephalic presentation with movable head above or in the pelvic inlet.

- Internal examination:
  - non-engaged head;
  - the sagittal suture lies straight in the pelvic axis at Hodge 1, −5 station, whereby the posterior fontanel is either anterior or posterior.

If the labor progresses past Hodge 1, −5 station, it is no longer a persistent occipital position. Increased flexion will cause the vertex to descend.

Labor Mechanism of Persistent Occipital Position from H1, −5 station, through the Birth of the Infant

In a delivery with the head in a persistent occipital position at H1 (Figure 2.53) the dilatation and engagement will often progress slowly.

If the sagittal suture still comes to lie in an oblique or transverse position, the labor and delivery will proceed as in an occiput OA or occiput OP delivery.

Hodge 1, −5 Station

The head lies in the persistent occipital anterior or posterior position at the level of the pelvic inlet.

The persistent occiput anterior position is the more favorable, since the brow is only blocked by the promontory. By turning a little to the left or to the right, the head can sometimes pass the promontory and then a vaginal delivery can take place. The persistent occiput posterior position is much less favorable. The broad forehead often gets stuck on the symphysis and the pubic bone. Frequently, labor does not progress in the persistent occiput posterior position and a cesarean section will be necessary (Figure 2.54).

Hodge 2, −2/−3 Station

With adequate contraction activity, the head will be able to engage through rotational movements and increased flexion.

Hodge 3, 0 Station

Through increased flexion, the head engages without internal rotation and passes through the birth canal in a forward direction.

Rotation

The rotation consists of zig-zagging motions. The head does not rotate. The entire passage through the birth canal takes place with the sagittal suture in an anteroposterior direction. The head is born in the same position as the position with which it entered the pelvic inlet.

After that, the labor proceeds in the same manner as the labor in occiput OA or occiput OP.

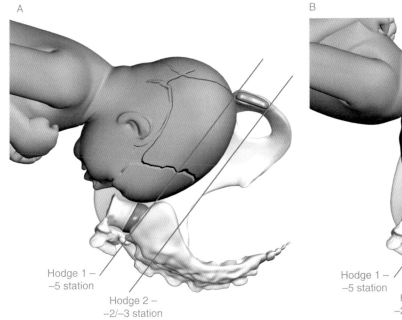
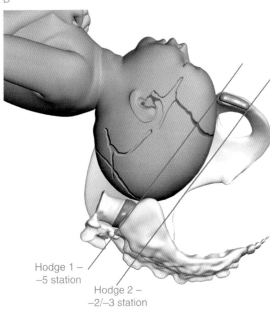

Hodge 1 –
−5 station

Hodge 2 –
−2/−3 station

Hodge 1 –
−5 station

Hodge 2 –
−2/−3 station

Figure 2.53A–B Persistent occiput position.

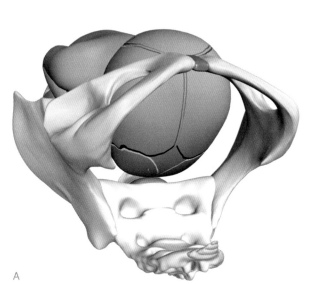
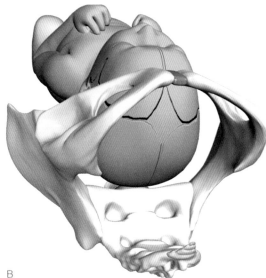

A

B

Figure 2.54A–B Persistent occiput anterior (A) and posterior (B).

Mechanism of Labor in Persistent Occiput Transverse Position

Characteristics

A persistent occiput transverse position is a position in which:

- the sagittal suture lies at or near the pelvic floor;
- the lie is a cephalic presentation;
- the presenting part is the head;
- the attitude is a flexion presentation, in which there is diminished flexion and both fontanels can be felt on palpation;
- the determining point is the occiput;

- the deepest point is the area around the sagittal suture, between the posterior and anterior fontanel, and therefore there is no eccentric pole;
- the dimensions of the head that pass through the pelvis are between those of the occiput presentation and the sinciput presentation (military attitude).

Incidence

The incidence is 1.5–1.9%.

Notation

Occiput presentation with the occiput (determining point: O) left or right transverse presentation (position: LOT or ROT).

Causes

Causes of a persistent occiput transverse position are:

- small or large fetus;
- dead fetus;
- little resistance of the birth canal (grand multiparity);
- android or platypelloid pelvis;
- insufficient contraction activity with or without the foregoing causes.

Diagnosis

- External examination:
  - cephalic presentation.
- Vaginal examination:
  - sagittal suture (nearly) transverse with the head on the pelvic floor;
  - both the anterior and the posterior fontanels can be felt.

Labor Mechanism of Persistent Transverse Position from H1, −5 Station, through the Birth of the Infant

A persistent transverse occiput position presents itself between Hodge 2, −2/−3 station and Hodge 4, +5 station. Until that moment, the descent proceeds as in an occiput presentation (Figure 2.55).

Rotation

In a normal pelvis, with or without stimulation of contractions, rotation can often still take place spontaneously and the infant can be born in occiput presentation. In case of a narrow pelvis, such as in a funnel-shaped android pelvis, there may not be enough room for rotation and often the head cannot engage.

Possible Interventions in Persistent Occiput Transverse Positions

The interventions are:

- stimulation of contractions;
- side-lying position of the mother on the side of the infant's back: this causes flexion of the head to be stimulated, allowing an eccentric pole to develop, rotation becomes possible and a normal occiput presentation occurs;
- if the conditions of an assisted delivery are satisfied:
  - digital correction (digital correction is done during a contraction; by placing two fingers on the side of the head, the head is flexed and rotated);
  - vacuum extraction.

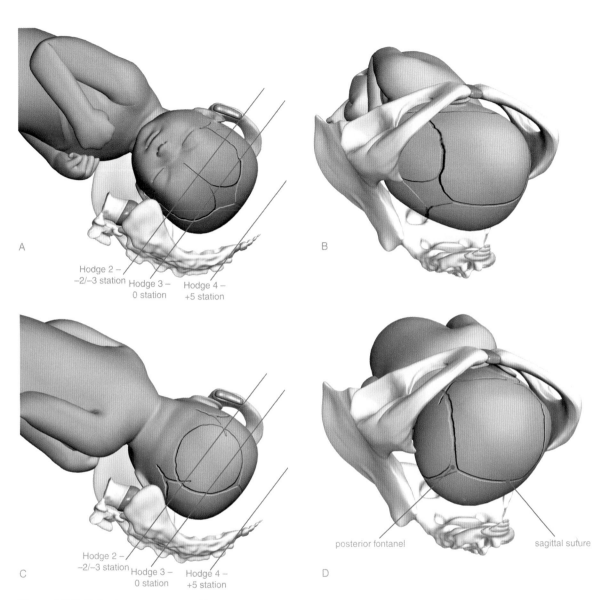

A

Hodge 2 –
–2/–3 station Hodge 3 –
0 station   Hodge 4 –
+5 station

B

C

Hodge 2 –
–2/–3 station Hodge 3 –
0 station   Hodge 4 –
+5 station

D

posterior fontanel   sagittal suture

Figure 2.55A–D Persistent transverse position.

Mechanism of Labor in Persistent Asynclitism

There are two types of persistent asynclitism:

- a persistent anterior asynclitism (Naegele's obliquity);
- a persistent posterior asynclitism (Litzmann's obliquity).

Characteristics

The contrast between physiological asynclitism and a persistent asynclitism is the degree of asynclitism. In a persistent asynclitism a fetal ear is felt.

In a persistent asynclitism:

- the lie is: cephalic presentation;
- the presenting part is: the parietal bone of the head;

- the attitude is: a flexion presentation (occiput or sinciput presentation);
- the determining part is: the occiput;
- the skull is often acutely deformed and the dimensions of the head that pass through the pelvis depend on the attitude.

Notation

Asynclitism anterior or posterior with the occiput (O) left (L) or right (R) transverse (T).

Causes

The causes of a persistent asynclitism could be:
- a tumor on the lateral side of the neck of the infant, torticollis;
- platypelloid pelvis.

Diagnosis

- External examination:
  - cephalic presentation.
- Vaginal examination:
  - In an anterior parietal bone presentation the fetal ear is anterior (under the symphysis) and the sagittal suture lies behind the pelvic axis.

- In a posterior parietal bone presentation the fetal ear is posterior and the sagittal suture lies in front of the pelvic axis (under the symphysis).

Labor Mechanism of Parietal Bone Presentation from H1, −5 Station through Birth

Hodge 1, −5 Station

- *Anterior asynclitism:* anterior asynclitism (Figure 2.56) is more favorable than posterior, since in anterior parietal bone presentation the posterior parietal bone upon engagement only needs to slide over the promontory and there is room in the sacral cavity. The risk of this presentation is overstretching at the front of the uterine segment by the protruding shoulder, with signs of a threatening uterus rupture.
- *Posterior asynclitism:* posterior asynclitism (Figure 2.57) is less favorable than anterior, since in posterior parietal bone presentation the anterior parietal bone becomes stuck on the promontory. The risk of this presentation is overstretching at the rear of the lower uterine segment by the protruding shoulder.

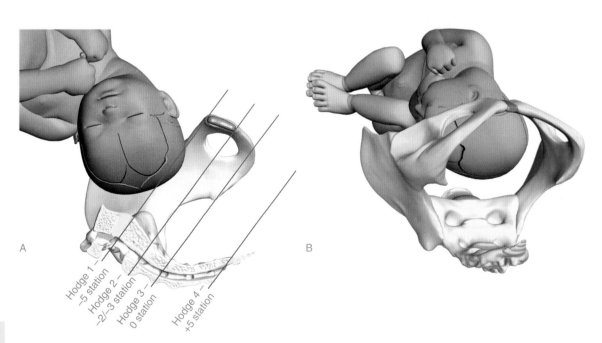

A

B

Figure 2.56A–B Anterior asynclitism.

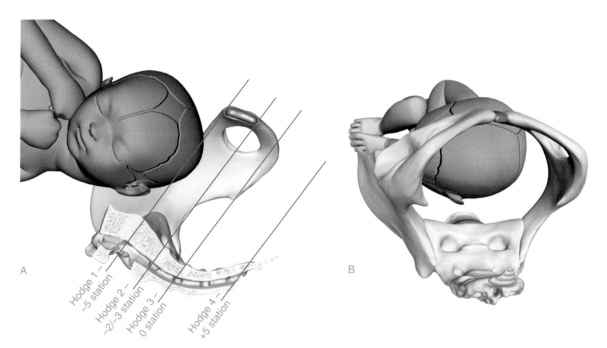

A   B

Hodge 1 – −5 station
Hodge 2 – −2/−3 station
Hodge 3 – 0 station
Hodge 4 – +5 station

Figure 2.57A–B Posterior asynclitism.

Hodge 2, −2/−3 Station

- *Anterior asynclitism:* if the posterior parietal bone was able to slide over the promontory, the head descends further and the labor proceeds as in an occiput OA delivery.
- *Posterior asynclitism:* frequently, a head in posterior parietal presentation does not pass Hodge 2, −2/−3 station and a cesarean section will have to be performed.

If the persistent asynclitism anterior presentation rotates to occiput OA, the rest of the delivery proceeds as in an occiput OA delivery.

Delivery of the Placenta

After the birth of the infant the height of the uterine fundus is determined. The fundus at that point is located at the level of the umbilicus.

Mechanism

The uterine volume becomes smaller after the birth of the infant. The reduction of the uterus takes place through retraction (passive) and contraction (active, afterbirth contractions). The afterbirth contractions usually start 5 to 10 minutes after the birth of the child. The placenta is unable to keep up with the reduction of the uterus. The placenta starts to pleat and behind these pleats the placenta tears away from the decidua and a hemorrhage appears behind the placenta.

After the placenta is completely or partially separated, it is expelled into the lower uterine segment and the vagina.

The placenta can be delivered via two different methods:

- *according to Schultze:* centrally behind the placenta a hematoma develops, whereupon the fetal side of the placenta is expelled first, followed by the (inside out) membranes and the hematoma ("Shiny Schultze") (Figure 2.58);
- *according to Duncan:* the hematoma develops on the lateral side of the placenta and discharges itself before the expulsion of the placenta, after which the placenta and the membranes along with the edge of the placenta are born first ("Dirty Duncan") (Figure 2.59).

The – due to retraction and contraction – compressed blood vessels of the placenta bed ensure that there is relatively little blood loss after the separation of the placenta.

Procedure

There are spontaneous and active management methods.

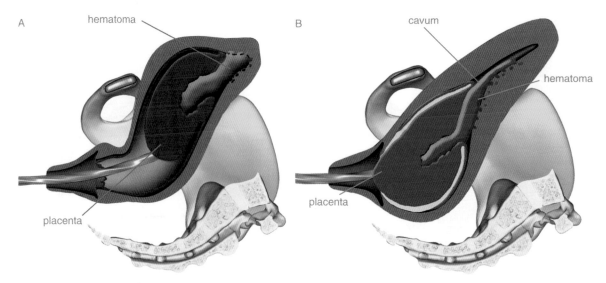

Figure 2.58A–B Delivery of the placenta according to Schultze.

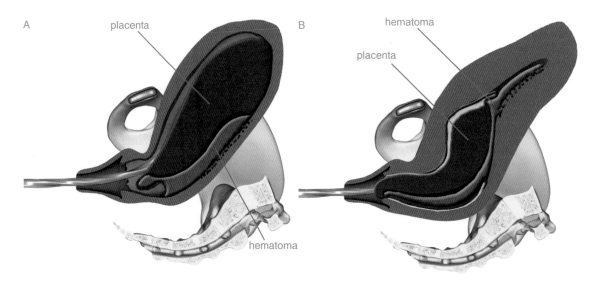

Figure 2.59A–B Delivery of the placenta according to Duncan.

In any of the maneuvers during the afterbirth, it must be borne in mind that they can only be applied if the uterus is properly contracted.

Spontaneous Management

Spontaneous management means that everybody waits until the placenta is spontaneously detached.

Signs indicating that the placenta is detached are:

- abdominal pain;
- more blood loss;
- the umbilical cord protrudes slightly out of the vulva (Ahlfeld's sign);
- the uterine fundus rises;
- the uterus veers to the right.

Check the foregoing points at regular intervals.

Aided by Küstner's maneuver, it can be ascertained whether the placenta lies in the lower uterine segment (the placenta is separated).

Küstner's maneuver is performed with a contracted uterus and a reclined woman.

A

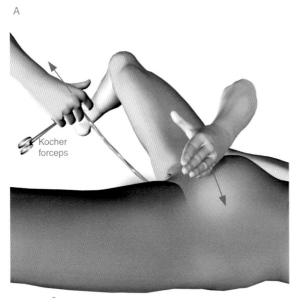

B

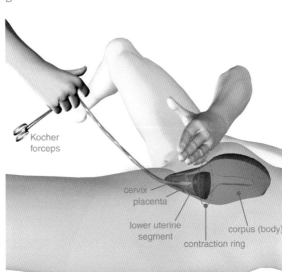

Figure 2.60A–B Küstner's maneuver.

The procedure works as follows (Figure 2.60):

- Take the end of the umbilical cord in one hand at the Kocher forceps and tighten the umbilical cord carefully.
- At the same time, press the abdominal wall with the ulnar side of the other hand at the location of the contraction ring (just above the symphysis pubis).

When the placenta lies detached in the lower uterine segment (LUS), the umbilical cord comes out (Küstner positive) or just stays in place. If the placenta is still in the body of the uterus, the umbilical cord will be pulled along to the inside (Küstner negative).

Only after the placenta is detached, apply the (modified) Baer's maneuver.

The Baer's maneuver works as follows (Figure 2.61):

- To support the abdominal muscles, place the palm of one hand slightly below the naval, at right angles to the direction of the rectus muscles.
- With the other hand, take the end of the umbilical cord at the Kocher forceps and carefully tighten the umbilical cord.
- Ask the mother to push along during a uterine contraction.
- Allow the placenta to be delivered in the direction of the birth canal.

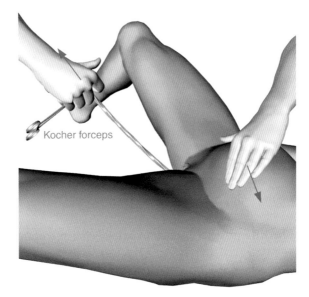

Figure 2.61 Baer's maneuver.

- Catch the placenta with the free hand and then let the membranes follow slowly.

Use the following procedure if the membranes do not follow:

- Put the placenta down.
- Place a Kocher forceps on the membranes at the level of the vaginal introitus. Massage the uterine

A

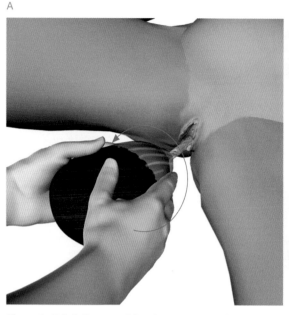

B

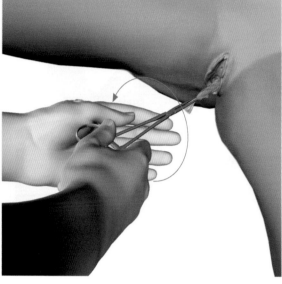

Figure 2.62A–B Rotation of the placenta (A) or Kocher (B).

fundus lightly and put slight traction on the membranes with the Kocher forceps.

- Or: rotate the placenta (or the Kocher) until the membranes let go (Figure 2.62).

Monitoring

After the placenta has been delivered, regularly check the mother for at least 1 hour after the birth, for:

- the position of the fundus (this may not rise);
- the contraction condition of the uterus;
- blood loss.

Check the placenta, including the following important points:

- whether the placenta and the membranes are complete;
- abnormalities of shape (lobes, membranacea);
- abnormalities of maternal and fetal surface (infarcts, chorioangioma, abrupt);
- cord abnormalities (the number of vessels, knots, velamantous insertion).

Then check:

- the total amount of blood loss (estimate and weigh if necessary);
- the vulva, the perineum, and the vagina for lacerations.

Active Management

Active management means that after the birth of the infant there is an active effort to cause the placenta to be expelled. Thus, there is no waiting for signs of detachment of the placenta.

The methodology is as follows (Figure 2.63):

- Administer 5 or 10 IU of oxytocin intramuscularly or intravenously immediately after the birth of the infant.
- Clamp the umbilical cord.
- Wait for a good contraction of the uterus.
- Place one hand above the symphysis pubis with the palm of the hand in the direction of the mother's navel. This hand provides counterpressure to the uterus.
- With the other hand, apply traction to the umbilical cord, either with the aid of a Kocher forceps or by wrapping the umbilical cord twice around several fingers. The traction is applied in the direction of the birth canal, first toward the perineum and upward when the placenta follows. This is called "controlled cord traction."
- The placenta must be delivered in a smooth motion.
- If this maneuver must be interrupted, it is important to first release the tension to the umbilical

A

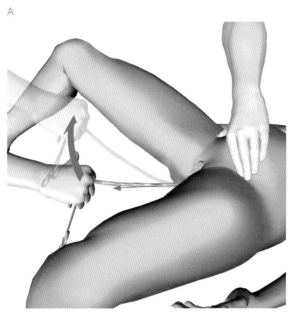

B

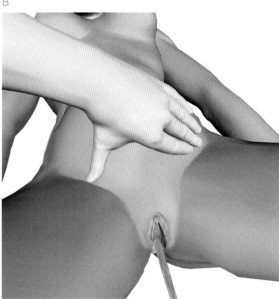

Figure 2.63A–B Active procedure.

cord and only let go of the counterpressure on the uterus after that.

- Check for blood loss and wait for a uterine contraction.

Active versus Spontaneous Management

Active management of the third stage of labor means a combination of the following actions[19]:

Administer oxytocin, 10 IU im/iv.

The umbilical cord is clamped soon after birth.

During the first contraction (after 3–5 minutes) birth of the placenta with controlled cord traction (CCT), followed by:

Massage of the uterus.

Active management of the third stage of labor using uterotonics is advised by the World Health Organization (WHO) because even women with a low risk for hemorrhage can have a hemorrhage post partum (HPP). Active management reduces the risk for severe hemorrhage (> 1000 ml) (RR 0.34; 95% CI 0.14–0.87) [LE A1]. Of all actions that are part of active management, giving oxytocin is the most important action.[20] For all other actions it is not evident whether they contribute to reducing HPP. Recent research shows that CCT contributes less to decreasing HPP [LE A2].[20] Massage of the uterus is an

effective way to prevent the use of uterus tonica, but there is less literature about method and duration of massage [LE B].[21,22] Also recent disadvantages of early cord clamping have been described: postponing cord clamping for at least 1 minute does not increase the risk for HPP.[23] For the baby, later clamping of the cord leads to a decrease in the risk of anemia. It can though lead to a light increase in the number of children with hyperbilirubinemia [LE A1].[24] A combination of active (administering oxytocin) and expectative (cord clamping between 1 and 3 minutes post partum using Baer) policy appears to give the best outcomes for mother and baby.[19]

Episiotomy and Perineal Lacerations (Grade 1 and 2)

Perineal lacerations are lacerations of the vagina, the vulva, and the perineum that may occur during childbirth. For a classification of perineal lacerations, we will use the international classification of perineal and sphincter lacerations proposed by Sultan in 2002 (Table 2.2).[25] In this section we will describe the first- and second-degree lacerations as well as episiotomies. Obstetric anal sphincter injuries (OASIS) are third- and fourth-degree lacerations which are discussed in Chapter 13 on sphincter lesions.

69

Table 2.2 Classification of lacerations according to Sultan

Grade 1	Skin laceration
Grade 2	Skin and perineal laceration without sphincter involvement
Grade 3	Perineal and anal sphincter laceration
Grade 3a	Laceration <50% of external anal sphincter
Grade 3b	Laceration >50% of external anal sphincter
Grade 3c	Laceration of both internal anal sphincter and external anal sphincter
Grade 4	Laceration of perineum, anal sphincter, and anal mucosa

Episiotomy

Episiotomies are probably the most frequently applied obstetric interventions. It is also one of the few surgical interventions for which patient consent is generally not requested. An episiotomy is an incision of the vagina, the perineum, and the underlying muscles. An episiotomy enlarges the outlet of the soft-tissue birth canal.[26]

A primary episiotomy is defined if the indication to perform episiotomy was already established before the labor with the idea of preventing extreme pressure to the pelvic floor or to the head of the infant. The indication for a secondary episiotomy is determined during the expulsion. Usually, a mediolateral episiotomy is employed (Figure 2.64). A midline episiotomy, in which an incision is made from the posterior commissure in the midline in the direction of the anal sphincter, is not often applied in the Netherlands, Flanders, and in China. This type of episiotomy is commonly used in the USA and Canada.[26]

Incidence

In the mid-twentieth century it was standard procedure in many countries to perform an episiotomy in nulliparous women. A more restrictive episiotomy policy, however, leads to less posterior perineal trauma than a policy in which an episiotomy is performed routinely (RR 0.88; 95% CI 0.84–0.92) and less OASIS (RR 0.67; 95% CI 0.49–0.91) [LE A1].[27] Moreover, by not performing an episiotomy there is a greater chance of an unblemished perineum: a routine episiotomy leads to 26% more need for suturing (RR 1.26; 95% CI 1.08–1.48) [LE A1].[28] Prenatal perineal massage, performed by the patient or partner once to twice a week from 35 weeks' pregnancy, appears to diminish the incidence of

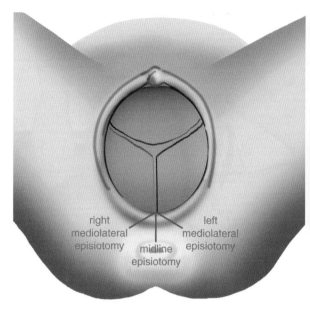

Figure 2.64 Midline and mediolateral episiotomies.

episiotomy in nulliparous women (RR 0.83; 95% CI 0.73–0.95) [LE A1].[29] Furthermore, hands off (or poised) versus hands on the perineum during the second stage of labor reduces the rate of episiotomy (RR 0.69; 95% CI 0.50–0.96) [LE A1].[16] Finally, comparing the position in the second stage of labor for women without epidural anesthesia, fewer episiotomies are performed in an upright position versus supine or lithotomy position (RR 0.79; 95% CI 0.70–0.90) [LE A1].[30] Delivery in an upright position increases the risk of perineal trauma (RR 1.35: 95% CI 1.20–1.51), but not for OASIS (RR 0.58; 95% CI 0.22–1.52).

Nevertheless, at present there are enormous international differences in episiotomy incidence, varying from 10% in Scandinavia to more than 90% in South America.[31] The incidence of episiotomy in the Netherlands is 26% and in Flanders 55% (nulliparous women 75%, multiparous women 41%).[32,33] Within the Netherlands there are also large differences in the incidence of episiotomy: of the nulliparous women who give birth in first-line care (midwife), 22% are given an episiotomy, while among the nulliparous women who give birth in second-line care (obstetrician), 51% are given an episiotomy. Among multiparous women giving birth in first-line care, 7% are given an episiotomy, compared to 17% of multiparous women giving birth in second-line care.[32] In Finland, the hospital-based lateral episiotomy rate ranges from 38% to 86% for primiparous and from 6% to 30% for multiparous women.[34]

Indications

The only real indication for performing an episiotomy is the reduction of delivery time for the infant (signs of fetal emergency) or the mother (fatigue, maternal illnesses).

A number of other indications have been reported for performing an episiotomy. Possible indications for performing an episiotomy are:

- fetal emergency;
- shoulder dystocia;
- vaginal assisted deliveries and breech deliveries;
- reduction of time of delivery in case of maternal illnesses;
- prolapse surgery or other vulvovaginal operation in the medical history.

The literature is not in complete agreement on the protective function of mediolateral episiotomy for the incidence of sphincter lesions. In a Cochrane review comparing routine episiotomy (episiotomy performed in 75% of participants) versus restrictive episiotomy (episiotomy performed in 28% of participants), a restrictive policy results in less severe perineal trauma (RR 0.67; 95% CI 0.49–0.91), especially in the group with mediolateral episiotomy (RR 0.55; 95% CI 0.31–0.96) [LE A1].[27] In a Finnish study, however, restricting lateral episiotomy use to lower incidences may result in higher rates of sphincter lesions and the optimal level of episiotomy is not yet known [LE B].[34]

It could be that the manner in which the episiotomy is placed, particularly the angle of the episiotomy relative to the midline, is of importance in the prevention of OASIS.[35] Based on a large observational study in the Netherlands, it seems that in an assisted vaginal delivery, sphincter lesions can be prevented by performing mediolateral episiotomies. This is true for both vacuum extractions (odds ratio [OR] 0.11; 95% CI 0.09–0.13) and forceps extractions (OR 0.08; 95% CI 0.07–0.11) [LE B].[36] A third- or fourth-degree laceration in the medical history is no indication for primary episiotomy [LE C].[25]

Technique for Episiotomy Placement

There is no international consensus on the definition of a mediolateral episiotomy.[37] In contrast with most Anglo-Saxon countries, in the Netherlands and

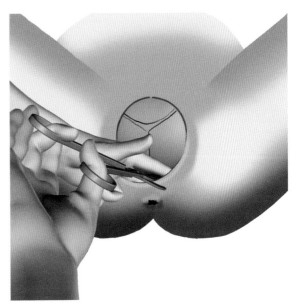

Figure 2.65 Open scissors are inserted as deeply as possible while guided by the fingers.

Flanders an episiotomy is placed at the left side of the patient. With respect to the episiotomy placement technique, this chapter will assume this location.

If tolerated by the labor, local anesthesia with 1% lidocaine is administered.[25] When the head is almost extended, the index and middle fingers of the left hand are placed between the skull and the pelvic floor. Then the open scissors are inserted as deeply as possible while guided by the fingers (Figure 2.65).

At the peak of the contraction, the skin, the subcutis, and the pelvic floor muscles are cut with a slightly pushing, yet smooth motion. The episiotomy starts from the center of the posterior commissure and is placed at an oblique angle in the direction of the left ischial tuberosity. Based on observational studies it appears that the average length of an episiotomy is 4 cm and the maximum length is 6 cm.[38,39] An insufficient angle increases the chance of sphincter injury and in order to obtain a postpartum angle of 45° the episiotomy must be placed at an approximate angle of 60° (Figures 2.66 and 2.67) [LE C].[40]

Preparation for Suturing

The preparation for suturing an episiotomy consists of[25,41]:

- explanation about the suturing;
- proper positioning and adequate lighting;

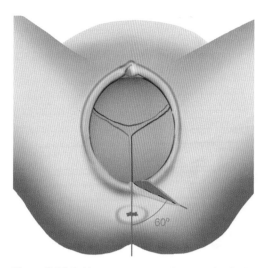

Figure 2.66 Episiotomy at an approximate angle of 60°.

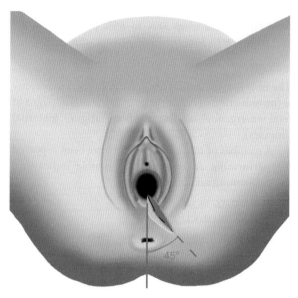

Figure 2.67 Postpartum angle of 45°.

- thorough inspection of the vagina and the perineum. Rectal examination is essential to ascertain whether a sphincter laceration developed and must take place in the inspection of each laceration. In a rectal examination the index finger is inserted in the anus, and the thumb is placed on the sphincter. The sphincter is palpated between the thumb and the index finger. In a study by Andrews et al., 56% of all sphincter lacerations were missed [LE C][42];
- suturing under aseptic circumstances;
- adequate anesthesia (10–20 ml lidocaine 1%);
- suturing must take place as soon as possible to prevent blood loss and infections. Suturing before the delivery of the placenta may lead to less blood loss [LE B], but carries the risk that the sutures may be removed if a manual placenta removal is still necessary.[43] If additional time is lost between the placement of the episiotomy and the suturing, the chance of bacterial contamination and thereby possibly also the chance of wound infection increases.

Suturing Technique

To suture an episiotomy, (atraumatic) synthetic absorbable suture material is used, such as polygalactin 910 (Vicryl) or polyglycolic acid (Surgicryl, Safyl, Dexon).

The repair of an episiotomy can be divided into three layers: vaginal trauma, deep and superficial perineal muscles, and the skin. Traditionally, repair was done according to these three layers, but nowadays, continuous suturing techniques are also often used.[44]

The first suture inside the vagina is placed above the upper margin of the incision to prevent the formation of a hematoma due to blood vessel retraction. Next, the vaginal mucosa is sutured with a continuous suture – possibly a mattress stitch – out to the hymenal ring (Figures 2.68 to 2.71).

Next, the pelvic floor muscles (the transverse perineal muscle, the bulbospongiosus muscle, and the urethrovaginal muscle) are sutured with a continuous stitch (Figure 2.72). However, some argue that the bulbospongiosus muscle should be deliberately sought and anchored by a separate suture primarily for anatomical correction but also for possibly preventing vaginal widening [LE D].

In practice, however, these muscles are usually not distinguishable and are approximated with the help of one or more sutures. Finally, the skin is closed with rapidly absorbable continuous intracutaneous sutures (Figures 2.73 and 2.74).[45] To suture an episiotomy, preference is given to a continuous suturing technique.

If all the layers are closed with a continuous suturing technique, there are significantly less pain symptoms compared to interrupted sutures during the first 10 days postpartum (RR 0.76; 95% CI 0.66–0.88) and an overall reduction in analgesia use (RR 0.70; 95% CI 0.59–0.84) [LE A1].[46]

Removal of suture material from the skin is considerably less frequently necessary if rapidly absorbable sutures are used (3-0 thickness Rapide)

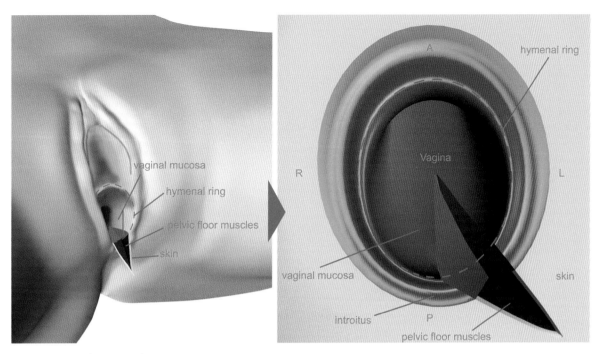

Figure 2.68 Initial situation when suturing.

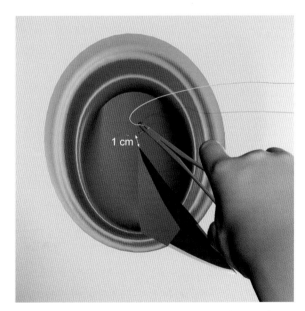

Figure 2.69 First suture inside the vagina is placed above the margin of the incision.

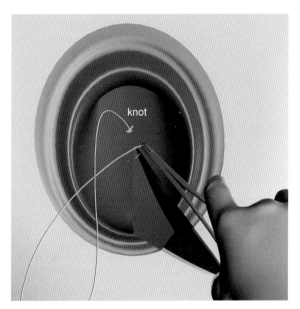

Figure 2.70 Suturing of the vaginal mucosa out to the hymenal ring.

compared to standard material (22/769 [3%] versus 98/770 [13%], p < 0.0001), and also in the continuous suturing technique compared to the interrupted suturing technique (24/770 [3%] versus 96/769 [12%], p < 0.0001) [LE A2].[45] However, rapidly

absorbable material may lead to more wound dehiscence.[38]

If after suturing the subcutis, the skin is properly positioned, it may be considered to withhold the intracutaneous suturing.[41] As an alternative to

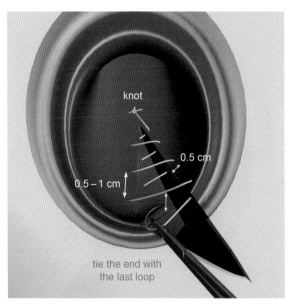

Figure 2.71 Continuous stitching of the vaginal mucosa out to the hymenal ring.

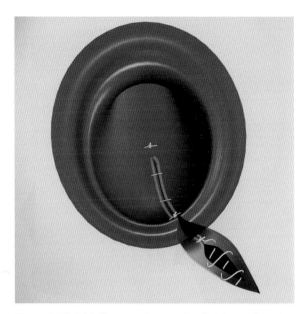

Figure 2.72 Pelvic floor muscles are sutured with a continuous stitch.

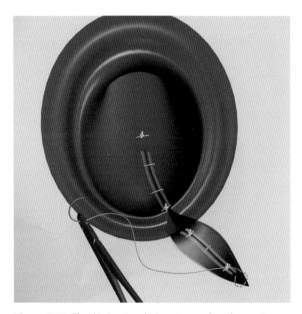

Figure 2.73 The skin is sutured intracutaneously with a continuous stitch.

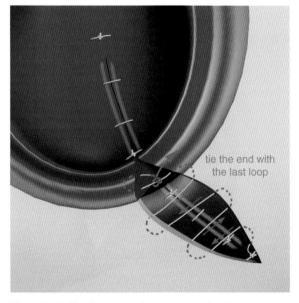

Figure 2.74 The skin is sutured intracutaneously with a continuous stitch (continuation phase Figure 2.73).

continuous sutures for each layer, the vaginal mucosa, the pelvic floor muscles, subcutis, and intracutaneous suturing can be done with one continuous suture.[41] After completing the suturing, a rectal examination must always be performed to ensure that no sutures were placed in the rectum. If this is the case, however, all of the sutures must be removed and the suturing must be done again.

Complications

The complications can be classified into short- and long-term complications. During the initial postpartum days the complications of an episiotomy are pain, infection, and bleeding. It appears that a spontaneous second-degree laceration causes less pain symptoms and dyspareunia than a mediolateral episiotomy [LE B].[47] A midline episiotomy is a recognized risk factor for sphincter lesions.[31] A *non-steroidal anti-inflammatory drug* (NSAID) such as indomethacin or diclofenac provides significant pain reduction during the first 24 hours postpartum and some argue that this should be standard treatment for all women after a laceration or an episiotomy, except in the case of contraindications [LE D].[25] Even though small quantities of this medication pass into the breast milk, in normal doses (indomethacin 25 mg three times a day, diclofenac 50 mg three times a day) no effect is expected in the infant.

Late complications of an episiotomy are pain and dyspareunia. There appears to be no difference in the incidence of urinary and/or fecal incontinence and genital prolapse after an episiotomy compared to an uninjured perineum or a first- and second-degree laceration [LE B].[47]

First- and Second-Degree Lacerations

Preparation and Technique for Suturing

The preparation for suturing a first- or second-degree laceration is comparable to that of an episiotomy (see Section: Episiotomy) (Figure 2.75).

Suturing a first- or second-degree laceration is comparable to suturing an episiotomy, with the exception that the wound margins are usually less sharp (see Section: Episiotomy).

Prevention of First- and Second-Degree Ruptures

There are no indications that perineal lacerations can be prevented through perineum massage during the expulsion or an episiotomy (see Section: Episiotomy).[25] Perineal injury can possibly be prevented through heat compression ([LE B]: nulli OR 0.7; 95% CI 0.4–1.0 and multi OR 0.6; 95% CI 0.3–0.9) and lidocaine spray for pain relief during the expulsion ([LE A2]: RR 0.63; 95% CI 0.42–0.93), but both outcomes are based on only one randomized study.[25] Although prenatal perineal massage in nulliparous women seems to diminish the chance of episiotomy (RR 0.83; 95% CI 0.73–0.95), there is no difference in the incidence of first- and second-degree laceration [LE A1].[29]

An observational study of almost 3000 spontaneous deliveries in Australia illustrates that lateral position deliveries produce the least amount of perineal lacerations (33.3%) and delivery in a sitting position has the greatest chance of perineal lacerations (58%). The study also demonstrated a significant difference in uninjured perinea if the delivery was guided by a gynecologist (31.9%) as compared to that by a midwife (56–61%) [LE B].[48] In a recent systematic review, Epi-No birth trainer (a device for training of the pelvic floor muscles with an inflatable balloon) did not reduce episiotomy rates and had no influence on reducing perineal tears [LE B].[49]

Essential Points and Recommendations

- Thorough inspection of each perineal laceration, including rectal examination, is important because (superficial) sphincter lesions can be missed (see Chapter 13 on sphincter lesions) [LE C].
- It is recommended to classify perineal lacerations according to the internationally accepted classification [LE D].
- Perineal laceration may be prevented through pain relief during the expulsion with the use of lidocaine spray [LE A2] or hot compresses [LE B]. Although prenatal perineal massage in nulliparous women seems to reduce the chance of episiotomy, there is no difference between the incidence of first- and second-degree laceration [LE A1].

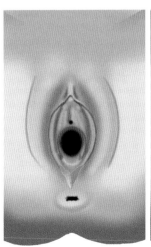 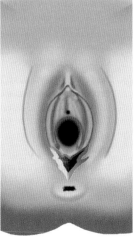

first-degree laceration   second-degree laceration

Figure 2.75 First- and second-degree lacerations.

- An episiotomy is an obstetric intervention that should only be performed on indication. The routine performance of an episiotomy does not prevent sphincter lesions [LE A1], leads to additional need for suturing the perineum [LE A1], and is probably coupled with increased pain and dyspareunia in the short and long term [LE B].
- If an episiotomy is needed, it must be performed adequately, from the center of the posterior commissure and in a bulging perineum at a 60° angle from the midline [LE C].
- Suturing an episiotomy must be performed under proper positioning, illumination, adequate local pain relief, and after careful inspection concerning the classification of the lesion, including a rectal examination [LE D].
- Preference is given to a continuous suturing technique with absorbable suturing material [LE A1].

References

1. Cunningham F, Leveno K, Bloom S, et al. Williams obstetrics. New York: McGraw-Hill, 2009.

2. Fraser DM, Cooper MA. Myles' textbook for midwives. London: Churchill Livingstone, 2003.

3. Hals E, Olan P, Pirhonen T, et al. A multicentre interventional program to reduce the incidence of anal sphincter tears. Obstet Gynecol. 2010; 116(4):901–8.

4. Heineman MJ, Evers JLH, Massuger LFAG, Steegers EAP. Obstetrie en Gynaecologie. De voortplanting van de mens. 7th edn. Amsterdam: Reed Business, 2012.

5. Henderson C, Macdonald S. Mayes' midwifery. London: Baillière Tindall, 2004.

6. Holmer AJM. Leerboek der verloskunde. Bussum: Van Dishoeck, Van Holkema & Warendorf NV, 1967.

7. Kloosterman GJ. De Voortplanting Van De Mens. Leerboek voor obstetrie en gynaecologie. Weesp: Centen, 1985.

8. Leidraad bij de studie der obstetrie en gynaecologie in drie delen. Deel I en III. Excerpta lectionum.

9. National Collaborating Centre for Women's Health. Intrapartum care of healthy women and their babies during childbirth. Clinical Guideline. 2009. http://www.guidance.nice.org.uk/CG55.

10. Dudenhausen JW. Praktische Geburtshilfe mit geburtshilflichen Operationen. Berlin/New York: Walter de Gruyter, 2011.

11. Reuwer P, Bruinse H, Franx A. Proactive support of labor. Cambridge: Cambridge University Press, 2009.

12. Stables D, Rankin J. Physiology in childbearing with anatomy and related biosciences. London: Baillière Tindall, 2005.

13. Tiran D. Baillière's midwives' dictionary. London: Baillière Tindall, 2003.

14. World Health Organization. Care in normal birth: a practical guide. Geneva: World Health Organization, Maternal and Newborn Health/Safe Motherhood Unit, 1996.

15. Stichting Perinatale Registratie Nederland. Perinatale zorg in Nederland: Jaarboeken 2003–2012. Utrecht: PRN, 2014. http://www.perinatreg.nl

16. Aasheim V, Nilsen ABV, Lukasse M, Reinar LM. Perineal techniques during the second stage of labour for reducing perineal trauma. Cochrane Database Syst Rev. 2011;12:CD006672.

17. Laine K, Skjeldestad FE, Sandvik L, et al. Incidence of obstetric anal sphincter injuries after training to protect the perineum: cohort study. BMJ Open. 2012;2: e001649.

18. Ponkey SE, Cohen AP, Heffner LJ, Lieberman E. Persistent fetal occiput posterior position: obstetric outcomes. Obstet Gynecol. 2003; 101(5 Pt 1):915–20.

19. Wereldgezondheidsorganisatie. Recommendations for the prevention and treatment of postpartum haemorrhage. Geneva: WHO, 2012.

20. Gülmezoglu AM, Lumbiganon P, Landoulsi S, et al. Active management of the third stage of labour with and without controlled cord traction: a randomized, controlled, non-inferiority trial. Lancet. 2012;379:1721–7.

21. Jangsten E, Mattsson LA, Lyckestam I, et al. A comparison of active management and expectant management of the third stage of labour: a Swedish randomised controlled trial. BJOG. 2011;118:362–9.

22. Hofmeyr GJ, Abdel-Aleem H, Abdel-Aleem MA. Uterine massage for preventing postpartum haemorrhage. Cochrane Database Syst Rev. 2008;(3):CD006431.

23. Begley CM, Gyte GM, Devane D, et al. Active versus expectant management for women in the third stage of labour. Cochrane Database Syst Rev. 2011;(11): CD007412.

24. McDonald SJ, Middleton P, Dowswell T, Morris PS. Effect of timing of umbilical cord clamping of term infants on maternal and neonatal outcomes. Cochrane Database Syst Rev. 2013;(7):CD004074.

25. National Institute for Health and Clinical Excellence. Intrapartum care: care of healthy women and their babies during childbirth. London: RCOG, 2007.

26. Kalis V, Laine K, de Leeuw JW, et al. Classification of episiotomy: towards standardization of terminology. BJOG. 2012;119:522–6.

27. Carroli G, Mignini L. Episiotomy for vaginal birth. Cochrane Database Syst Rev. 2009;(1):CD000081. doi: 10.1002/14651858.CD000081.pub2.

28. Hartmann K, Viswanathan M, Palmieri R, et al. Outcomes of routine episiotomy: a systematic review. JAMA. 2005;293:2141–8.

29. Beckmann MM, Garrett AJ. Antenatal perineal massage for reducing perineal trauma. Cochrane Database Syst Rev. 2006;(1):CD005123. doi: 10.1002/14651858.CD005123.pub2

30. Gupta JK, Hofmeyr GJ, Shehmar M. Position in the second stage of labour for women without epidural anaesthesia. Cochrane Database Syst Rev. 2012;5: CD002006. doi:1002/14652858.CD002002.pub3.

31. Graham ID, Carroli G, Davies C, et al. Episiotomy rates around the world: an update. Birth. 2005;32:219–23.

32. Stichting Perinatal Registratie Nederland. Perinatale zorg in Nederland 2012. Utrecht: PRN, 2013.

33. Christiaens W, Nieuwenhuijze MJ, de Vries R. Trends in medicalisation of childbirth in Flanders and the Netherlands. Midwifery. 2013;29:e1–8.

34. Räisänen S, Vehviläinen-Julkunen K, Gissler M, Heinonen S. Hospital based lateral episiotomy and obstetric anal sphincter injury rates: a retrospective population based register study. Am J Obstet Gynecol. 2012;206(4):347.e1–6. doi: 10.1016/j.ajog.2012.02.019. Epub 2012 Feb 28.

35. Eogan M, Daly L, O'Connell PR, et al. Does the angle of episiotomy affect the incidence of anal sphincter injury? BJOG. 2006;113:190–4.

36. de Leeuw JW, de Wit C, Kuijken JP, et al. Mediolateral episiotomy reduces the risk for anal sphincter injury during operative vaginal delivery. BJOG. 2008;115:104–8.

37. Kalis V, Stepan Jr J, Horak M, et al. Definitions of mediolateral episiotomy in Europe. Int J Gynecol Obstet. 2008;100(2):188–9.

38. Verspyck E, Sentilhes L, Roman H, et al. Episiotomy techniques. J Gynecol Obstet Biol Reprod. 2006;35:1540–51.

39. van Dillen J, Spaans M, van Keijsteren W, et al. A prospective multicenter audit of labor-room episiotomy and anal sphincter injury assessment in the Netherlands. Int J Gynecol Obstet. 2010;108:97–100.

40. Kalis V, Karbanova J, Horak M, et al. The incision angle of mediolateral episiotomy before delivery and after repair. Int J Gynecol Obstet. 2008;103:5–8.

41. Sultan AH, Thakar R. Lower genital track and anal sphincter trauma. Best Pract Res Clin Obstet Gynaecol. 2002;16:99–115.

42. Andrews V, Sultan A, Thakar R, et al. Risk factor for obstetric anal sphincter injury: a prospective study. Birth. 2006;33:117–22.

43. Baksu B, Davas I, Akyol A, et al. Effect of timing of episiotomy repair on peripartum blood loss. Gynecol Obstet Invest. 2008;65:169–73.

44. Kettle C, Fenner D. Repair of episiotomy, first and second degree tears. In: Sultan AH. Perineal and anal sphincter trauma. Springer: London, 2008, pp. 20–32.

45. Kettle C, Hills R, Jones P, et al. Continuous versus interrupted perineal repair with standard or rapidly absorbed sutures after spontaneous vaginal birth: a randomised controlled trial. Lancet. 2002;359:2217–23.

46. Kettle C, Hills RK, Ismail KMK. Continuous versus interrupted sutures for repair of episiotomy or second degree tears. Cochrane Database Syst Rev. 2007(4): CD000947. doi: 10.1002/14651858.CD000947.pub2.

47. Sartore A, de Seta F, Maso G, et al. The effects of mediolateral episiotomy on pelvic floor function after vaginal delivery. Obstet Gynecol. 2004;103:669–73.

48. Shorten A, Donsante J, Shorten B. Birth position, accoucheur, and perineal outcomes: informing women about choices for vaginal birth. Birth. 2002;29:18–27.

49. Brito LG, Ferreira CH, Duarte G, Noguera AA, Marcolin AC. Antepartum use of Epi-No birth trainer for preventing perineal trauma: systematic review. In Urogynecol J. 2015;10:1429–36.

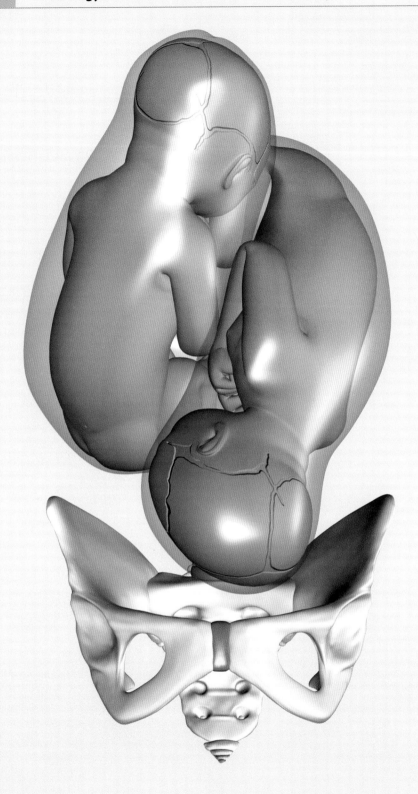

Compound Presentation and Umbilical Cord Prolapse

A.J. Schneider and J.J. Duvekot

General Information

Introduction

In this chapter we discuss the obstetric aspects of compound presentation (extremity prolapse) and umbilical cord prolapse of an infant in cephalic or breech presentation.

The recommendations made in this chapter are based on the opinion of experts [LE D], except where indicated otherwise.[1]

Definition

The extremities and umbilical cord are *presenting* if they are positioned next to or lower than the fetal head with unruptured membranes. If the membranes are ruptured, we speak of *prolapsed* extremities or umbilical cord in those cases (Figures 3.1 and 3.2).

Prolapsed Extremities

Incidence

A cephalic presentation with a presenting or prolapsed hand or arm is a rare occurrence. The incidence varies between 0.4 and 1.3 in 1000 childbirths.[2–5] Prolapsed extremities are quite frequently combined with a prolapsed umbilical cord. It is prudent to be aware of this and to conduct a specific examination for this.

Diagnosis

A diagnosis of *presenting* extremities can be made by internal examination and especially by means of ultrasound. In the event of *prolapsed* small parts, the

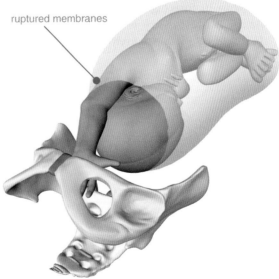

ruptured membranes

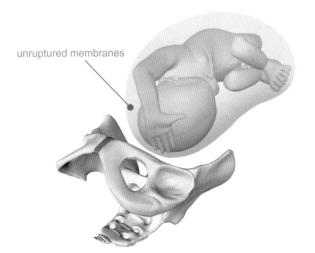

unruptured membranes

Figure 3.1 Presenting hand.

Figure 3.2 Prolapsed hand.

Obstetric Interventions, ed. P. Joep Dörr, Vincent M. Khouw, Frank A. Chervenak, Amos Grunebaum, Yves Jacquemyn, and Jan G. Nijhuis. Published by Cambridge University Press. © Cambridge University Press 2017.

diagnosis can usually be established more precisely by internal examination.

A hand can be differentiated from a foot because, if the clasping reflex is still intact, the hand will grasp the examination finger. Moreover, the foot is usually located at a right angle to the lower leg, in contrast with the position of the hand to the lower arm.

If a knee or elbow is palpable, it is important to indicate whether this is positioned deeper than the largest diameter of the head. A knee and an elbow can be difficult to distinguish, therefore the accompanying hand or foot must always be sought.

The need to distinguish a prolapsed arm from a prolapsed hand is to ascertain whether the wrist joint is located lower than the largest diameter of the head. We can also speak of a complete or incomplete arm presentation.[5]

Causes and Risk Factors

Extremities may prolapse due to insufficient closure of the pelvic inlet by the presenting part. Predisposing factors for this phenomenon are as follows.

- *Parity:* In primiparous women the head generally descends during the last weeks of pregnancy and closes off the pelvic inlet. In multiparous women the presenting part sometimes remains above the pelvic inlet until the start of contractions. The chance of presenting/prolapsed parts is therefore 10 times higher in multiparous women.[5]
- *Anatomical discrepancy between head and pelvis:* In the event of a relatively large head and/or a relatively small pelvis, engagement does not take place. This discrepancy is most prevalent in small women (<1.60 m) with a large infant in the first pregnancy.
- *Head not engaged:* This occurs after spontaneous membrane rupture or by inducing labor by artificially rupturing of the membranes in a situation of a not (yet) engaged presenting part.
- *Rupturing of the membranes in case of polyhydramnios:* After rupturing of the membranes, the small parts may flow out next to the head that is not (yet) in close contact with the pelvic inlet.
- *Small, premature (dead, macerated) infant.*
- *Space-occupying process in the true pelvis:* In a low-lying myoma in the true pelvis or with a marginal placenta previa or low-lying placenta. Frequently an oblique lie will be present.
- *Second of a set of twins:* After the birth of the first infant, the second infant often engages so rapidly that the chance of presenting/prolapsed extremities or umbilical cord is increased.

Therapy
Vaginal Delivery Impossibility

There is a (relative) impossibility of vaginal delivery in case of the following prolapsed small extremities in combination with a cephalic presentation[2,6]:

- head and two hands (Figure 3.3);
- head and arm (Figure 3.4);

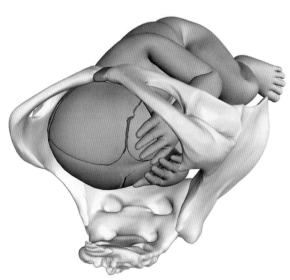

Figure 3.3 Head and two hands.

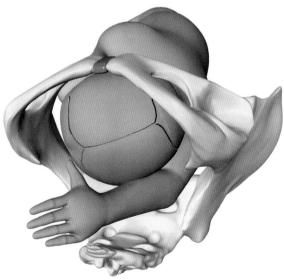

Figure 3.4 Head and one arm.

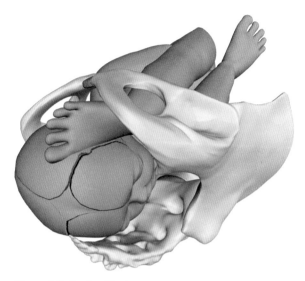

Figure 3.5 Head and foot.

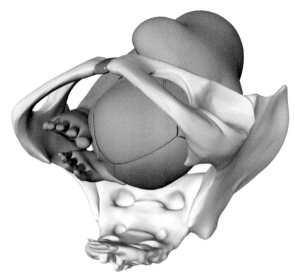

Figure 3.6 Head with hand and foot.

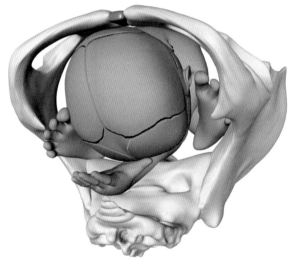

Figure 3.7 Head with hand and two feet.

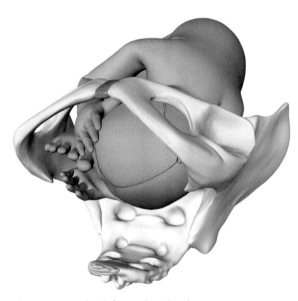

Figure 3.8 Head with foot and two hands.

- head and foot (Figure 3.5);
- head with one arm and one foot (Figure 3.6);
- head with one hand and two feet (Figure 3.7);
- head with one foot and two hands (Figure 3.8).

Vaginal delivery in these situations will only be possible in case of a very small or dead infant. In case of a living infant, it makes no sense to wait for improvement in the situation and a cesarean section will be necessary.

Presenting Hand or Arm

In case of a presenting hand or arm, the membranes should not be ruptured artificially. During the early dilation phase, the woman can be positioned on the opposite side of the presenting hand or arm, whereby space is created so that the hand or arm can pull back spontaneously.

Prolapsed Hand or Arm

See Animations 3.1 and 3.2.

The clinical procedure is determined by ascertaining whether the wrist joint and/or the elbow joint are located below the largest diameter of the head (Figure 3.9). Anatomically, the wrist forms the

A

B

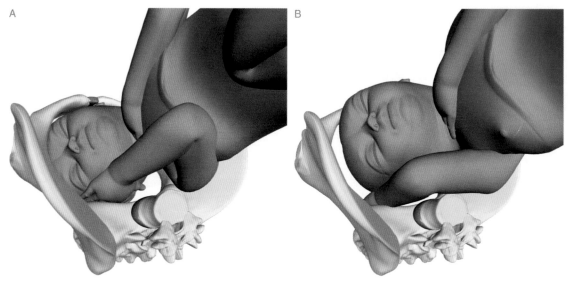

Figure 3.9A–B Prolapsed hand (A) and prolapsed arm (B).

thickest part between the fingers and the lower arm with the shape of a double wedge. If we look at this merely mechanically, the arm – if the wrist is positioned lower than the head at the start of the labor – slides in front of the head as it gets deeper into the true pelvis.

If the head and the hand have not yet engaged very much, a repositioning of the hand can be attempted by stimulating the infant to pull the arm back by softly squeezing the hand. If this is not effective and the wrist remains deeper than the head, we have a case of a prolapsed arm or a complete arm presentation. Because of the lack of space and an unconquerable obstacle, the delivery comes to a sudden halt. Waiting until complete dilation is reached may cause a uterine rupture due to excessive stretching.[7] In addition to the fact that the delivery cannot proceed because of this, this presentation is further complicated in one-third of the cases due to the simultaneous prolapse of the umbilical cord.[5]

It would be different if the head engages and the wrist is not situated below the largest diameter of the head, which would prevent the arm from prolapsing further. This presentation does not present clinical problems.[5]

If, in addition to the wrist, the elbow is also palpably lower than the largest diameter of the head, we have a case of absolute delivery obstruction due to the presenting part.

Special Situations

Repositioning of a Prolapsed Arm

A method recommended by WHO to use in case of a prolapsed arm – only to be used in situations with lack of modern facilities – is as follows (see Animation 3.3). Repositioning of a prolapsed arm can be attempted in a motivated patient: after positioning the woman in a knee–elbow position, the arm is pushed past the head to above the pelvic inlet and held there until the head has occupied the vacated space (Figure 3.10). In the western world it is recommended that this procedure be performed in an operating room. In case of failure of this maneuver or if the umbilical cord prolapses, a cesarean section can then be performed immediately. If the procedure is successful, the rest would be a normal delivery.[8]

Internal Version and Extraction

In addition to the above-mentioned repositioning of the arm, internal version can be performed only on the second of a set of twins with a presenting arm and only when the obstetrician has experience with this procedure: after locating the back by ultrasound, search for the foot with your hand on the abdominal side of the fetus, grasp the ankle between the index and middle fingers, and pull the leg firmly down (see Chapter 6 on delivery in breech presentation) (see Animation 3.4). If possible, pull the second foot

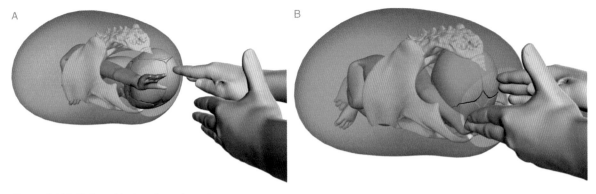

A B

Figure 3.10A–B Repositioning of a prolapsed arm.

down at the same time so that the infant can be delivered vaginally (Figure 3.11) (see Animation 3.5). Internal version and extraction is best performed under locoregional or general anesthesia in the operating theatre.

Adjacent or Occult Hand

In the case of vacuum extractions it is reported that more force is needed to extract the head in the presence of an occult hand (Figure 3.12) [LE B].[9]

Prognosis and Therapy

The prognosis of a prolapsed hand or arm depends on any simultaneously existing disorders (for instance, a prolapsed umbilical cord). In most instances of a prolapsed arm, the problem will have to be solved by performing an emergency cesarean section.

Complications

Complications in the event of presenting or prolapsed extremities are rare.

In a stagnated dilation there is a chance of overstretching and rupture of the uterus with a prolapsed arm.

A very rare complication (three published cases) is necrosis of a prolapsed arm due to the circulation being cut off by the head. This is so uncommon that in those cases an investigation should be performed into the increased coagulation tendency in the neonate.[10] Less serious consequences of impingement are hematomas on the arm or the hand.

Prevention

In general, prevention is not very successful. There are, however, some situations in which the presenting part does not close off the pelvic inlet very well and caution is

called for. An example of this is a non-engaged head in combination with unruptured membranes. It is better to rupture the membranes only while at the same time the head is pressed down into the pelvic inlet by a helper. The bladder should be emptied beforehand.

In case of ruptured membranes and a non-engaged presenting part, clinical bed rest may be prescribed. If, in the case of a non-engaged head, the membranes rupture outside the hospital, it is prudent to instruct the patient to come to the hospital as soon as possible. In most cases this will be faster than waiting for an ambulance and certainly if the contractions have not yet started, instances of prolapsed extremities or umbilical cord will not present a problem.

Important Points and Recommendations

- In case of a smoothly progressing dilation and engagement, all combinations of cephalic presentation with presenting or prolapsed extremities can in principle be monitored to see how the further development of the labor and delivery progresses [LE D].
- By softly squeezing a finger of a presenting or prolapsed hand the infant may be inclined to retract the hand [LE D].
- If the infant does not retract the arm after stimulation, the location of the thickest part – the double wedge formed by the wrist – is an indicator of the prognosis. If the wedge is located below the head, it will be pushed along on further engagement and constitute an obstacle. Delivery must then be done by cesarean section [LE D].
- A vaginal delivery with a prolapsed arm is only possible if the fetus is very small or if it is dead. In other situations, contractions will reduce when pushing. After reaching complete dilation, there is a risk of uterine rupture [LE D].

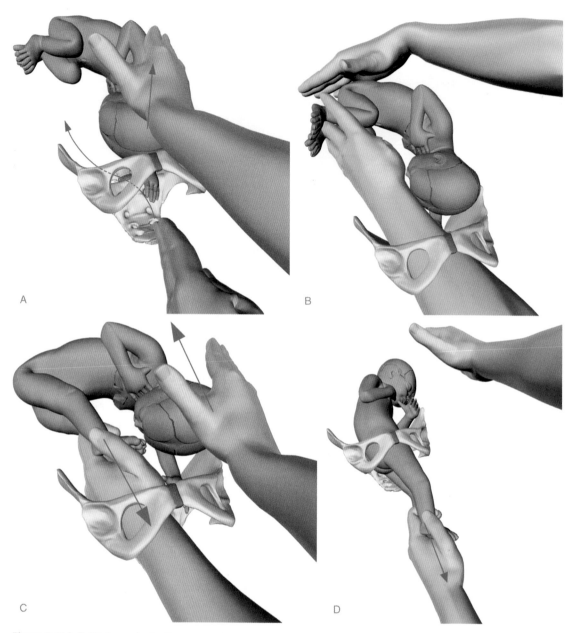

Figure 3.11A–D Version and extraction.

Prolapsed Umbilical Cord

Definition

The umbilical cord is *presenting* if, with unruptured membranes, the umbilical cord is palpably lower than the presenting part.

If the membranes are ruptured, then there is a case of *prolapsed* umbilical cord (Figure 3.13).

If the umbilical cord is situated alongside the presenting part during labor, it is called an *occult* umbilical cord prolapse.

Incidence

The incidence of a prolapsed umbilical cord in cephalic presentations varies between 1 and 6 per 1000 births.[11,12] In breech presentations the incidence

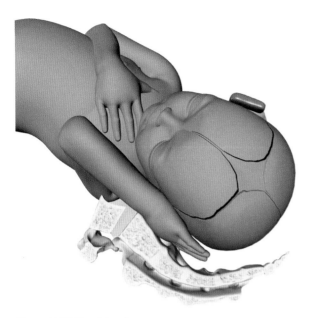

Figure 3.12 Occult hand.

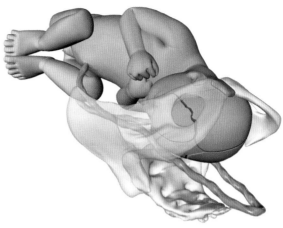

Figure 3.13 Prolapsed umbilical cord.

ranges from 4% to 6% and is lower with a complete breech presentation than with a footling breech.[12,13] In preterm deliveries with a fetus in breech presentation the incidence is even higher. The longer the umbilical cord, the greater the chance of prolapse. A prolapsed umbilical cord occurs more in male fetuses, who on average have longer umbilical cords than female fetuses.

The exact frequency of occult umbilical cord prolapses is not known, but it probably occurs more than is clinically acknowledged.

Diagnosis

A *presenting* umbilical cord diagnosis can be made by internal examination and especially by means of an ultrasound examination. A presenting umbilical cord is difficult to detect by palpation; ultrasound (color flow Doppler) examination can therefore be helpful.

In case of a *prolapsed* umbilical cord, the diagnosis can often be made very well through internal examination. Often the umbilical cord is still pulsating and is therefore easy to detect. The fetal heart rhythm pattern can still be normal with a prolapsed umbilical cord, but the majority of cases present with bradycardia or variable decelerations.[14,15] Especially when fetal heart rhythm disorders develop after spontaneous or assisted rupturing of the membranes, a prolapsed umbilical cord must be ruled out by means of internal or speculum examination. In case of preterm ruptured membranes, in which it is the rule to perform as few internal examinations as possible, this situation forms the exception to the rule.

In an *occult* umbilical cord, because of the pinching of the umbilical cord between the presenting part and the cervix, decelerations will develop on the cardiotocogram (CTG) and thereby provide an initial indication. The definitive diagnosis is usually only made during a cesarean section.

Causes and Risk Factors

The risk factors for developing a prolapsed umbilical cord are listed in Table 3.1. A distinction is made between general and procedure-related risk factors. At least 50% of all prolapsed umbilical cord cases are preceded by an obstetric procedure.[13]

Therapy

A prolapsed umbilical cord constitutes an emergency that demands immediate action. The danger of a prolapsed umbilical cord is twofold, i.e., mechanical: the impingement of the umbilical cord between the infant and the wall of the birth canal, and vasospasm: the contraction of blood vessels in the umbilical cord through cooling and manipulation. This will, in both cases, lead to a decrease in the blood flow to the fetus with asphyxia as a result.

In the event of a prolapsed umbilical cord, the procedure must be aimed at having the delivery take

Table 3.1 Risk factors for umbilical cord prolapse[11,12]

General risk factors	Procedure-related risk factors
Multiparity	Artificial rupturing of membranes
Low birthweight (<2500 g)	Vaginal manipulation of fetus in case of ruptured membranes
Premature birth	Version and extraction
Congenital fetal disorders	Insertion of intrauterine pressure catheter
Breech presentation	Insertion of skull electrode
Transverse lie or oblique lie	External version
Second of set of twins	Application of forceps or vacuum cup
Polyhydramnios	
Non-engaged presenting part	
Low-lying placenta	
Extremely long umbilical cord (>80 cm)	
Anencephaly	

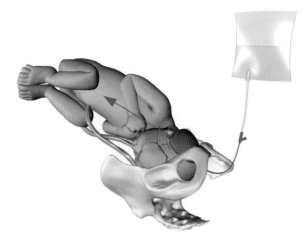

Figure 3.14 Filling of the bladder with saline solution.

place as soon as possible and in the following manner:

- Call for help: in addition to extra obstetricians/gynecologists and nurses, a pediatrician and anesthesiologist should be notified.
- Determine the fetal heart rhythm:
  - In the absence of *fetal heart action*, this must be determined by ultrasound. It may at times be difficult to determine if indeed no pulsations can be felt in the umbilical cord. In case of fetal death, the policy must follow local protocol.
  - In case of a *normal fetal heart rhythm pattern*, the choice between an emergency cesarean section and an assisted vaginal delivery will depend on the degree of dilation and the nature of the engagement of the presenting part.
    - If it is decided to proceed with an assisted vaginal delivery, the outlet position must be such that the delivery can take place quickly and without problems. The conditions must be the same here as with an operative vaginal delivery in other indications. This is not a situation in which extra risks should have to be taken. A total breech extraction or version and extraction should only be performed under favorable circumstances.
    - If it is decided to perform a cesarean section, acute tocolysis can be considered. With

a pregnancy duration before viability (24–25 weeks) an expectative approach may be chosen. As a rule, cesarean sections are not performed before this time in the Netherlands due to the moderate neonatal prognosis at this early stage. This situation is different in other countries.

- In case of an *abnormal fetal heart rhythm pattern*, the choice is also between an emergency cesarean section or an operative vaginal delivery, depending on the degree of dilation, the nature of the presenting part, and the engagement. If it is decided to proceed with an assisted vaginal delivery, the outlet position must be such that the delivery can take place quickly and without problems.
  - If it is decided to do an emergency cesarean section, it is useful to push the presenting part upward. This can be done through the retrograde filling of the bladder with 500–750 ml saline solution via a 16-G Foley catheter, which is then clamped off (see Animation 3.6). A possible side effect of this could be a decrease in the contraction activity. Naturally, the balloon of the catheter must be inflated to hold it in place. Only at the moment of the incision, the Kocher forceps are released from the indwelling catheter. For this reason, every delivery room should be equipped with an indwelling catheter, a bag of infusion liquid, Kocher forceps, and an inflator (Figure 3.14).

– A second possibility is to push the presenting part up with the examining hand. This uncomfortable procedure can best be done with half of the hand (three fingers) or the entire hand. An alternative to this is internally pushing the presenting part out of the pelvis and then suprapubically fix the presenting part with the other hand. After the presenting part has been fixed externally, the internal hand may be removed and the presenting part should remain in the pushed-up position until arrival in the operating room.[15]

– A third method is to place the patient in a knee–elbow position. An alternative to this is the *head-down* or Trendelenburg position. The latter position is combined with a left side lie. Improvement of the fetal condition after the presenting part has been pushed up should not be a reason to slow down or change the procedure that was set in motion.

Pushing the umbilical cord back into the uterus must be avoided [LE D]. This has never appeared to be very beneficial. There is only one publication in which this method has been applied with reasonable success. Touching or cooling of the umbilical cord must be avoided to prevent vasospasm. Whether actively keeping the umbilical cord warm helps is a question that still needs to be answered. One possibility is to place an umbilical cord that is hanging outside the vagina back into the vagina.

In the past, if dilation was not complete yet, an assisted vaginal delivery was attempted by means of Dührssen's incisions in the cervix (Figure 3.15). Nowadays this method must be used for emergency cases only.

Of all indications for a cesarean section, a prolapsed umbilical cord is one of the few real emergency indications. Prognostically there is no clear relationship with the time elapsed between the decision to do a cesarean section and the delivery of the infant. This is probably because in publications with many patients, this *decision-delivery-time* does not amount to more than 30 minutes and is therefore already very short.

Training of the obstetrics team in the handling of emergencies, such as a prolapsed umbilical cord, probably leads to a decline in the perinatal death and morbidity rate.

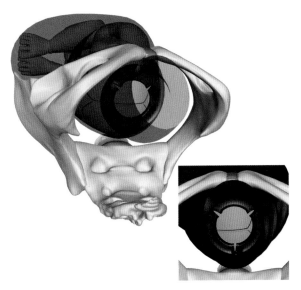

Figure 3.15 Dührssen's incisions.

Complications

Perinatal death due to a prolapsed umbilical cord appears to be on the decrease. During the first half of the twentieth century the death rate was still 32–47%. In the last 20 years the death rate has gone down to less than 10%.[12,16,17] The liberal performance of cesarean sections and improvements in neonatal care has contributed greatly to this decline.

The location in which a prolapse of the umbilical cord occurs is prognostically one of the most important factors. If the umbilical cord prolapse occurs outside the hospital, the perinatal death rate is 10 times higher than when this occurs in the hospital.[11]

The literature sporadically reports on the successful outcome of conservative treatment of an umbilical cord prolapse in a pregnancy duration of less than 24 weeks.[14] Usually, however, these cases result in fetal death within a few hours.

Prevention

Just as in the case of a prolapsed arm or hand, prevention is not very successful. There are, however, some situations in which the presenting part does not block the pelvic inlet completely and caution must be exercised. In that case, we would offer the same advice as in the prevention of a prolapsed arm or hand.

For women with an infant in an oblique lie or with a non-engaged presenting part it may be suggested to hospitalize them for observation at a certain point in pregnancy and, if possible, introduce labor and delivery in a controlled manner after external version. Nethertheless, this does not prevent compound presentation or umbilical cord prolapse after spontaneous rupture of the membranes. These women must always be properly instructed to come immediately to the hospital after spontaneous rupture of the membranes. The recommendation to be transported in a reclined position is obsolete and leads to unnecessary delays.

When obstetric procedures are necessary in the event of a non-engaged presenting part, there must be the possibility to perform an emergency cesarean section. In this situation, artificial rupturing of the membranes should be avoided.

In the Netherlands, patients with preterm prelabor rupture of membranes are usually admitted to the hospital. Especially in the case of a breech presentation there is a greater chance of a prolapsed umbilical cord.

It is difficult to predict this type of emergency. Routine ultrasound examination to locate the umbilical cord beforehand is not very effective for predicting a prolapsed umbilical cord [LE B].[18]

Important Points and Recommendations

- Anyone who guides labor and deliveries must be aware of the risk factors that can lead to umbilical cord prolapse [LE D].
- In the event of a prolapsed umbilical cord, the fastest way to deliver must be sought [LE D].
- A case of a prolapsed umbilical cord can be delivered vaginally if the delivery can be performed quickly and safely [LE D].
- Pushing the presenting part back is essential in the treatment of the prolapsed umbilical cord with an abnormal fetal heart rhythm pattern [LE D].
- Pushing the presenting part up can be done manually, by filling the bladder or through a different reclining position of the woman [LE D].

References

1 van Everdingen JE, Burgers JS, Assendelft WJJ, et al. Evidence-based richtlijn ontwikkeling. Houten: Bohn Stafleu Van Loghum, 2004.

2 Bhose L. Compound presentation. A review of 91 cases. Br J Obstet Gynaecol. 1961;68:307–14.

3 El-Mowafi D. Geneva Foundation for Medical Education and Research. Complex and breech presentation. http://www.gfmer.ch

4 Perkins R. Compound presentations. eMedicine, 2015. http://emedicine.medscape.com/article/262444-overview.

5 Martius G. Pathologie der Geburt. In: Martius G (ed). Lehrbuch der Geburtshilfe. Stuttgart: Georg Thieme Verlag, 1971, pp. 374–6.

6 Asimakopulos N. Compound presentation: prolapse of three extremities with the head. Can Med Assoc J. 1965;92:929–31.

7 Newton P. Foetal arm prolapse and presumed maternal death in a wild hanuman langur (Presbytis entellus). Primates. 1990;31:143–5.

8 World Health Organization, UNFPA, UNICEF, World Bank (eds). Compound presentation. In: Managing complications in pregnancy and childbirth. A guide for midwives and doctors. Geneva: WHO, 2003. http://www.who.int/reproductive-health/impact/index.html

9 Vacca A. The 'sacral hand wedge'; a cause of arrest of descent of the fetal head during vacuum assisted delivery. BJOG. 2002;109:1063–5.

10 Tebes CC, Mehta P, Calhoun DA, et al. Congenital ischemic forearm necrosis associated with a compound presentation. J Matern Fetal Med. 1999;8:231–3.

11 Siassakos D, Fox R, Draycott TJ. Umbilical cord prolapse. Green-top Guideline No 50. RCOG, April 2008.

12 Lin MG. Umbilical cord prolapse. Obstet Gynecol Surv. 2006;61:269–77.

13 Barclay M. Umbilical cord prolapse and other cord accidents. In: Sciarra JJ (ed). Gynecology and obstetrics. Philadelphia, PA: Lippincott, 1989, p. 1.

14 Koonings PP, Paul RH, Campbell K. Umbilical cord prolapse. A contemporary look. J Reprod Med. 1990;35:690–2.

15 Usta JM, Mercer BM, Sibai BM. Current obstetrical practice and umbilical cord prolapse. Am J Perinatol. 1999;16:479–84.

16 World Health Organization, UNFPA, UNICEF, World Bank (eds). Prolapsed cord. In: Managing complications in pregnancy and childbirth. A guide for midwives and doctors. Geneva: WHO, 2003. http://www.who.int/reproductive-health/impact/index.html

17 Carlin A, Alfirevic Z. Intrapartum fetal emergencies. Semin Fetal Neonatal Med. 2006;11:150–7.

18 Ezra Y, Strasberg SR, Farine D. Does cord presentation on ultrasound predict cord prolapse? Gynecol Obstet Invest. 2005;56:6–9.

Delivery of Twins

M. Laubach and Y. Jacquemyn

General Information

Introduction

A twin pregnancy is an obstetrically high-risk pregnancy that is characterized by a higher perinatal morbidity and mortality in comparison with singleton pregnancies. This is due, among other things, to an increased incidence of intrauterine growth restriction and premature birth. More than 50% of all twins are born before the 37th week of pregnancy. The average gestational age at birth is 36.7 ± 2.7 weeks.[1]

Therefore, the peripartum approach surrounding the delivery of twins must, on the one hand, take these factors into account and, on the other hand, contemplate some additional specific elements, such as an abnormal fetal lie before and during the labor and delivery.

See Animation 4.1.

Incidence

The incidence of twin pregnancies in the western world has continued to rise since the 1970s and currently fluctuates between 16 and 24 per 1000 pregnancies.[2,3] This may be attributed to the use of assisted reproduction techniques, but could also be the result of the rise in maternal age.[2]

Timing of Delivery

For twin pregnancies beyond 36 weeks of gestational age an attempt has to be made to plan the delivery in such a way that perinatal mortality and morbidity continue to be as low as possible.

Epidemiological studies have shown that the perinatal death rate of twins is five to seven times higher than that of singleton pregnancies with the same pregnancy duration.[4] The lowest incidence of perinatal death was encountered during the 38th week of the pregnancy. After 38 weeks, the perinatal death rate increases comparably to the rise in post-term singleton pregnancies after 41 weeks. Considering both the birthweight and the pregnancy duration, the lowest *perinatal mortality rate* (PMR) (3.9/1000) was reported in neonates weighing between 2.5 and 2.9 kg and between 36 and 39 weeks of pregnancy duration [LE B].

There is little good evidence on optimum timing of delivery taking chorionicity into account. In uncomplicated monochorionic diamniotic twin pregnancies early delivery between 34 and 36 weeks is recommended in order to reduce the risk of stillbirth [LE B].[5-7] Monochorionic diamniotic twins with successfully treated twin-to-twin transfusion syndrome require close observation throughout pregnancy [LE C].[8]

The risk for intrauterine fetal death in monochorionic diamniotic twin pregnancies beyond 34 weeks of gestational age is 1.5–1.7%.[9-11] This incidence is even three times lower in dichorionic twin pregnancies (0.5%). The perinatal mortality drops from 8% to 1% in dichorionic twins between 36 and 38 weeks. (LE B)

The perinatal morbidity seems to remain high in all twin pregnancies even after 34 weeks, suggesting potential benefits of prolonging pregnancy beyond 36 weeks. Additionally, neonatal morbidity (especially respiratory distress syndrome) is significantly increased in case of an elective induction of labor prior to 37 weeks and neonatal intensive care hospitalization has been reported more frequently. This increase is even greater in the case of twins born by cesarean section (13% before 37 weeks compared to 2% after this term) [LE B].[12]

Today, one sufficiently powered randomized controlled trial (RCT) has demonstrated that, in uncomplicated twin pregnancies, elective induction

Obstetric Interventions, ed. P. Joep Dörr, Vincent M. Khouw, Frank A. Chervenak, Amos Grunebaum, Yves Jacquemyn, and Jan G. Nijhuis. Published by Cambridge University Press. © Cambridge University Press 2017.

of labor at 37 weeks versus an expectant management results in significantly less adverse neonatal outcome without an increased number of complications. [LE A2].[13]

Optimum timing for delivery in uncomplicated monochorionic twin pregnancies after 35 completed weeks of pregnancy has to be discussed with the parents, taking the consequences of a late intrauterine fetal death in these cases into account compared to potential respiratory complications of premature induced delivery [LE B].[6,7]

Cesarean Section

Indications for Planned Cesarean Delivery

In twin pregnancies, certain indications for cesarean delivery are similar to those among singleton pregnancies and include placenta previa, placental abruption, abnormal fetal evaluation, breech, and intrauterine growth restriction.

There is growing evidence in the literature that there is no indication for a routine policy of scheduled cesarean delivery in all twin pregnancies.[14–17] The results of a large randomized multicenter study (Twin Birth Study) demonstrated no significant improvement in neonatal outcome for cesarean section after 32 gestational weeks in cases where the presenting twin is in a vertex position [LE A2].[18]

Indications for delivering twins in a planned cesarean section are:

- *conjoined twins*, except in an extremely immature delivery [LE D];
- monochorionic monoamniotic twins [LE D][19];
- first twin in breech or transverse presentation. [LE D]

Considerations

- During labor, in 19% of cases the first twin is not presenting in a vertex position (non-vertex). Historically, these pregnancies have been resolved by means of cesarean delivery. This policy is inspired by the fear of being confronted with the so-called *locked twins* phenomenon. This occurs when delivery of the head of the first twin is prevented by the presenting part of the second twin when the body of the first twin has already been delivered. The initial evidence for this comes from a compilation of 145 case reports, from which an incidence of locked twins of between 1/645 and

1/817 births was deduced. The reported mortality rate was between 30% and 43%. Actually only eight observational studies have been published, which were analyzed in a recent systematic review.[20] No benefit was found supporting cesarean delivery in pregnancy with non-vertex first twins after 32 weeks and with a birthweight of >1500 g. These conclusions pertain to both twins. Considering the Term Breech Trial[21] and the lack of experience in vaginal breech deliveries in many centers, it appears that currently an elective cesarean section is the recommended delivery method of twins with the first fetus in breech presentation [LE D]. In a transverse presentation of the presenting twin, a planned cesarean delivery is always indicated.

- Some authors have proposed elective cesarean delivery in all cases in which at least one of the twins has an estimated birthweight of <1500 g. There are no prospective randomized studies. Numerous observational studies have not been able to demonstrate a difference in perinatal results [LE B].[22–24] Only one study indicates a significantly better perinatal survival after cesarean delivery of infants with a birthweight of <1000 g [LE B].[25] It can be concluded that the discussion on whether or not a cesarean delivery should be performed on the basis of the estimated birthweight is not fully crystallized.

- The gestational age as such is no indication for a cesarean delivery and birthweight is more predictive in terms of intrapartum complications [LE B].[23,24]

- No study exists that investigates the influence of an elective cesarean delivery on the perinatal result in the presence of a weight difference of >25% between the twins. A difference in estimated weight is currently no indication for a cesarean delivery [LE C].[25,26]

- A scarred uterus after a cesarean delivery with an incision in the lower uterine segment from a previous pregnancy does not imply an increased risk of uterine rupture in a twin pregnancy, compared to a singleton pregnancy (90/10 000 deliveries). The chance of success in a vaginal delivery lies between 65% and 85% [LE C].[27]

Vaginal Delivery

During labor, in 81% of cases the first twin is in vertex presentation (vertex twin A). In 40% to 50% of cases, both fetuses are in vertex presentation and in 30% to

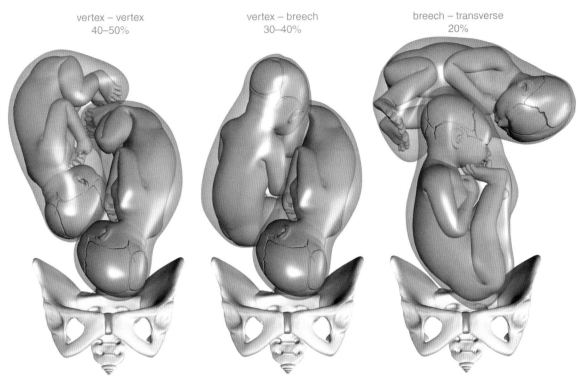

vertex – vertex
40–50%

vertex – breech
30–40%

breech – transverse
20%

Figure 4.1 Most prevalent combinations of presentations.

40% of cases there is a combination of vertex twin A and non-vertex twin B (Figure 4.1).[3]

In the literature, vaginal delivery of sets of twins is (still) universally accepted.[3,15–17] But in clinical reality, it appears that only 50% of twins are born spontaneously by vaginal delivery. Epidemiological research shows that between 40% and 45% of sets of twins are born by planned cesarean delivery and 8% by assisted vaginal delivery.[2]

The choice of a planned cesarean delivery is primarily dictated by the indication of increased risk (RR 1.62) of perinatal morbidity for the second child after vaginal delivery. The reported increase is independent of the prelabor lie and chorionicity, but is associated with a long interval between the twins (intertwin interval) in a planned vaginal delivery [LE B].[22,28,29]

Since a secondary cesarean delivery has higher maternal and neonatal morbidity, it is important to select the twin that would be the most likely candidate for vaginal delivery. This may also be decided on the basis of the obstetric history. The literature shows that the probability of a successful vaginal delivery decreases if antepartum maternal pathology exists,

such as diabetes or hypertension. At term, malpresentation of the second twin sometimes is associated with the failure of vaginal delivery [LE B].[30] It seems advisable to take these factors into consideration when determining the delivery mode of term twin pregnancies.

Labor and Delivery Management in Vaginal Deliveries[3,8,31,32]

Vaginal delivery of twins is considered a high-risk birth in terms of the risk of peripartal complications. Therefore, these deliveries should be conducted in centers with adequate infrastructure to react rapidly to complications.

General guidelines for a vaginal delivery of twins are as follows:

- All women pregnant with twins should receive information about the possible obstetrical attitudes concerning twin delivery.
- For each woman who is pregnant with twins there should be an individual plan that anticipates all possible scenarios during the first (dilatation) and second (expulsion) stage of labor.

- The presence of an experienced gynecologist with sufficient assistants, such as a resident or midwife, is of utmost importance.
- An operating room with a surgical team and the possibility of neonatal resuscitation must be available.
- On admission, an ultrasound evaluation of the fetal position must be made.
- An intravenous line is needed during the dilation stage. A blood cross-match is made and blood must be available.
- Fetal heart tones are recorded by cardiotocography (CTG) that is equipped for recording twins. As soon as the membranes of the presenting twin are ruptured, a CTG by (scalp) electrode of the fetus is recommended.
- Contraction stimulation with oxytocin is not always necessary during the delivery of the first infant, but is started after delivery of the first infant to prevent weak contractions.
- From the time of complete dilation and until the delivery of the second infant a pediatrician must be present near the delivery room. A resident, midwife, or a second gynecologist experienced in conducting ultrasound examinations and helping in assisted vaginal deliveries and cesarean sections must also be present in the delivery room. It is the aim to have an anesthesiologist present at the hospital during the second and third stage of labor.
- After the birth of the first infant, the position of twin B is determined by ultrasound, as well as the location of the fetal heart. After that, the CTG registration is continued.
- Active management of the third stage of labor is pursued during the third phase.

Intertwin Time Interval

There is insufficient evidence in the literature on the maximum duration of the intertwin interval. The notion that the intertwin time interval should not be more than 30 minutes is based on a study dating back to the time before the systematic use of CTG.[33] Later publications do not report an increase in neonatal complications in longer intertwin time intervals as long as fetal heart rate is reassuring.[29,34,35] It appears that with a longer duration of the intertwin time interval the risk in a cesarean delivery for the second twin increases by a factor of 6 to 8. Studies from recent years also show that the peripartal complications for

the second twin increase as the delivery takes longer. Limiting the intertwin time interval to less than 15 minutes is linked to a significant decrease in the number of cases of low Apgar scores and metabolic acidosis, compared to a time interval of more than 60 minutes. [29,34,35] It seems prudent therefore to limit the duration of the intertwin time interval. Recent literature recommends an intertwin time interval of a maximum of 15 to 30 minutes [LE C].[3,36]

Delivery of Vertex–Vertex Twins

After the birth of the first twin, one in every five twins – depending on the pregnancy duration – will change its presentation.[23] Therefore, an ultrasound confirmation of the presentation of the second fetus is recommended before the intravenous oxytocin infusion is started or increased. The uterine activity is evaluated manually. Initial pushing takes place with unruptured membranes. An amniotomy is only performed if the head is sufficiently connected to the completely dilated cervix. Owing to complications, such as umbilical cord prolapse or a lack of engagement progress, in 4% to 10% of the cases the procedure will change to an assisted delivery with vacuum or forceps, a cesarean section, or internal version, followed by breech extraction (Figure 4.2).[35,37]

Delivery of Vertex–Non-vertex Twins

Technically, there are various options when performing these deliveries:

- vaginal breech delivery;
- breech extraction (possibly preceded by internal version in case of transverse presentation);

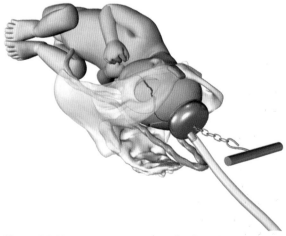

Figure 4.2 Vacuum extraction in case of prolapsed umbilical cord.

Table 4.1 Non-vertex twin 2: way of delivery and neonatal results

	N	Breech extraction (BE) (N)	Vaginal delivery (%)	Fetal emergency	ECV (N)	Vaginal delivery (%)	Fetal emergency	C-section ratio
Gocke et al.[39]	96[a]	55	96	0/55	41	70	16/41	$p < 0.001$
Wells et al.[40]	66	43	98	0/43	23	48	11/23	$p < 0.001$
Chauhan et al.[38]	44	23	96	0/23	21	52	10/21	$p = 0.001$
Smith et al.[41]	76	43	97	1/43	33	76	13/33	$p = 0.008$
Barrett& Ritchie[42]	206	183	98.8	11/183	23	26+12 (2ary BE)	7/23	$p = 0.001$
Total	523	347		12/347 (3.5%)	176		57/176 (32%)	$p < 0.001$
								$p < 0.001$

[a] The publication also includes the study of women with a planned cesarean delivery. This subgroup was not included in the table.
BE = breech extraction.

- external cephalic version (ECV) and vaginal delivery in vertex presentation;
- cesarean delivery of the second twin.

After a breech extraction, as confirmed in several studies, more infants are delivered vaginally than after ECV. This is not linked to a greater risk of fetal emergency (Table 4.1). For this reason, breech extraction is preferred with regard to vaginal delivery in this situation [LE B].[38–44]

A combined vaginal delivery (twin A) and cesarean section (twin B) has the greatest risk of perinatal asphyxia, defined as an Apgar score of <4 after 5 minutes. This was determined in comparison with a vaginal delivery of both infants and in comparison with a planned cesarean delivery. Therefore, it is best to avoid this situation [LE C].[22,37,44] At centers with insufficient experience in vaginal breech delivery or breech extraction, it is best to handle these pregnancies by planned cesarean section or to refer them to another medical center [LE D].

The techniques of external version and breech extraction do not differ from the techniques used in single births and are described in Chapters 5 and 6.

Internal version and extraction are reserved in modern-day obstetrics for the delivery of the second twin and for some cases of cesarean delivery (see Animation 4.2). This procedure can be performed on the condition that the cervix is completely effaced and dilated and that the presenting part has not engaged yet. Adequate anesthesia (epidural, midazolam, or general anesthesia) is also necessary.

The presentation of the fetus is determined by ultrasound prior to the extraction. The fetal breech and the position of the feet and of the fetal back should be clearly identified.

In order to rotate a transverse or non-engaging vertex presentation internally into a breech presentation and then to proceed with a breech extraction, one hand is entered into the uterus along the anterior side of the fetal abdomen. Through the unruptured membranes, one or both feet are grasped at the level of the ankle and guided with mild traction through the cervix to the pelvic outlet. At the same time, the obstetrician's external hand may be able to support the rotation of the body. As soon as the fetus is in a longitudinal lie and the feet are at the level of the vulva, the membranes are ruptured manually. After that the breech extraction takes place (see Chapter 6).

Specific Situations

Monochorionic Diamniotic Twins

In the absence of specific complications such as a *twin-to-twin transfusion syndrome* (TTTS), the manner of delivery does not differ between monochorionic and dichorionic twins. The above-indicated problems of fetal presentation determine the procedure.[45,46]

The mode of delivery in monochorionic diamniotic (MCBA) pregnancies complicated by TTTS has to be evaluated case by case. Yet, in the absence of complications after laser treatment, planned delivery is recommended from 34 weeks and no later than 37 weeks [LE C].[8]

Monoamniotic Twins

Delivery with a planned cesarean section between 32 and 34 weeks is recommended [LE B].[47–49]

Acute Intrapartum Tocolysis

If uterine relaxation is needed to perform a breech extraction or other maneuvers, general anesthesia with short-term administration of anesthetic gases can be used. As an alternative, intravenous administration of nitroglycerin can be used. The dose is 0.1 to 0.2 mg per 10 kg body weight and rarely leads to a serious decrease in blood pressure in the mother.[50] The clinical experience reports that the use of ritodrine or atosiban is equally effective, but usage of these agents is not explicitly mentioned in the literature; ritodrine is no longer available.

Locked Twin

As mentioned above, the locked twin phenomenon is primarily known from historical publications (Figure 4.3). In this unusual situation, the diagnosis is made during the expulsion stage. The techniques are used after stopping the oxytocics and under acute tocolysis. In practice, an attempt is made to push the head of the second twin up and out of the pelvis, so that the following head of the first twin can enter the pelvis, which can then be born by means of the necessary maneuvers or by forceps extraction. Zavanelli's maneuver followed by an emergency cesarean section has also been reported.

Important Points and Recommendations

- The average gestation period of a twin pregnancy is 36.7 weeks [LE B].
- If spontaneous labor is delayed, the delivery of twins can be discussed with the parents as from 37 weeks but should not be postponed beyond 38 weeks [LE A2].
- The delivery will be by planned cesarean section in the following situations (Figure 4.4):
  - Non-vertex presentation of the presenting fetus [LE B];
  - Non-vertex presentation of one of the twins if a gynecologist with experience in vaginal breech deliveries and breech extraction is not available [LE C];
  - monochorionic monoamniotic twins [LE B];
  - conjoined twins [LEC];
  - obstetric reasons (placenta previa, fetal emergency on the CTG, TTTS, etc.);
  - maternal contraindications for a vaginal delivery.

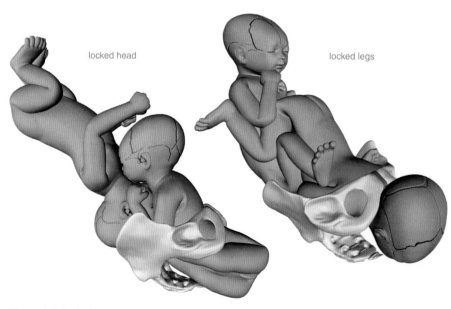

locked head   locked legs

Figure 4.3 Locked twins.

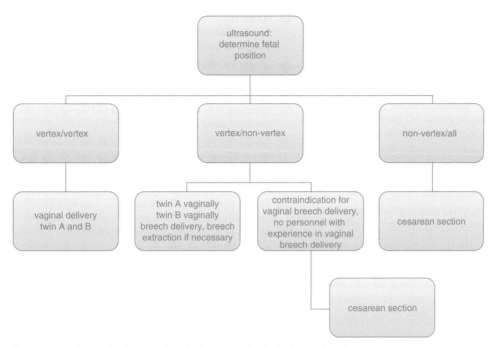

Figure 4.4 Delivery of dichorionic diamniotic or monochorionic diamniotic twins.

- All other sets of twins can (in anticipation of the results of a randomized study) be delivered vaginally, provided enough experienced personnel are present [LE B].
- In a planned vaginal delivery, the presence of personnel with experience in vaginal twin delivery, vaginal breech delivery, and breech extraction is mandatory [LE B].
- After the birth of the first infant and ultrasound monitoring of the fetal position, intravenous oxytocics are administered in order to limit the inter-twin time interval to less than 30 minutes [LE B].
- If the second child is in a longitudinal lie (vertex or breech), a spontaneous delivery is attempted [LE B].
- In the case of a lack of progress in the delivery of the second twin in breech position, a breech extraction – in experienced hands – is the best delivery method [LE B].
- If the second twin is in a transverse position, breech extraction, preceded by internal version – in experienced hands – is the best delivery method for the second twin in non-vertex presentation [LE B].
- Active management is practiced during the third stage. Immediately after the birth of the second twin (intravenous or intramuscular) oxytocin must be administered to the mother [LE B].

References

1 Loos RJF, Derom C, Eeckels R, et al. Length of gestation and birthweight in dizygotic twins. Lancet. 2001;**358**:560–1.

2 Breart G, Barros H, Wagener Y, et al. Characteristics of the childbearing population in Europe. Eur J Obstet Gynecol Reprod Biol. 2003;**111**:S45–52.

3 Cruikshank DP. Intrapartum management of twin gestations. Obstet Gynecol. 2007;**109**:1167–76.

4 Cheung YB, Yip P, Karlberg L. Mortality of twins and singletons by gestational age: a varying-coefficient approach. Am J Epidemiol. 2000;**152**:1107–16.

5 Lee YM, Wylie B, Simpson L, D'Alton ME. Twin chorionicity and the risk of stillbirth. Obstet Gynecol. 2008;**111**:301–8.

6 Hack KE, Derks JB, Elias SG, et al. Increased perinatal mortality and morbidity in monochorionic versus dichorionic twin pregnancies: clinical implications of a large Dutch cohort study. BJOG. 2008;**115**:58–67.

7 Vergani P, Russo FM, Follesa I, et al. Perinatal complications in twin pregnancies after 34 weeks: effects of gestational age at delivery and chorionicity. Am J Perinatol. 2013;**30**(7):545–50.

8 Vayssière C, Benoist G, Blondel B, et al. Twin pregnancies: guidelines for clinical practice from the French College of Gynaecologists and Obstetricians (CNGOF). Eur J Obstet Gynecol Reprod Biol. 2011;**156**(1):12–17. DOI: 10.1016/j.ejogrb.2010.12.045

9   Hack KE, Derks JB, Elias SG, et al Perinatal mortality and mode of delivery in monochorionic diamniotic twin pregnancies >32 weeks of gestation: a multicenter retrospective cohort study. BJOG. 2011;118:1090–7.

10 Breathnach FM, McAuliffe FM, Geary M, et al. Optimum timing for planned delivery of uncomplicated monochorionic and dichorionic twin pregnancies. Obstet Gynecol. 2012;119:50–9.

11 Sullivan AE, Hopkins PN, Hsoin-Yi W, et al. Delivery of monochorionic diamniotic twins in the absence of complications: analysis of neonatal outcome and costs. Am J Obstet Gynecol. 2012;206:257e1–7.

12 Bakr AF, Karkour T. What is the optimal gestational age for twin delivery. BMC Pregnancy Childbirth. 2006;6:3.

13 Dodd JM, Crowther CA, Haslam RR, Robinson JDS; Twins Timing of Birth Study group. Elective birth at 37 weeks of gestation versus standard care for women with an uncomplicated twin pregnancy near term: the Twins Timing of Birth Randomized Trial. BJOG. 2012; 119:964–73.

14 Carroll MA, Yeomans ER. Vaginal delivery of twins. Clin Obstet Gynecol. 2006;49:154–66.

15 Rossi AC, Mullin PM, Chmait RH. Neonatal outcomes of twins according to birth order, presentation and mode of delivery: a systematic review and meta-analysis. BJOG. 2011;118 (5):523–32.

16 Hofmeyr GJ, Barrett JF, Crowther CA. Planned caesarean section for women with a twin pregnancy. Cochrane Database Syst Rev. 2011;12: CD006553.

17 Vendetelli F, Rivière O, Crenn-Hébert C, et al. Is a planned cesarean necessary in twin pregnancies? Acta Obstet Gynecol Scand. 2011;90:1147–58.

18 Barrett JFR, Hannah ME, Hutton EK, et al. Twin Birth Study Collaborative Group: a randomized trial of planned cesarean or vaginal delivery for twin pregnancy. N Engl J Med. 2013;369:1295–305.

19 Griffith HB. Monoamniotic twin pregnancy. Br J Clin Pract. 1996;40:294–7.

20 Steins Bisschop CN, Vogelvang TE, May AM, Schuitemaker NW. Mode of delivery in non-cephalic presenting twins: a systematic review. Arch Gynecol Obstet. 2012;286(1):237–47.

21 Hannah ME, Hannah WJ, Hewson SA, et al. Planned caesarean section versus planned vaginal birth for breech presentation at term: a randomised multicentre trial. Lancet. 2000;356:1375–83.

22 Schmitz T, de Carnavalet C, Azria E, et al. Neonatal outcomes of twin pregnancy according to the planned mode of delivery. Obstet Gynecol. 2008;111:695–703.

23 Armson BA, O'Connell C, Persa V, et al. Determinants of perinatal mortality and serious morbidity in the second twin. Obstet Gynecol. 2006;108:556–64.

24 Zhang J, Bowes WA Jr, Grey TW, et al. Twin delivery and neonatal and infant mortality: a population-based study. Obstet Gynecol. 1996;88:593–8.

25 Ginsberg NA, Levine EM. Delivery of the second twin. Int J Gynaecol Obstet. 2005;91:217–20.

26 Amaru RC, Bush MC, Berkowitz RL, et al. Is discordant growth in twins an independent risk factor for adverse neonatal outcome? Obstet Gynecol. 2004;103:71–6.

27 Ford AA, Bateman BT, Simpson L. Vaginal birth after cesarean delivery in twin gestations: a large, nationwide sample of deliveries. Am J Obstet Gynecol. 2006;195(4):1138–42.

28 Yang Q, Walker MC, Chen XK, et al. Impacts of operative delivery for the first twin on neonatal outcomes in the second twin. Am J Perinatol. 2006;23(7):381–6.

29 Edris F, Oppenheimer L, Yang Q, et al. Relationship between intertwin delivery interval and metabolic acidosis in the second twin. Am J Perinatol. 2006;23(8):481–5.

30 Wen SW, Fung Kee Fung K, Oppenheimer L, et al. Neonatal mortality in second twin according to cause of death, gestational age, and mode of delivery. Am J Obstet Gynecol. 2004;191(3):778–83.

31 Barrett J, Bocking A. The SOGC Consensus Statement: management of twin pregnancies. Part 2. J Soc Obstet Gynecol Can. 2000;22:623.

32 Robinson C, Chauhan SP. Intrapartum management of twins. Clin Obstet Gynaecol. 2004;47:248–62.

33 Rayburn WF, Lavin JP Jr, Miodovnik M, et al. Multiple gestation: time interval between delivery of first and second twins. Obstet Gynecol. 1984;63:502–5.

34 Brown HL, Miller JM Jr, Neumann DE, et al. Umbilical cord blood gas assessment of twins. Obstet Gynecol 1990;75:826–9.

35 Stein W, Misselwitz B, Schmidt S. Twin-to-twin delivery time interval: influencing factors and effect on short-term outcome of the second twin. Acta Obstet Gynecol Scand. 2008;87:346–53.

36 Sentilhes L, Bonhours AC, Biquard F, et al. Mode d'accouchement des grosses gemellaires. Gynecol Obstet Fertil. 2009;37:432–41.

37 Usta IM, Nassar AH, Awwad JT, et al. Comparison of the perinatal morbidity and mortality of the presenting twin and its co-twin. J Perinatol. 2002;22:391–6.

38 Chauhan SP, Roberts WE, McLaren RA, et al. Delivery of the nonvertex second twin: breech extraction versus external cephalic version. Am J Obstet Gynecol. 1995;173:1015–20.

39 Gocke SE, Nageotte MP, Garite T, et al. Management of the nonvertex second twin: primary cesarean section, external version, or primary breech extraction. Am J Obstet Gynecol. 1989;**161**:111–14.

40 Wells SR, Thorp JM Jr, Bowes WA Jr. Management of the nonvertex second twin. Surg Gynecol Obstet. 1991;**172**:383–5.

41 Smith SJ, Zebrowitz J, Latta RA. Method of delivery of the nonvertex second twin: a community hospital experience. J Matern Fetal Med. 1997;**6**:146–50.

42 Barrett JF, Ritchie WK. Twin delivery. Best Pract Res Clin Obstet Gynaecol. 2002;**16**:43–56.

43 Rabinovici J, Barkai G, Reichmann B, et al. Internal podalic version with unruptured membranes for the second twin in transverse lie. Obstet Gynecol. 1988;**71**:428–30.

44 Caukwell S, Murphy DJ. The effect of mode of delivery and gestational age on neonatal outcome of the non-cephalic-presenting second twin. Am J Obstet Gynecol. 2002;**187**:1356–61.

45 Baghdadi S, Gee H, Whittle MJ. Twin pregnancy outcome and chorionicity. Acta Obstet Gynecol Scand. 2003;**82**:18–21.

46 Sau A, Chalmers S, Shennan AH, et al. Vaginal delivery can be considered in monochorionic diamniotic twins. BJOG. 2006;**113**:602–4.

47 Riethmuller D, Lantheaume S, Teffaud O, et al. [Obstetrical and neonatal prognosis of monoamniotic twin gestations.] J Gynecol Obstet Biol Reprod (Paris). 2004;**33**(7):632–6.

48 Sau AK, Langford K, Elliott C, et al. Monoamniotic twins, what should be the optimal antenatal management. Twin Res. 2003;**6**:270–4.

49 Kurzel RB. Twin entanglement revisited. Twin Res. 1998;**1**(3):138–41.

50 Dufour P, Vinatyier D, Vanderstichele S, et al. Intravenous nitroglycerin for internal podalic version of the second twin in transverse lie. Obstet Gynecol. 1998;**92**:416–19.

External Cephalic Version

E. Roets, M. Hanssens, and M. Kok

General Information

Introduction

External cephalic version (ECV) or external rotation refers to the abdominal manipulation of the fetus from a transverse, oblique, or breech presentation to a cephalic presentation. During recent years, especially since the publication of the Term Breech Trial, there has been a tendency in breech presentations to deliver by cesarean section in order to diminish direct fetal complications associated with vaginal breech delivery.[1] Through ECV, an attempt is made to reduce the incidence of term breech presentations, resulting in a decreased number of cesarean deliveries due to breech presentations. Since the number of cesarean sections in breech presentation is on the increase, ECV is gaining in importance.

Prevalence and Success Rate

Approximately 3% to 4% of term fetuses (and a larger proportion of preterm fetuses) present in breech presentation. The success rate of ECV differs drastically depending on who is doing the reporting, and varies between 29% and 97%.[2] The most recent meta-analysis included 84 studies and reported a success rate of 16–100% (95% CI 56–57) [LE A1].[3]

Contraindications and Factors Influencing ECV

There are several opinions on the question of whether a particular factor constitutes a contraindication for ECV.[4,5] A recent review on this topic showed there is no general consensus on the eligibility of patients for external cephalic version, and proposed to limit contraindications to clear empirical evidence or to a clear pathophysiological relevance. The proposed list of contraindications is all based on level D evidence[6]:

- placental abruption in history or signs of placental abruption;
- severe preeclampsia or HELLP syndrome;
- signs of fetal distress (abnormal CTG and/or abnormal Doppler flow).

The following factors are not contraindications in so many words, but they may influence the success rate of an external cephalic version procedure to a greater or lesser extent. The following division between maternal and fetal factors is somewhat artificial, since some factors cannot be classified simply under one or the other (e.g., amniotic fluid quantity).

Maternal Factors

- *Uterine tonicity*: The extent to which the uterus is relaxed will increase the success rate of ECV (OR 1.8, 95% CI 1.2–2.9) [LE A1].[7]
- *Multiparity*: This is closely related to uterine tonicity: a multiparous uterus is often more relaxed (OR 2.5, 95% CI 2.3–2.8) [LE A1].[8]
- *Nature of the abdominal wall* (obesity – muscle tone): These are factors that influence the ease of palpability of the fetus. Obesity lessens the success rate of ECV (OR 1.8 in the absence of obesity, 95% CI 1.2–2.6) [LE A1].[8] Also with increasing muscular tone of the abdominal wall muscles (in case of maternal anxiety or stress) the fetus is more difficult to manipulate, which will lower the success rate of version [LE D].

Obstetric Interventions, ed. P. Joep Dörr, Vincent M. Khouw, Frank A. Chervenak, Amos Grunebaum, Yves Jacquemyn, and Jan G. Nijhuis. Published by Cambridge University Press. © Cambridge University Press 2017.

- *Ethnicity*: In African women the presenting part engages later in the pelvic inlet than in Caucasian women. This increases the probability of success (see Section: Fetal factors [engagement of the presenting part]).[9]

Fetal Factors

- *Amniotic fluid quantity*: Although not statistically significant, there appears to be a greater probability of success of ECV in the clinical presence of a sufficient quantity of amniotic fluid.[10] In an ultrasound evaluation, an Amniotic Fluid Index (AFI) ≥10 leads to a greater probability of success of the ECV (OR 1.8, 95% CI 1.5–2.1) [LE A1].[11]
- *Palpability of (the head of) the fetus*: To the extent that the fetal head is more easily palpable, the probability of success of an ECV increases (OR 6.3, 95% CI 4.3–9.2) [LE A1].[8] Naturally, this is related in part to the uterine tonicity, but also to maternal obesity and abdominal wall muscular tonicity (see Section: Maternal factors [uterine tonicity and nature of the abdominal wall]). The position of the placenta also determines the palpability of the fetus: a posteriorly located placenta is related to a greater probability of success (OR 1.9, 95% CI 1.5–2.4) than an anterior placenta or a fundally located placenta [LE A1].[11]
- *Engagement of the presenting part*: The probability of success increases if the presenting part has not engaged (OR 9.4, 95% CI 6.3–14) [LE A1].[8]
- *Nature of the breech presentation*: Complete breech presentation (*complete breech*: hips and knees in flexion) has a greater probability of success with ECV than incomplete breech (*frank breech*: hips in flexion, knees in extension) (OR 1.8, 95% CI 1.1–1.7) [LE A1].[11]
- *Fetal weight*: Experienced practitioners agree that a fetus of ≥4000 g is more difficult to turn than a fetus of ≤3000 g. However, no specific cut-off values are available on this [LE D].

Operator-Related Factors

Although it has never been the subject of a randomized study, it seems logical that ECV has a greater chance of success if performed by an experienced practitioner [LE D].

Technique

Technical Execution of ECV[2,12–14]

In advance of an ECV, cardiotocography and a (repeated) ultrasonography (to determine the position of the fetal spine) should be performed.

External cephalic version of the fetus is achieved by subjecting the infant to a somersault. This can be a forward roll or a back flip. The pregnant woman is placed in a supine position.

It is easiest to turn a fetus that is lying with its back to the side (left or right). A fetus with the back forward is preferably first turned to a side-lying position. Next, the following maneuvers are applied:

- *Forward roll (see Animation 5.1)*
  - The fetal buttocks are lifted out of the pelvis and pushed with one hand to the side (the side of the fetal back) and gently cranially (Figure 5.1).
  - With the other hand, the fetal head is brought into flexion, so that the head and the buttocks are encompassed by both hands (Figure 5.2).
  - The head is pressed gently contralaterally (the side of the fetal abdomen) and gently caudally (Figure 5.3).

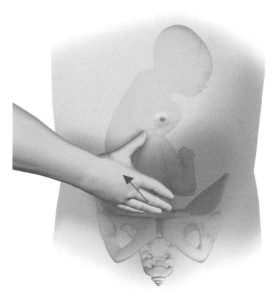

Figure 5.1 Mobilization of the buttocks.

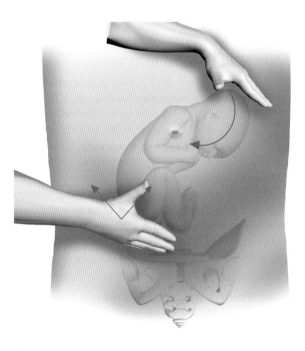

Figure 5.2 Head is brought into flexion.

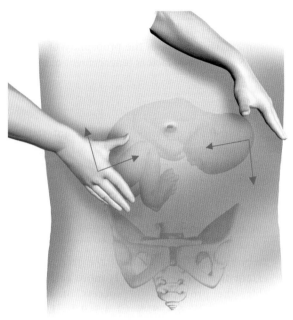

Figure 5.3 Forward roll.

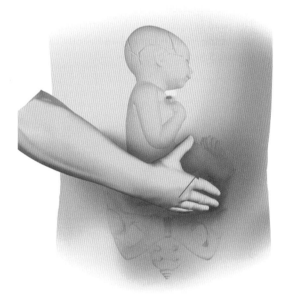

Figure 5.4 Mobilization of the buttocks.

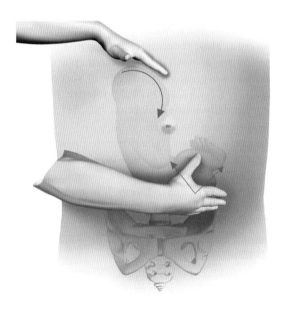

Figure 5.5 Head is brought into flexion.

- *Back flip (see Animation 5.2)*
  - The fetal buttocks are lifted out of the pelvis and pushed with one hand to the side (the side of the fetal abdomen) and gently cranially (Figure 5.4).

  - With the other hand, the fetal head is brought into flexion, so that the head and the buttocks are encompassed by both hands (Figure 5.5).
  - The head is pressed gently contralaterally (the side of the fetal back) and gently caudally (Figure 5.6).

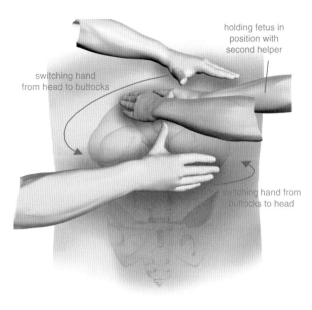

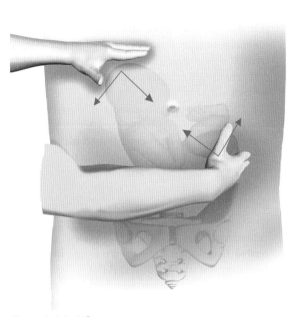

Figure 5.7 Switching hands.

Figure 5.6 Back flip.

When a transverse position is achieved in this manner, it is recommended to pause a moment and hold the fetus in this position. At this point an assistant can hold the fetus stable, so that the operator can switch hands (Figure 5.7).

Frequently, the rest of the version is enacted "almost spontaneously" by the fetus, provided it is properly guided.

The entire procedure is performed with jerking (intermittent) motions. It is important not to use excessive force. The movements can best be performed by ballottement, i.e., with alternating pressure between the head and the buttocks [LE D].

A maximum of three attempts is recommended [LE D].[15]

It is especially important to provide ample explanation to the pregnant woman and try to provide maximum maternal relaxation through reassurance.

Measures for Increasing the Success Rate

- *Tocolysis*: The use of betamimetics is associated with an increased chance of success of an ECV attempt (OR 0.74 for failure with the use of betamimetics; 95% CI 0.64–0.87) [LE A1].[16] Blinding is not practical in these types of studies. In a randomized, double-blind, placebo-controlled study with 310 patients, the administration of oral nifedipine did not prove to lead to more success in attempted ECV (RR 1.1, 95% CI 0.85–1.5) [LE A1].[17]
- *Epidural/spinal analgesia*: A significantly higher chance of success is reported in a Cochrane review with the use of epidural, but not with spinal analgesia [LE A1].[16] Still, we have to warn against the possible danger of using too much force when using epidural analgesia, since the pain sensation of the mother is eliminated.[2] Additionally, the risks and extra cost of this type of analgesia must be taken into consideration.

As for other methods, such as the use of vibroacoustic stimulation or amnioinfusion, there is insufficient evidence in terms of practical recommendations.

Timing

The success rate of ECV is evidently larger when performed earlier during the pregnancy (smaller fetus, less chance of engaging). However, in case of complications such as ruptured membranes or placental abruption the consequences for the neonate are greater due to preterm delivery. A randomized trial reporting on 1543 women randomly assigned to having a first ECV procedure between the gestational ages of 34(0/7) and 35(6/7) weeks of gestation (early ECV) or at or after 37(0/7) weeks of gestation (delayed ECV group) showed fewer fetuses in a non-cephalic presentation at birth in the early ECV group (41.1%) versus (49.1%) in the delayed ECV group (RR 0.84, 95% CI 0.75, 0.94, p = 0.002). There were no differences in rates of C-section (52.0% versus 56.0%) (RR 0.93, 95% CI 0.85, 1.02, p = 0.12) or in risk of preterm birth (6.5% versus 4.4%) (RR 1.48, 95% CI 0.97, 2.26, p = 0.07) in early versus delayed ECV. It was concluded that ECV at 34–35 weeks versus 37 or more weeks of gestation increases the likelihood of cephalic presentation at birth but does not reduce the rate of cesarean section and may increase the rate of preterm birth [LE A1].[18]

There is no upper time limit on the appropriate gestation for ECV. Successes have been reported at 42 weeks of gestation and can be performed in early labor provided that the membranes are intact [LE C].[19]

Complications

During/Soon After ECV

ECV is a safe procedure. Nevertheless, (rare) complications such as fetal death have been reported. Transitory changes in the heartbeat pattern, abruptio placentae, fetomaternal transfusion, and umbilical cord accidents constitute the more frequently mentioned complications.

In a meta-analysis with 12 955 versions, a complication ratio of 6.1% (95% CI 4.7–7.8) was found, including 0.24% serious complications (95% CI 0.17–0.34) and 0.35% emergency C-sections (95% CI 0.26–0.47). Complications were not related to the result of the version (OR 1.2, 95% CI 0.93–1.7).[3]

- *Fetal death and placental abruption*: In the meta-analysis of Grootscholten et al. fetal death and placenta detachment are defined as serious complications.[3] Only 2 out of the 12 (0.09%) fetal deaths in a total of 12 955 version attempts were attributed to the (attempted) ECV. Abruptio placentae occurred in 11 cases (0.08%), which is not significantly different from a normal term population.
- *Umbilical cord accidents*: In several studies, *umbilical cord entwinement* is reported as a complication of ECV. But it appears from a large cohort study

that this is not associated with an inferior perinatal result and is therefore irrelevant to clinical practice [LE B].[20] In the above-mentioned meta-analysis, *umbilical cord prolapse* was studied in five clinical trials; it occurred in eight cases (0.06%) [LE A1].[3]

- *CTG changes*: Transitory changes in the heartbeat pattern occur in 4% of the cases of term ECV [LE B].[2] This especially concerns bradycardia or decelerations, which disappear after stopping the manipulation. The aforementioned meta-analysis reports an abnormal CTG pattern in 6.1% (95% CI 5.7–6.5) of the version attempts, which led to an emergency C-section in 0.2% (95% CI 0.1–0.3) of the cases.[3] The end result in all of these cases was good.
- *Fetomaternal transfusion*: In a review on ECV-related risks, seven studies were found in which a Kleihauer test was performed [LE A1].[14] Significant fetomaternal transfusion was found in 3.7%, but massive fetal hemorrhage was not reported.
- *Other complications*: Other reported complications are limited to case reports and they are rare. There are two known cases of spinal cord trauma, one of which had a fatal outcome (1978) and the other one had a complete neurological recovery.[2,21] This could be caused by traction on the fetal spinal cord when the head is abruptly moved from hyperextension to flexion. For that reason, despite little evidence, hyperextension of the fetal head is considered to be a contraindication for attempted version. One case of ECV-related hip fracture is known.[19]

In a Vaginal Delivery After Successful ECV

Patients who underwent successful ECV still appear to have an increased susceptibility to cesarean section. In a meta-analysis of 11 studies there was a C-section rate of 21% in the post-ECV group versus 11% in members of the control group. The combined relative risks (95% CI) were 2.21 (1.64–2.97) for dystocia and 2.16 (1.62–2.88) for threatened fetal well-being [LE B].[22] The incidence of assisted delivery also remains high: OR 1.37 (1.11–1.68) [LE B].[23]

Possible explanations for this are an anomalous maternal pelvic shape (predisposing for breech presentation) or factors inherent to the fetus in breech presentation (other configuration of the head, lower birthweight, lower fetoplacental ratio).[22,23]

Measures for Preventing Complications

Based on the foregoing, several recommendations can be made for keeping the chance of complications as small as possible:

- preceding ultrasound: to confirm position and rule out the existence of hyperextension of the fetal head;
- preceding CTG: to discover already existing fetal heart arrhythmias;
- administration of anti-D immunoglobulin to rhesus D negative pregnant women;
- quantification of possible fetomaternal transfusion with the Kleihauer–Betke test has not been proven effective in preventing complications; it is, however, informative on the approximately 4% of the cases with fetomaternal transfusion.
- post-version cardiotocography and monitoring fetal movements during the first days.

Important Points and Recommendations

- Breech presentation occurs in 3% to 4% of term pregnancies, and even more in preterm.
- Owing to the increasing number of cesarean sections for term breech presentations and the low complication risk of an ECV, an attempt at ECV must be proposed to every pregnant woman with a fetus in breech presentation in the absence of absolute contraindications [LE A1].
- After a successful ECV, the chance of a cesarean section and/or assisted delivery is still higher than for pregnancies with a fetus in "spontaneous cephalic presentation" [LE B].
- For a trained practitioner, the success rate of ECV is around 50% [LE B]. The success rate can be individualized for the patient by taking into account the variables in Table 5.1.
- An ECV is effective in reducing the number of term breech presentations starting at 34 weeks of gestation [LE A1]. Before 36 weeks there seems however a slightly higher risk of preterm delivery with no difference in cesarean deliveries compared to ECV after 36 weeks [LE A1].
- ECV is a safe procedure, with few significant complications [LE A1]. Women must be informed of the (rare) possibility of

Table 5.1 Success rate of ECV varies according to a number of variables

Decreases the chance of success	Increases the chance of success
Maternal	
Term	Preterm
Strong uterine tonicity	Slight uterine tonicity
Primigravida	Multigravida
Obesity	Bodyweight <65 kg
Tense abdominal wall	Relaxed abdominal wall
Caucasian	African
Fetal	
Incomplete breech	Complete breech
Anterior placenta	Posterior placenta
Complete engagement	No engagement
Decreased amniotic fluid	Normal amniotic fluid
>4000 g	<3000 g

complications. In 0.4% (95% CI 0.3–0.5) of all versions an emergency cesarean section must be performed due to alleged fetal distress. With each ECV the following measures can be taken to increase the chance of success and to decrease the chance of complications:

- preceding ultrasound;
- preceding CTG;
- administration of betamimetics [LE A1];
- administration of anti-D gammaglobulin in rhesus D negative women, in doses dictated by the result of the Kleihauer–Betke test. In Flanders and the Netherlands they administer such a high dose of anti-D that you have to ask yourself if the systematic quantification of fetomaternal transfusion is actually worthwhile.
- post-version cardiotocography and monitoring fetal movements during the first days.

References

1 Hannah ME, Hannah WJ, Hewson SA, et al; Term Breech Trial Collaborative Group. Planned cesarean section versus planned vaginal birth for breech presentation at term: a randomised multicentre trial. Lancet. 2000;**356**:1375–83.

2 Hanssens M, Claerhout F, Corremans A, et al. Beleid en techniek bij uitwendige kering. In: Slager E, Fauser BCJM, Devroey P, et al. (ed). Infertiliteit, gynaecologie en obstetrie anno 2001 (Nederland) – Congress Proceedings, 2001:300–7.

3 Grootscholten K, Kok M, Oei SG, et al. External cephalic version-related risks: a meta-analysis. Obstet Gynecol. 2008;**112**(5):1143–51.

4 Feitsma AH, Middeldorp JM, Oepkes D. De uitwendige versie bij de aterme stuit: een inventariserend onderzoek. Ned Tijdschr Obstet Gynaecol. 2007;**120**:4–7.

5 Kok M, van der Steeg JW, Mol BW, et al. Which factors play a role in clinical decision-making in external cephalic version? Acta Obstet Gynecol Scand. 2008;**87**(1):31–5.

6 Rosman AN, Guijt A, Vlemmix F, et al. Contraindications for external cephalic version in breech position at term: a systematic review. Acta Obstet Gynecol Scand. 2013;**92**(2):137–42.

7 Hutton EK, Hofmeyr GJ. External cephalic version for breech presentation before term. Cochrane Database Syst Rev. 2006;**1**:CD000084.

8 Kok M, Cnossen J, Gravendeel L, et al. Clinical factors to predict the outcome of external cephalic version: a meta-analysis. Am J Obstet Gynecol. 2008;**199**(6):630.e1–7.

9 Briggs ND. Engagement of the fetal head in the negro primigravida. Br J Obstet Gynaecol. 1981;**88**(11): 1086–9.

10 Haas DM, Magann EF. External cephalic version with an amniotic fluid index < or = 10: a systematic review. J Matern Fetal Neonatal Med. 2005;**18**(4):249–52.

11 Kok M, Cnossen J, Gravendeel L, et al. Ultrasound factors to predict the outcome of external cephalic version: a meta-analysis. Ultrasound Obstet Gynecol. 2009;**33**(1):76–84.

12 Rovinsky JJ. Abnormalities of position, lie, presentation and rotation. In: Kaminetsky HA, Iffy L (eds). Principles and practice of obstetrics and perinatology. 1st edition. New York: John Wiley & Sons, 1981: Chapter 49.

13 Percival R. Obstetric operations. In: Percival R (ed). Holland & Brews' manual of obstetrics. 14th edition. Edinburgh: Churchill Livingstone, 1980:614–740.

14 Collaris RJ, Oei SG. External cephalic version: a safe procedure? A systematic review of version-related risks. Acta Obstet Gynecol Scand. 2004;**83**(6):511–18.

15 WHO. The WHO Reproductive Health Library. 1997;8. http://apps.who.int/rhl/archives/cd000083_leder_com/en/

16 Hofmeyr GJ, Gyte GML. Interventions to help external cephalic version for breech presentation at term. Cochrane Database Syst Rev. 2004;**1**:CD000184.

17 Kok M, Bais JM, van Lith JM, et al. Nifedipine as uterine relaxant for external cephalic version: a randomized controlled trial. Obstet Gynecol. 2008;**112**(2Pt1):271–6.

18 Hutton EK, Hannah ME, Ross SJ, et al. Early ECV2 Trial Collaborative Group. The Early External Cephalic Version (ECV) 2 Trial: an international multicentre randomised controlled trial of timing of ECV for breech pregnancies. BJOG. 2011;**118**(5):564–77.

19 Ferguson JE, Dyson DC. Intrapartum external cephalic version. Am J Obstet Gynecol. 1985;**152**:297–8.

20 Sheiner E, Abramowicz JS, Levy A, et al. Nuchal cord is not associated with adverse perinatal outcome. Arch Gynecol Obstet. 2006;**274**(2):81–3.

21 Chapman GP, Weller RO, Normand IC, et al. Spinal cord transsection in utero. Br Med J. 1978;**2**:398.

22 de Hundt M, Velzel J, de Groot CJ, et al. Mode of delivery after successful external cephalic version: a systematic review and meta-analysis. Obstet Gynecol. 2014;**123**:1327–34.

23 Corremans A, Hanssens M, Gabriëls K. Arbeid en bevalling na een geslaagde uitwendige kering à terme. Gunaekeia. 2004;**9**(2):47–50.

Vaginal Breech Delivery

A.T.M. Verhoeven, J.P. de Leeuw, H.W. Bruinse, H.C.J. Scheepers, and B. Wibbens

General Information

Introduction

Possessing and maintaining the skills for vaginal breech delivery is becoming increasingly more important as the number of cesarean sections due to breech presentation has increased drastically during recent years. There are no randomized trials on the best maneuvers used in vaginal breech birth. The best materials we have been able to find with regard to vaginal breech delivery maneuvers are the following:

- original descriptions of the maneuvers by their "inventors";
- authoritative textbooks produced during the past century[1–6];
- manikin simulation instructions by Dutch, Belgian, and German medical school faculties;
- dissertations in Dutch;
- expertise of the authors.

The practice of *evidence-based medicine* implies the integration of the best evidence together with individual expertise.

This chapter deals with term breech deliveries, except where specifically mentioned otherwise.

Definition

A breech presentation is a longitudinal lie with the buttocks and/or foot (feet), and rarely the knees, as the presenting part.

Classification of Breech Presentations

The following breech presentations are differentiated (Figure 6.1):

- *frank breech presentation*: the legs lie alongside the body, flexed at the hips and extended at the knees: the term incidence is 2.25%;
- *complete breech presentation*: the feet are next to the breech, the legs are flexed at the hips and at the knees: the term incidence is 0.75%;
- *footling presentation*: one or both legs are extended at the hips or knees and lie below the breech.

Incidence

The incidence of term breech presentation is 3% to 4%. At a gestational age of approximately 32 weeks, the incidence is 10% to 15% [LE C].[7]

Causes

Causes of breech presentation are:

- premature birth;
- fetal growth restriction;
- congenital disorders (e.g., anencephaly, hydrocephaly, and neuromuscular disorders);
- multifetal pregnancy;
- umbilical cord problems (short umbilical cord, entwinement);
- oligo- or polyhydramnios;
- placenta previa;
- congenital uterine anomalies, myomas;
- pelvic tumors;
- contracted pelvis.

The cause for a breech presentation is usually not found.

Congenital disorders occur two to three times more in children born in breech presentation than children born in cephalic presentation [LE B].[8] Hyperextension of the fetal neck can be a sign of a congenital disorder [LE C].[9]

Obstetric Interventions, ed. P. Joep Dörr, Vincent M. Khouw, Frank A. Chervenak, Amos Grunebaum, Yves Jacquemyn, and Jan G. Nijhuis. Published by Cambridge University Press. © Cambridge University Press 2017.

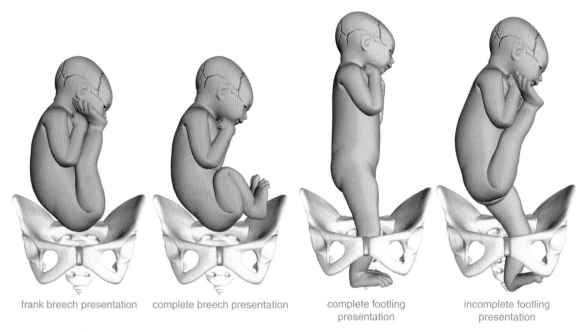

frank breech presentation   complete breech presentation   complete footling   incomplete footling
                                                                     presentation   presentation

Figure 6.1 Types of breech presentations.

Complications

In breech births there is a greater chance of complications during the delivery than in cephalic presentation births. The following complications can occur:

- *Prolapse of the umbilical cord*: In breech presentations there is a greater chance of umbilical cord prolapse: 5% in a complete breech presentation, 15% in a footling presentation, and 0.5% in frank breech presentation.[10] The risk of an umbilical cord prolapse is 1% in all forms of term breech births and 0.4% in cephalic presentations.[11]

- *Asphyxia* can occur during the second stage of labor in case of a prolonged compression of the umbilical cord between the head and the pelvis. Compression of the umbilical cord occurs from the moment the anterior scapula point is visible.[2,3] In a breech presentation – in contrast with a cephalic presentation – the umbilical cord is always compressed during the second stage because of its insertion below the head. The incidence of an arterial umbilical cord pH of <7.10 is from 4% to 10% in breech deliveries and ±1% in cephalic presentations [LE B].[12–15] After adequate resuscitation, short-term asphyxia does not usually have long-term consequences.[3,16,17]

- *Mechanical lesions* can occur in a non-progressive breech delivery, when (partial) extraction is

needed. In a planned term vaginal delivery, the chance of mostly short-term injury (cerebral, brachial plexus injury, hemorrhaging, and ruptures of internal organs) is 0.92%: 9 in 1000. These traumas occur just as often in assisted vaginal deliveries in cephalic presentation and rarely result in a permanent handicap.[18]

- *Perinatal mortality*: The perinatal death rate of breech presentations is 0.39% in planned vaginal deliveries and 0.17% in planned cesarean sections. That is a difference of 0.22%: 2 in 1000 infants.[18,19] In a recent French/Belgian prospective study there was no difference between perinatal mortality and morbidity [LE B].[20]

The Choice of Vaginal Delivery versus Cesarean Section

The choice between a vaginal delivery and an elective cesarean section must be made together with the pregnant woman in a conversation in which all of the pros and cons of both delivery methods are discussed. The decision must also take into account the expertise of the gynecologist and the logistics of the clinic. The considerations must not only contemplate the perinatal and maternal risks of the current delivery, but also those of the previous and possible future deliveries (increased chance of uterus rupture, placenta previa, placenta accreta). Bringing one extra full term live birth into the world requires approximately 380 extra cesarean sections [LE C].[21]

Individual desires are important: the situation of a completed family or of a first pregnancy at a higher age, in which a future pregnancy is unlikely, differs substantially from that of a young primigravida, who may have the ability or the desire to become pregnant again.[18,22]

The mode of delivery of preterm breech babies is still up for debate.[23] There are, however, some specific things to watch out for in managing the labor. A relatively large head increases the risk of the head being impacted at the cervix. It should therefore be remembered that the use of forceps would not be the first choice in this case, but that the procedure should proceed with a Dührssen's incision. A breech presentation of the second of a set of twins does not require special counseling. For this, a vaginal birth can be pursued (see Chapter 4).[24]

Contraindications

The type of breech presentation, the estimated birthweight, and the position of the fetal head are determined by means of external and ultrasound examinations.

Contraindications for a vaginal breech birth are:

- contraindications for a vaginal delivery, such as poor fetal condition, congenital abnormalities that make a vaginal birth impossible (hydrocephaly), placenta previa, presenting umbilical cord;
- footling or knee presentation, except when the infant is ready to be born [LE D]. Note: a footling presentation is rare in a normal size fetus at term with a closed cervix and unruptured membranes, but this can occur during the delivery after the rupturing of the membranes;
- suspected contracted pelvis, such as after a difficult or failed assisted delivery, or during an internal pelvic examination [LE D];
- hyperextension of the fetal head (thus, any position other than a neutral or flexed position constitutes a contraindication [LE D]);
- macrosomia: estimated weight >4000 g [LE D] and intrauterine growth restriction: estimated weight <2500 g [LE A];[17,19,25,26]
- absence of an experienced gynecologist [LE A2].[26]

Prevention

External version at 36 weeks seems to lead to a significant reduction (50%) in the incidence of breech deliveries and therefore of the number of cesarean sections (see Chapter 5 on external version).

History

In the description of the different maneuvers and methods we took the Dutch and Flemish obstetric traditions as the point of departure. For an adequate understanding, the history is important.

Before 1936, the policy in breech deliveries was to wait until the first scapula point was born. If, despite forceful pushing, the rest did not follow during a contraction, the arms were delivered according to the "classic" method (posterior arm first) or according to Müller[27] (anterior arm first) (1898), and then the head according to Mauriceau.[28] The Bracht maneuver was introduced in 1935.[29–33] Løvset published his maneuver during the same period.[34–37] During the 1940s, the preference gradually moved to the Bracht maneuver in Dutch obstetric training for infants with normal tonicity and a normal estimated birthweight. If this failed, one of the three methods was used to deliver the arms.

Delivery Methods in Breech Presentations

General Points of Interest in Breech Presentation Births

- The circumference of the breech is irregular and smaller than that of the head. In a premature or dysmature infant there is a chance for the head to get impacted at the cervix. Consequently, Dührssen's incisions may be necessary (see Chapter 3). For the sake of visibility, it may be decided to perform this only at the 12 o'clock position, which would minimize the chance of bladder lesions.[38]
- The breech closes the pelvic inlet less effectively than the head. This creates a greater chance of umbilical cord prolapse.[11]
- The ratio between the head and the pelvis cannot be ascertained beforehand. If a disproportion becomes evident during the delivery of a cephalic presentation, a vaginal delivery can usually be cancelled on time; in a breech presentation there is usually no way back.[39]
- A thorough (internal) pelvic examination during the pregnancy may provide early revelation of the "pelvic factor" in case of a disproportion between the head and the pelvis (see Chapter 1) [LE C].

- A pelvic examination with *magnetic resonance pelvimetry* offers no added value in a term breech presentation [LE A2].[40]
- In a complete breech presentation there are fewer clear internal rotations (rotations around the longitudinal axis) than with a frank breech presentation. For that reason, in a complete breech presentation the back will rotate to the back (dorsal side of the mother) more often than in a frank breech presentation. In that case, it is recommended when using the Bracht maneuver to turn – even before the umbilicus is visible – the back forward (ventral side of the mother).
- By performing an adequate episiotomy (at the right moment), more room becomes available for the necessary procedures involved in a (partial) breech extraction. Furthermore, the head can be delivered more evenly and there is less chance of a grade 3 or 4 sphincter rupture resulting from the rapid stretching of the perineum [LE B].[41]
- CTG monitoring is recommended: in case of unruptured membranes with external registration; in case of ruptured membranes with an electrode on one buttock. In comparison with a birth in cephalic presentation, the heart rate is higher in a breech delivery, there are more decelerations due to umbilical cord compression when the breech reaches the pelvic floor, the variability is decreased, and there are fewer accelerations [LE C].[42,43]
- Micro blood testing can be performed on the buttocks on the same indication as in a cephalic presentation. The validation of this is limited: the reliability of the measurements was good, but it concerned only a small group of patients.[44]
- In a vaginal breech delivery, the progress of the delivery must be assessed carefully. In a non-progressing engagement, dilation, or expulsion, a cesarean section must be performed despite adequate contractions.
- From the moment the scapula point becomes visible, the birth of an infant that is in good condition and in a frank breech presentation may take approximately another 4 minutes before an Apgar score of <7 appears after 5 minutes [LE C].[10,45] A hurried extraction contributes to the arms being outstretched beside the head [LE D].

Preparations for Breech Delivery

If the breech delivery does not progress spontaneously or smoothly according to the Bracht maneuver, rapid response must be available to prevent asphyxia. In a breech delivery everything has to be ready for a possible partial breech extraction, a forceps extraction of the aftercoming head, or an emergency cesarean section.

Conditions for a breech delivery are as follows:

- discussion of the pros and cons of a vaginal breech delivery and an elective cesarean section;
- explanation of the procedure and clear instructions to the woman;
- properly instructed assistance;
- birthing bed with the possibility of a low bed position;
- empty bladder;
- open intravenous infusion port;
- readily available forceps;
- emergency plan: if a spontaneous birth or Bracht maneuver is not successful, know what the next step will be and make sure that step can be performed rapidly;
- availability of operating room and surgical team;
- availability of a pediatrician and possibility for neonatal resuscitation.

Steps to Follow in a Breech Birth

The order of the maneuvers in a breech birth is as follows:

1 With the Bracht maneuver, the arms, shoulders, and head are born in one motion.
2 If the arms do not follow, delivery is done with the Müller maneuver, according to the "classic" maneuver or the one according to Løvset, after which the head is delivered as in Point 3 below. In principle, all three methods can be applied to deliver the arms: the choice is partially determined on the basis of the experience of the gynecologist and partially on the pros and cons of each maneuver.
3 If the head does not follow, the procedure goes over to Mauriceau, De Snoo, or forceps.

Breech Delivery According to Bracht

Conducting a Breech Delivery

To conduct a breech delivery according to the Bracht method (see Animation 6.1), good tonicity of the infant is essential: good muscle tone is a condition for the lordosis of the back, which supports the rotation of the fetus over the symphysis, as well as to maintain the mosaic of the extremities and the chin on the chest. If an asphyctic infant is expected, it is better to make a choice for a partial breech extraction.

The birth of an infant in breech presentation has a slow and a rapid phase. First of all, a complete dilation and a gradual engagement of the breech into the pelvic floor are aimed for. The rapid phase takes place during the contraction after the breech has "crowned" and an episiotomy is performed. The infant should be delivered during this contraction.

The essence of the method is that the natural movement of the fetal body is supported into the direction of the extension of the birth canal. Instead of a downward traction (caudally and dorsally) pressure is performed from above through uterine contractions, supported by fundus pressure. The helper performs the most important work by applying fundus pressure: the gynecologist, by moving the infant toward the mother's abdomen, essentially ensures that the infant does not fall to the ground! Furthermore, delivery is enhanced since the maneuver of encompassing the breech maintains the mosaic of the "smooth fetal cylinder," which keeps this mosaic of extremities and chin on the chest from "disintegrating," by which expulsion could be further complicated.[31,33]

Applying pressure from the moment the umbilicus is born is important for the following reasons: it prevents lifting of the arms, it strengthens the flexion of the head, and enhances all forms of partial extraction.[2,4] Applying pressure is inherent in the Bracht maneuver: he considered an episiotomy "essentially unnecessary."[26] Presently there are clinics where the method is practiced in a modified manner: that means, pressure is applied only on indication of insufficient expulsion progress, but always with the application of an episiotomy. (In 1928, Covjanov introduced a comparable method in Russia[47]).

Methodology of Breech Delivery According to Bracht

- Instruct the mother not to push until there is complete dilatation and a clear urge to push.
- Allow the breech to engage as far down as possible before starting active pushing by the mother.
- Perform an episiotomy at the end of the contraction that precedes the contraction in which the birth is expected to take place. This is the case when the breech threatens to crown, i.e., when both trochanters are visible. Prevent the breech from crowning at the end of the contraction by letting the mother breathe during part of the contraction.
- Instruct the mother to push forcefully during the next contraction.
- To support the contraction have a helper apply pressure with both hands to the fundus of the uterus during that contraction (Figure 6.2).

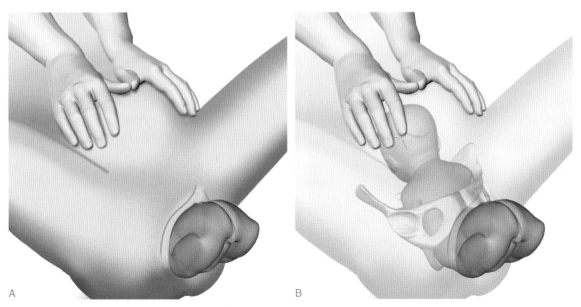

A   B

Figure 6.2 Fundus pressure according to Kristeller.[1]

111

- Make sure that when the torso is born the back turns to the front (ventral) (Figure 6.3A). If this does not occur spontaneously, turn the back to ventral without applying traction.
- Loosen the umbilical cord as soon as the umbilicus is born to prevent it from being under pressure.
- After the umbilicus is born, apply the Bracht maneuver (Figure 6.3B). That means that the fingers will encompass the breech, and the thumbs the upper legs (Figure 6.3C).

- Support and guide the infant's torso without applying traction toward the mother's abdomen until the arms are born and the posterior hairline becomes visible. With the posterior hairline as the point of rotation, turn the infant over the symphysis toward the abdomen of the mother (Figure 6.4). The woman keeps pushing and the helper continues to apply pressure to the fundus, possibly even with a fist if the fundus has become too small to apply pressure with two hands (Figure 6.5).

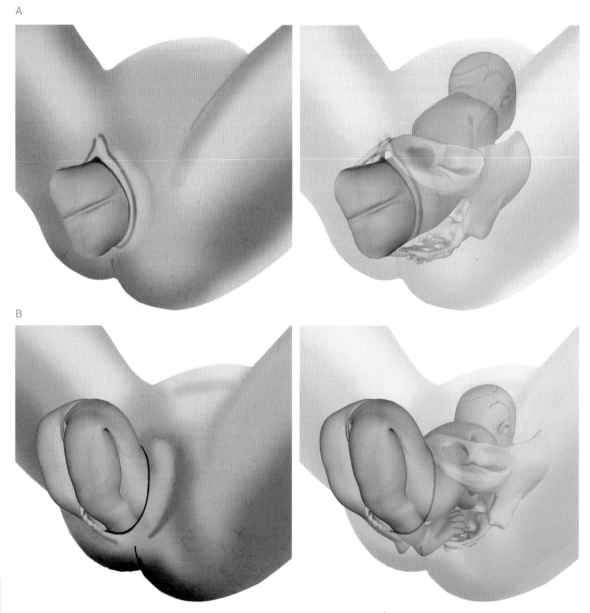

A

B

Figure 6.3 Start of the Bracht maneuver (A); then the hands guide the back forward (B).[1]

C

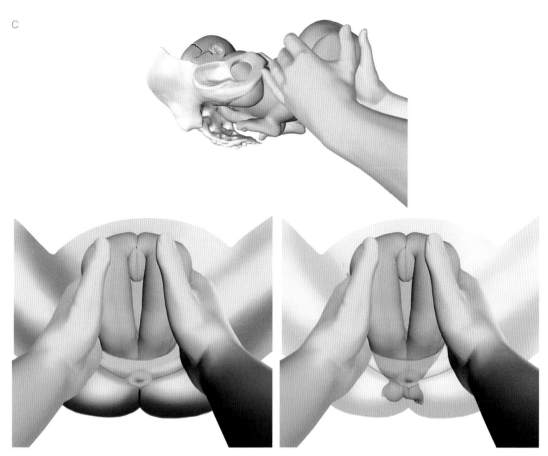

Figure 6.3 (cont.)

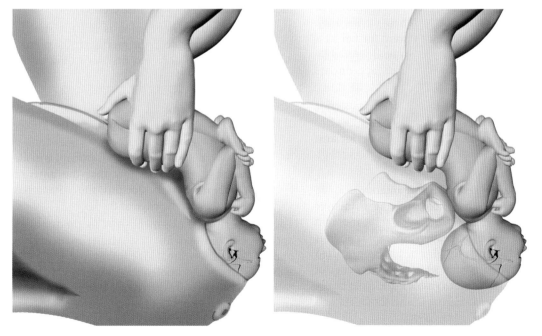

Figure 6.4 Rotation over the symphysis; meanwhile an assistant applies pressure to reinforce the abdominal pushing and the contractions.[1]

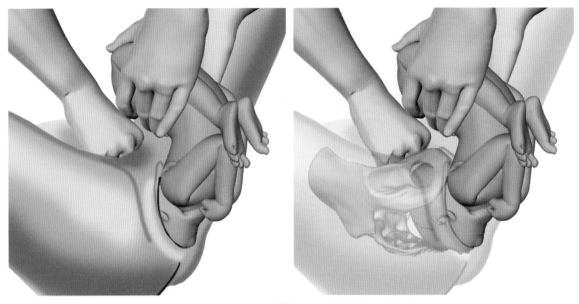

Figure 6.5 Pressure applied by the helper (from Bracht's article[31,33]).

If the Bracht maneuver fails – considered to be the case if there is still no progress after 1 minute of applying the Bracht maneuver – then the delivery continues with the help of a partial breech extraction.

Partial Breech Extraction

If the infant is hypotonic, e.g., due to the mother's (pain) medication or asphyxia, entrapment of the fetal arms behind the neck may occur. These nuchal arms may impact the pelvic inlet and prevent further descent of the fetus. The arms can then be delivered by applying one of the following three appropriate maneuvers:

- the "classical" maneuver to deliver the posterior arm first;
- the Müller maneuver to deliver the anterior arm first;
- the Løvset maneuver.

If the Bracht maneuver fails, the anterior scapula point is usually already visible and the maneuver stagnates at the shoulders. If, however, at the moment of the Bracht maneuver stagnation the scapula point is not yet visible, the torso must first be further extracted (Figure 6.6). This moment at which the lower edge of the anterior scapula becomes visible is the most favorable for the subsequent freeing of the shoulders and arms. If pulling shallower, the arms are more difficult to reach. If pulling deeper, the head may obstruct the delivery of the arms.[6]

Methodology

The breech is grasped with both hands so that the thumbs are next to each other on the sacrum and the index fingers reach over the iliac crest.

1 The direction of the traction is initially straight upward (ventral side of the mother) if the posterior arm is to be delivered first according to the classical method (Figure 6.6).

2 The traction is initially directed straight downward (dorsal side of the mother) if the anterior arm is to be delivered first according to the Müller method (see Figure 6.10).

3 If the Løvset method is applied, an attempt is made to get the shoulders so low that the anterior scapula point is visible. For this, the woman has to lie slightly past the edge of the bed.

Each of the three above-mentioned methods has its specific use and benefits. The Müller maneuver is appropriate in a normal size infant and a normal pelvis, in which no problems are expected.[27,48] The following benefits are listed against the classical method: the speed and simplicity of the maneuver,

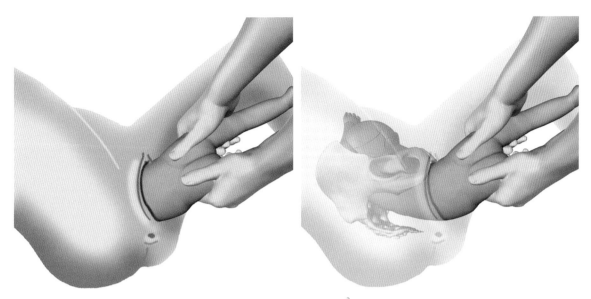

Figure 6.6 Extraction in ventral direction to deliver the posterior shoulder first.[2]

the minimum risk of clavicle and humerus fractures, and the lower incidence of infection. The classical method is useful as a last resort in more difficult cases, that is, in case the Müller or Løvset methods fail, and it is also appropriate for a hypotonic infant. The Løvset maneuver is only appropriate in the case of good muscle tonicity and in a large, rather than dysmature, infant. This is because in hypotonia, the 180° rotation of the torso will be followed less well by the pectoral girdle than in the case of healthy tonicity. The method is also appropriate if the arms are embedded in the neck, i.e., nuchal arms [LE D].[37]

In principle, any of the three methods can be applied. Which method to apply is, on the one hand, determined by personal experience and, on the other hand, by the above-mentioned disadvantages and benefits for the individual patient. In all three methods, the application of fundus pressure by a helper is essential to the success.

Delivery of the Arms
Posterior Arm First ("Classical" Method)

See Animation 6.2.

Methodology

1   Take the lower legs of the infant in a forked grip with the hand that coincides with the abdominal side of the infant.

2   Bend the torso firmly in a ventral direction (abdominal side of the mother) and to the groin that coincides with the abdominal side of the infant (Figure 6.7A).

3   Insert the index and middle fingers of the other hand alongside the posterior shoulder and upper arm of the infant, up to the crease in the elbow (Figure 6.7B).

4   Using the two outstretched fingers like a splint, move the fetal upper arm toward the abdominal side of the infant, sweeping it past the face. Continue this until the arm is born (Figure 6.7C).

5   Take the lower legs of the infant in a forked grip with the hand that coincides with the dorsal side of the infant (Figure 6.8).

6   Move the infant's torso as far dorsally as possible (dorsal side toward the mother) and diametrically opposite to the previous position (thus from left anterior to right posterior or from right anterior to left posterior), whereby the anterior arm is delivered with the other hand in the same way as the delivery of the posterior arm (Figure 6.8).

The method mentioned in Point 6 for delivering the anterior arm is the French variant of the classical method, which is usually taught in the Netherlands, and is also called the "combined arm delivery."[6]

If this does not resolve the delivery of the anterior arm, the original German method can be applied by

A

B

C

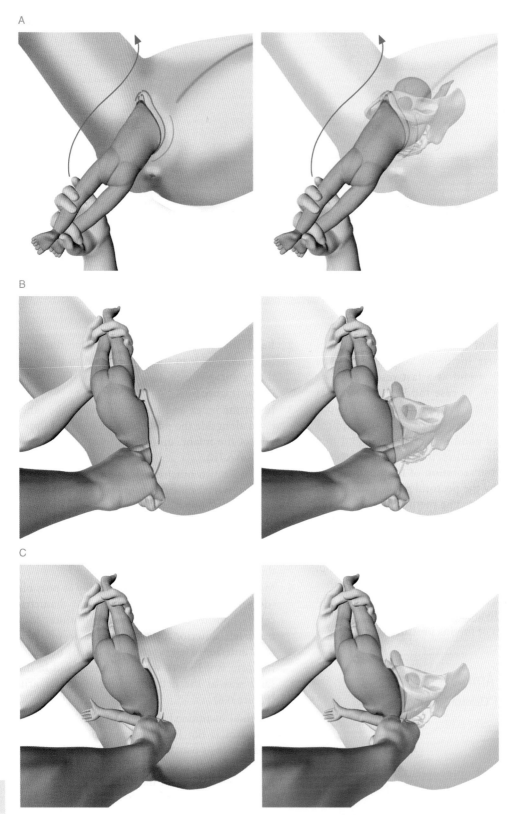

Figure 6.7 Delivery of the posterior arm according to the "classical" method.[2,46]

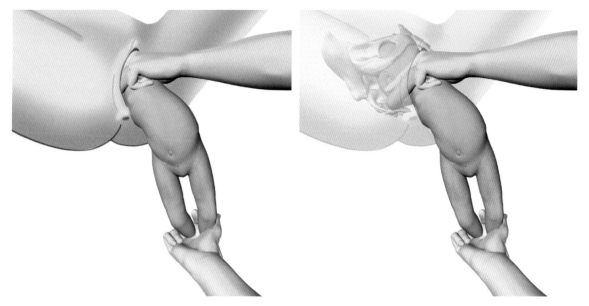

Figure 6.8 French variant of the classical method.

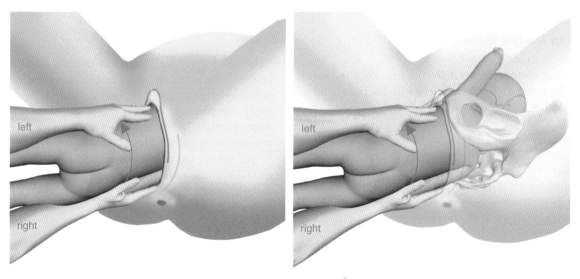

Figure 6.9 Stopfen: 180° rotation, the anterior arm becomes the posterior arm.[2]

having the anterior arm become the posterior arm, and then proceed as described above.

For this, the torso is grasped with both stretched out hands, which function as splints. The already delivered arm is included in this and pressed against the body. The rotation is done in such a way that the dorsum that is located laterally after the delivery of the posterior arm always passes under the symphysis,

thus along the ventral side, and turned to the other side. The 180° rotation of the torso then follows with "stop and go" movements: meaning, the infant is not turned in one single maneuver, but with a series of short turning motions, whereby the torso is pushed up each time toward the sacrum and then pulled back again (*stopfen* = as in plugging a pipe) (Figure 6.9).

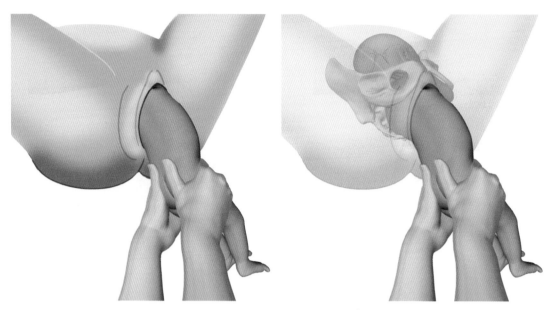

Figure 6.10 Extraction on the buttocks until the anterior scapula becomes visible.[1]

Anterior Arm First (Müller Maneuver)

See Animation 6.3.

If the anterior arm is delivered first, then in that case the right arm is also delivered with the right hand and the left arm with the left hand.

Here it is also the case that if at the moment of stagnation of the Bracht maneuver the anterior scapula is not yet visible, the torso must first be further extracted (Figure 6.10). The breech is grasped with both hands so that the thumbs are next to each other and the index fingers reach over the iliac crest. Then the infant is pulled firmly and straight down, i.e., in the direction of the gynecologist's feet, until the first shoulder follows. For this, the woman must lie slightly past the edge of the bed.

The Müller maneuver is an imitation of the natural, spontaneous breech birth, in which the anterior shoulder and arm are the first to appear under the symphysis.

Methodology

1 Grasp the breech firmly with the thumbs parallel on the buttocks and the index fingers over the iliac crest; the other fingers surround the thighs. First, apply continuous traction, slowly, constantly down (dorsally) until the anterior shoulder and arm are out (Figure 6.11A). If the shoulder width is not yet in the anteroposterior diameter, the shoulder girdle must be turned in that direction during the extraction.

2 Then pull straight in a ventral direction. Pull the infant firmly against the mother's body until the posterior arm and shoulder appear (Figure 6.11B). Sometimes, one of the arms does not appear spontaneously and becomes trapped in the vulva. Then, sweep the arm out with two fingers that splint the humerus (Figure 6.11C).

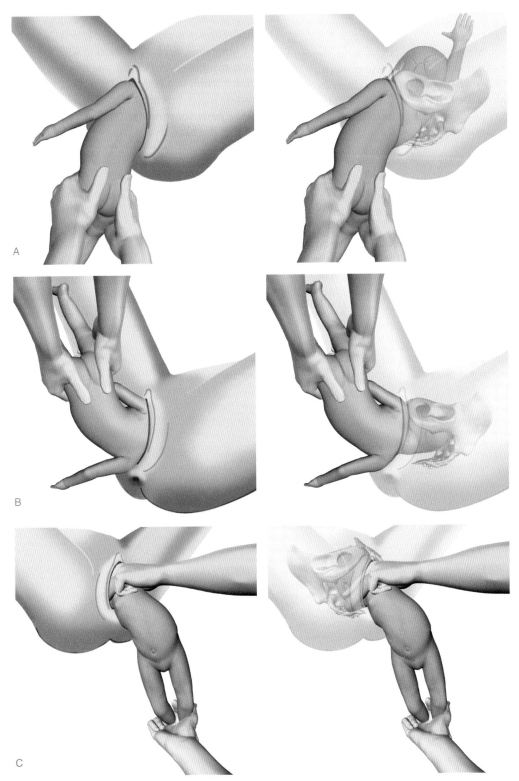

Figure 6.11 Delivery of the anterior arm according to Müller, spontaneous dropping of the anterior arm (A); posterior arm through traction to dorsal and ventral, respectively (B); sweeping of the anterior arm with two, humerus splinting, fingers (C).[1,2]

Løvset Maneuver

See Animation 6.4.

Initially, Løvset himself always began with the Müller maneuver. Only after this maneuver failed, would he apply his own maneuver. Therefore, he had already tried as best he could to bring the shoulders as low as possible through extraction, but without the lower edge of the anterior scapula becoming visible in this way.

The Løvset maneuver is not appropriate with hypotonia, as muscle tonicity is needed for this maneuver to be successful. In a hypotonic and/or dysmature infant, rotations of the torso will lead less well to having the shoulder girdle follow.

Therefore, it is better to apply the classic method on a hypotonic infant. The Løvset method has greater success in a large child than in a dysmature child. The method is also appropriate if the arms are embedded in the neck, i.e., nuchal arms.

Methodology

1   Grasp the infant with the thumbs on the sacrum, and the index fingers over the iliac crests. The remaining fingers surround the upper legs from the back (Figure 6.12).

2   At the same time, apply light traction with the 180° rotation mentioned in Point 3: the first 90° of the rotation traction in a horizontal direction, followed by traction in the direction of the gynecologist's feet.

3   Turn the posterior shoulder 180° forward, in such a way that the back always passes by the mother's symphysis. Sometimes the forward turned arm falls out by itself (Figure 6.13).

4   If the arm does not fall out, take the index and middle fingers of the same-sided hand (thus the left hand for the left shoulder) over the shoulder like a trough alongside the upper arm up to the elbow.

5   Apply pressure to the elbow and sweep the arm past the face and the torso to the outside (Figure 6.14).

6   Grasp the infant again as in Points 1 and 2.

7   Turn the infant 180° back again, in which the back appears alongside the symphysis again (Figure 6.15).

8   Repeat the procedures in Points 4 and 5.

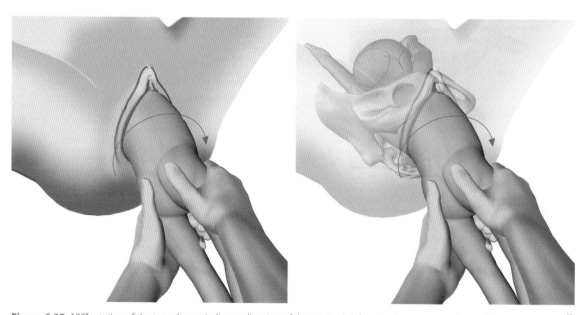

Figure 6.12 180° rotation of the torso (arrow indicates direction of the rotation): left posterior arm comes forward; Løvset maneuver.[49]

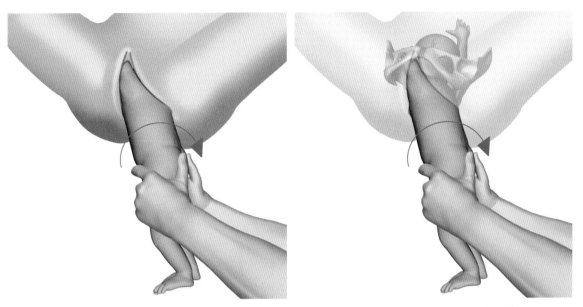

Figure 6.13 Torso is rotated 180° (arrow indicates the direction of the turn): posterior arm is now under the symphysis.[49]

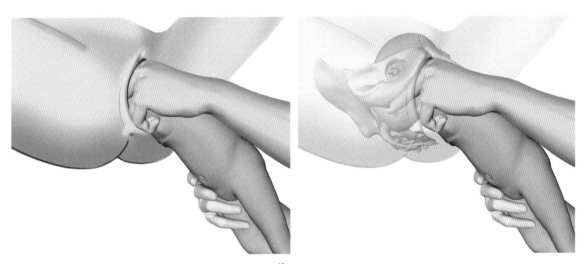

Figure 6.14 Delivery/"sweeping" of left arm; Løvset maneuver.[49]

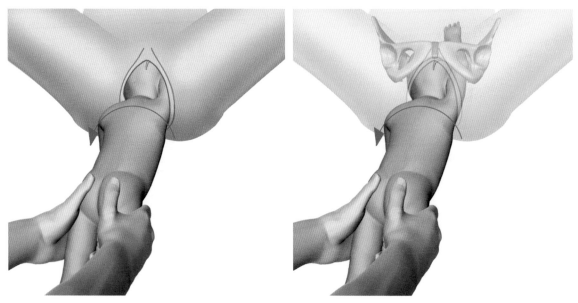

Figure 6.15 180° reverse rotation of the torso (arrow indicates direction of the turn).[49]

A   B

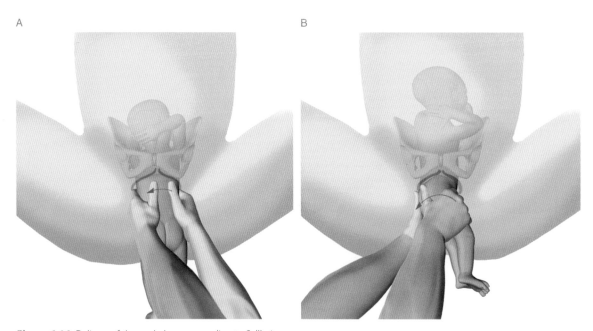

Figure 6.16 Delivery of the nuchal arms according to Sellheim.

Sellheim Maneuver[50]

In the event of embedded arms, the embedded arm is prepared for being brought down by turning the infant's torso 180° around its longitudinal axis (Figure 6.16A). The torso is turned 180° in stages by means of several rapid, short turn motions. Thus, the turning of the torso by 180° is done in

"halting" movements; i.e., the child is not turned all at once, but by means of a series of short turns, in which the torso is repeatedly pushed up sacrally and then pulled back down again (*stopfen*) (see Figure 6.9).

The direction of the rotation is dictated by the direction in which the hand of the corresponding embedded arm of the infant is pointing (Figure 6.16A,B). In a sense, the infant indicates the direction. Afterwards, the torso has to be turned back by 180°, otherwise the spine will be turned to the back![50]

Delivery of the Aftercoming Head

The aftercoming head will have to be delivered as in the Bracht maneuver or if after the delivery of the arms in a partial breech extraction the head is not born. In that case, the Mauriceau and De Snoo maneuvers can be applied, as well as the forceps.

For the delivery of the head it is important that the occiput is under the symphysis and is (maximally) flexed.

In all three methods, careful fundus pressure remains important for success.

Mauriceau Maneuver[28,46]

See Animations 6.5 and 6.6.

Methodology

1 Grasp the legs with a forked grip and lift up the torso.
2 Place the middle finger of the other hand (the right hand if the posterior fontanel is in the right half of the pelvis; the left hand if on the left side)

in the mouth of the fetus, the thumb against the lower jaw, and the index and ring fingers on the maxilla.

3 Let the infant "ride" with the belly and spread legs on the lower arm, i.e., with the legs hanging down on each side.
4 Maneuver (rotate) the head with the inserted fingers in such a way that the posterior fontanel comes to lie under the symphysis and is held in flexion at the same time (Figure 6.17A).
5 Place two forked fingers of the other hand from the back around the neck and apply traction to the shoulders of the infant (Figure 6.17C). Avoid hooking the shoulders because of the risk of a plexus injury.
6 Caution: traction may not be applied with the finger that is placed inside the mouth!
7 The exterior hand pulls the infant down (dorsally), i.e., in the direction of the gynecologist's feet, until the posterior hairline is visible.
8 Have an assistant carefully apply fundus pressure to the head above the symphysis, so that less traction force is applied via the neck.
9 When the posterior hairline becomes visible, move the torso gradually in a ventral and cranial direction, whereby the symphysis functions as the rotation point and allow the head to be born gradually (Figure 6.17B).

A

B

C

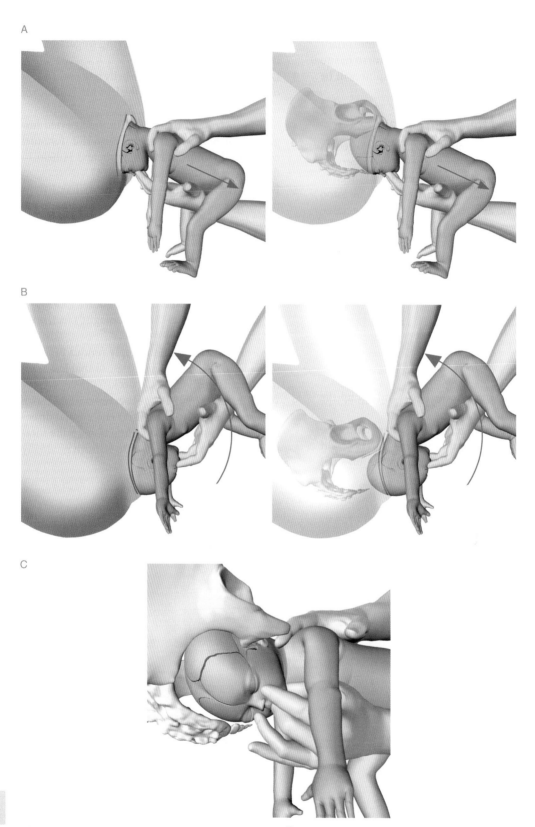

Figure 6.17 Mauriceau maneuver (A, B) with detail graphic (C).[46]

The De Snoo Maneuver[51,52]

See Animations 6.7 and 6.8.

Methodology

1 Grasp the legs with a forked grip and lift up the torso.
2 Insert the index and middle fingers of the left hand alongside the downturned chest and neck of the infant.
3 Check by vaginal examination whether the chin is turned to the back (dorsal), which will usually be the case in a ventrally turned back. If not, the chin can be turned to the back with the fingers inserted in the mouth.
4 From the front, grasp the neck of the infant with the left index and middle fingers over the shoulders.

5 Lay the torso of the infant on the left arm ("as in riding").
6 Place the right hand above the symphysis (Figure 6.18A).
7 Pull with the left hand on the shoulder girdle and simultaneously apply pressure with the right hand to the head above the symphysis (Figure 6.18B).
8 With the left hand, pull in the direction of the axis of the birth canal, thus increasingly toward ventral as the head gets deeper into the pelvis.

Forceps on Aftercoming Head[53–57]

By using forceps on the aftercoming head it is not so much the (ex)traction, but the enhancement of the flexion of the head through the action of the forceps

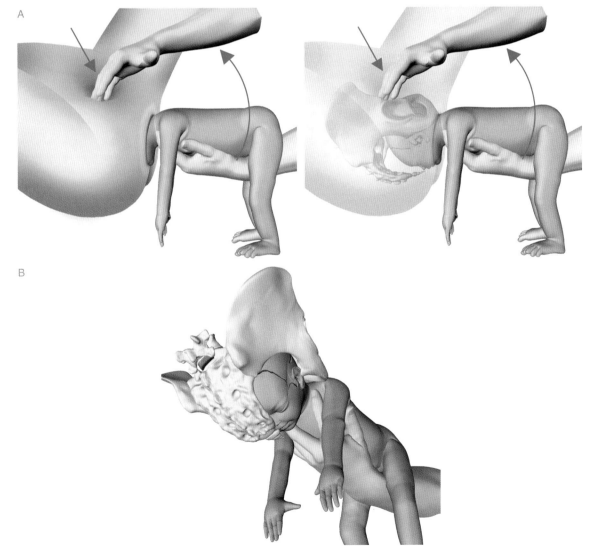

Figure 6.18 The De Snoo maneuver.

that is the most important aspect of the delivery. Naegele's forceps (the large size), the forceps according to Kielland, and the Piper forceps are all appropriate. The most important part is that the neck is long enough and that the pulling is performed in the proper direction. It is crucial to always have the forceps ready that were used for practicing on the dummy.

A condition for using forceps on the aftercoming head is that the occiput is in anterior position and engaged.

Methodology

See Animations 6.9 and 6.10.

1 An assistant holds the child with a hollow back and the arms out of the way. This can be done by:

- holding the infant from above with a warm towel under the torso; or
- taking the legs in a forked grip and holding the infant above the horizontal plane and at the same time holding the hands on the back of the infant with the other hand (the best place for the assistant to stand would be on the left side of the woman) (Figure 6.19A). The blades of the forceps are inserted as described in Chapter 7 on vaginal assisted deliveries.

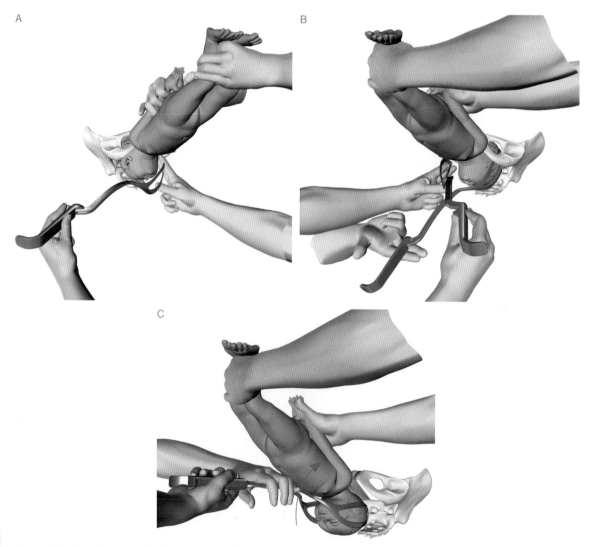

A

B

C

Figure 6.19 Piper forceps on the aftercoming head.[3]

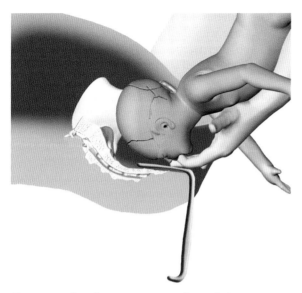

Figure 6.20 Speculum maneuver according to DeLee.

2 Ensure that the blades are inserted from a plane that lies below the horizontal line of the obstetric bed, thus from dorsal to ventral (Figure 6.19B).

3 The blades will be lying around the infant's head, along the mento-occipital circumference (= in the chin-occiput line) (Figure 6.19C).

4 First, maximum flexion of the head is realized with the forceps, then traction is applied in the direction of the pelvic axis. The rotation point is the infant's neck.

If the head does not follow, a Doyen vaginal speculum (24 cm, 180 × 60 mm) can be used according to DeLee, to suction the infant and to allow it to breathe and a symphysiotomy can be considered (Figure 6.20).[58]

Complete Breech Extraction

The only still undisputed indication for a complete breech extraction is the necessity for assisted delivery of the second member of a set of twins as part of the version and extraction in a transverse presentation that cannot be corrected [EL A2].[59–61]

Also if for the second twin in breech presentation an indication arises to terminate, a choice for a breech extraction can be made if the estimated weight of this infant is not much greater than that of the first infant.[62] A combined vaginal delivery (twin A) and cesarean section (twin B) carries with it the greatest risk of perinatal asphyxia (of twin B), defined as Apgar score of <4 after 5 minutes. This is true in comparison with a vaginal delivery of both infants and in comparison with a planned cesarean section [LE C].[63,64]

If there is an indication to terminate a breech delivery of a singleton delivery even before the torso is born, an emergency C-section is performed, since the total breech extraction is susceptible to a high mortality (14%) and morbidity rate. Breech extraction then becomes only an alternative if a cesarean section is no longer possible.[2,22,25,46,62]

Complete Breech Presentation

See Animation 6.11.

Methodology

1 While the external hand supports the fundus of the uterus, the hand that coincides with the abdominal side of the infant is inserted.

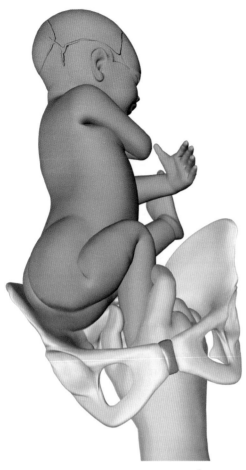

Figure 6.21 Bringing down the anterior foot.[2]

2 The anterior leg is brought down by grasping the ankle with the forked grip and by placing the thumb after traction on the posterior side of the lower leg, the calf (Figure 6.21). It is important that the posterior side of the leg points to the front or is brought to the front by turning it, since that prevents the back from turning backwards. Bringing down the anterior leg prevents the breech from getting stuck on the symphysis, as is possible when the posterior leg is brought down first.

3 After that, the other fingers surround the entire lower leg. Then the most important aspect is the direction of the traction: straight down (dorsally), to the gynecologist's feet (Figure 6.22). After that, the other hand grasps the upper leg as high as possible and pulls it straight down until the hip is delivered. The thumb of this hand rests on the buttock; the other fingers firmly surround the upper leg (Figure 6.23).

4 After the anterior trochanter has been passed (Figure 6.24), stand at the abdominal side of the infant. Surround the upper leg as high as possible with the entire hand (with the right hand if the back is to the right; with the left hand if the back is to the left). With the wrist of the hand, which

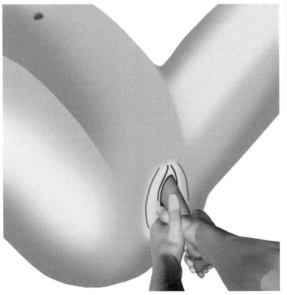
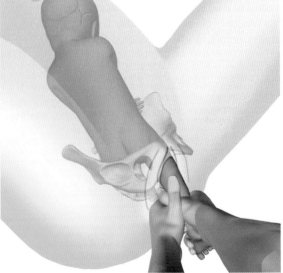

Figure 6.22 Grasping the lower leg, traction downward.[1]

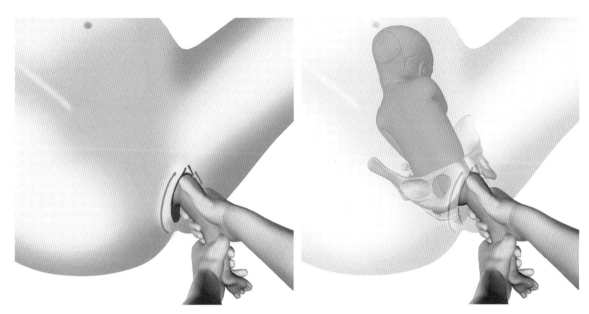

Figure 6.23 Traction on the lower leg in dorsal direction.[1]

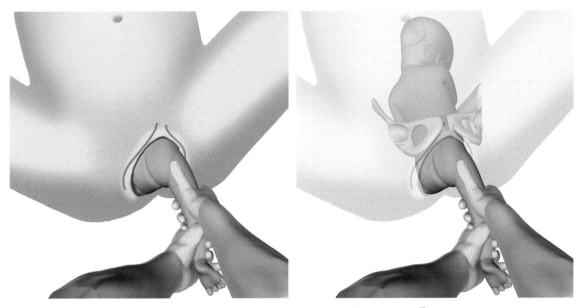

Figure 6.24 Traction on the anterior leg in dorsal direction until the anterior trochanter is visible.[49]

surrounds the upper leg and rests on the symphysis, rotate the posterior buttock over the perineum by moving the anterior leg into a vertical position (Figure 6.25). After the anterior trochanter has been passed, pull forward (ventrally) and finally completely upward to allow the posterior hip to be born (Figure 6.25).

5 As soon as possible, hook the index finger of the other hand into the posterior hip. Do not do this with two fingers, as this could increase the possibility of femur fracture! The thumb will naturally rest on the buttock, so that both thumbs will be situated parallel on the sacrum (Figure 6.26).

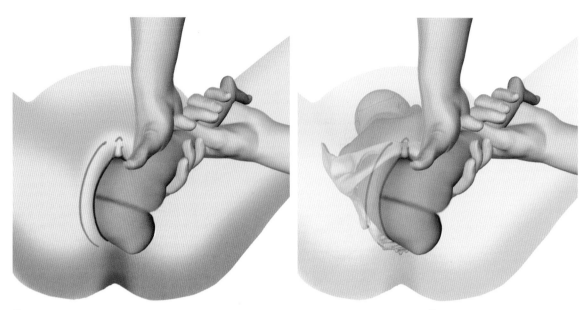

Figure 6.25 Traction on the anterior leg in ventral direction until the posterior trochanter is visible.[49]

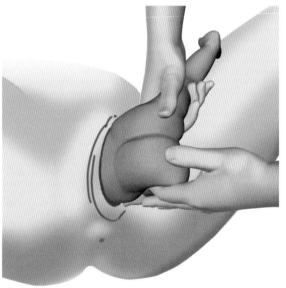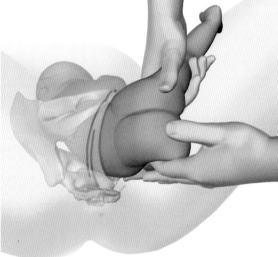

Figure 6.26 Hooking the posterior hip with a finger.[49]

6 Then the breech is grasped firmly with both hands and pulled first to the front (ventrally), if you want to deliver the posterior arm first according to the classical method (Figure 6.27), or straight down (dorsally) until the lower edge of the anterior scapula point is visible and palpable, if you want to deliver the anterior arm first according to the Müller maneuver (Figure 6.28).

This is followed by delivery of the arms and delivery of the head (see Animation 6.14), as in Section: Partial breech extraction.

Advice: if upon the appearance of the lower edge of the shoulder a posterior foot that is elevated against the abdomen does not fall out yet and becomes stuck in the vagina, that leg should never be pulled. By turning the torso in the direction of the back of the infant, the leg will fall out by itself!

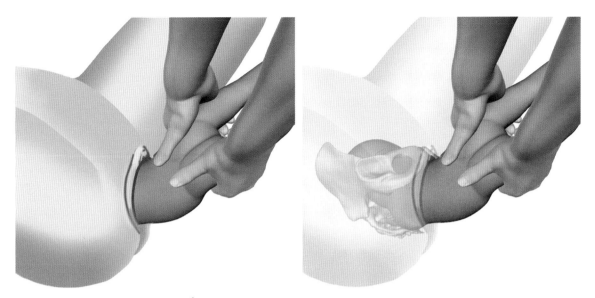

Figure 6.27 Traction in ventral direction.[2]

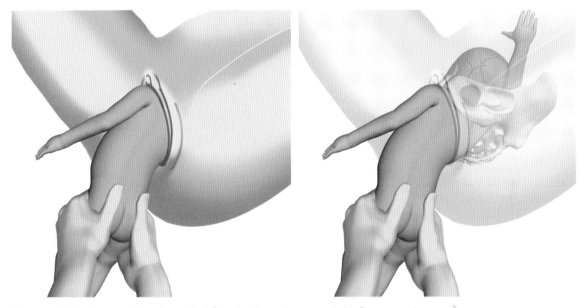

Figure 6.28 Traction toward the obstetrician's feet: thumbs on the sacrum; index fingers over the crests.[2]

Frank Breech Presentation

There are two possibilities: the not yet completely engaged breech and the deeply engaged breech.

Not Yet Completely Engaged Breech

In frank breech presentation, the anterior leg can only be brought down if the breech has not engaged very far yet. In case of an engaged breech, this can sometimes be pushed above the pelvic inlet in order to bring down the anterior foot with the Pinard maneuver (see Animation 6.12). The breech is pushed up above the pelvic inlet and placed on the iliac fossa, which coincides with the dorsal side of the infant.

Insert the index and middle fingers of the inserted full hand on the side of the extremities (thus, the left index finger if the back is to the left and vice versa) with stretched fingers until the finger

A　　　　　　　　　　　　　　　B

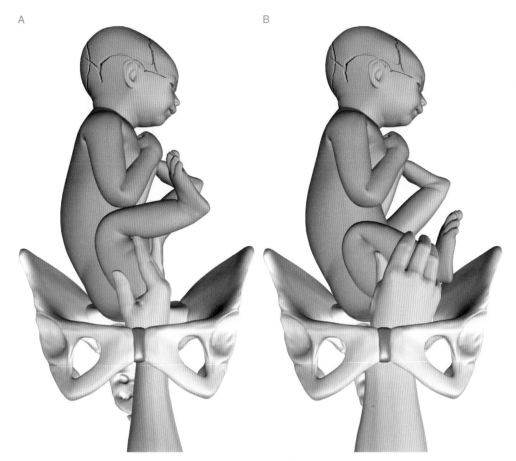

Figure 6.29 Pinard maneuver: bringing down the anterior foot.[1]

tips arrive at the back of the knee of the anterior leg: this is abducted, which creates space to bend the lower leg and bring down the foot. First, grasp the entire lower leg. If the lower leg is bent, take the ankle between the index and middle fingers and place the thumb on the dorsum of the foot, after which the entire foot is pulled out (Figure 6.29).

Deeply Engaged Breech

If the breech is already firmly on the pelvic floor, pushing it up to bring down a leg is sometimes no longer possible. Then you have to pull on the breech itself until it is outside the vulva. That is difficult and risky: therefore, extraction of a deeply engaged frank breech (see Animation 6.13) can best be accomplished by first pushing up the breech so far in a cranial direction that a leg can be brought down by

means of the Pinard maneuver (Figure 6.29). For this, a uterus relaxing inhalation anesthesia (sevoflurane) is recommended. If the anesthetist has not yet arrived, midazolam (Dormicum) is recommended.

The technique of the extraction of the unborn breech is as follows. As in all assisted deliveries, insert the left hand into the right half of the pelvis and the right hand into the left half of the pelvis. Point the palm of the hand to the infant's abdomen. Then insert the index finger from the side into the groin against the iliac crest, and the thumb on the sacrum. Since it is difficult to pull hard with one finger, place the other hand around the wrist of the inserted hand. Pull the anterior buttock down and under (Figure 6.30). When the anterior buttock is visible in the vulva, insert the index finger of the second hand into the posterior groin crease. By

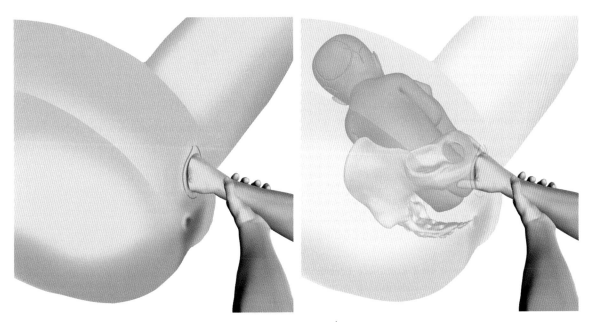

Figure 6.30 Extraction on the anterior groin in the direction of the dorsum.[1]

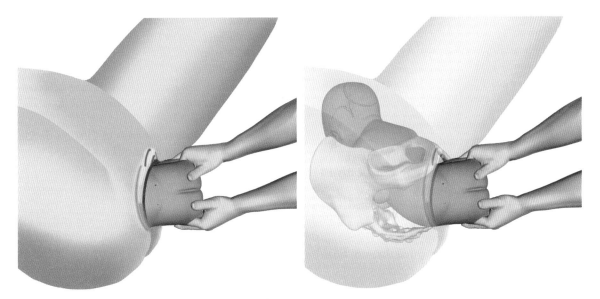

Figure 6.31 Extraction on both groins in ventral direction.[1]

pulling the breech firmly upward, it is now always possible to make the posterior buttock appear over the perineum (Figure 6.31). Maintaining fundus pressure remains essential in this maneuver!

Note

Frequent errors in breech extraction are:

- traction direction insufficiently straight to dorsal or ventral;
- two fingers instead of one finger in the hip, which carries a greater risk of hip fracture;
- starting too early with arm delivery: deliver the arms only after the anterior scapula point is visible/palpable.

Important Points and Recommendations[17]

Before the Delivery

- If there is no contraindication to an external version or a vaginal breech delivery, recommend an external version. If an external version is not successful or refused, the options are vaginal delivery or an elective cesarean section.
- Discuss the pros and cons of a vaginal breech delivery versus an elective cesarean section and record the outcome of the discussion in the file.
- Perform an ultrasound examination before delivery.

  - Determine whether it is a complete breech presentation, a frank presentation, or a footling presentation.
  - A cesarean section is recommended in case of a footling presentation, unless delivery is unavoidable.
  - Determine the position of the head relative to the torso.
  - If the head is hyperextended a cesarean section is recommended.
  - Perform a cesarean section in case of a presenting umbilical cord [LE A2].

- Perform external and ultrasound examinations to estimate the birthweight (the error margin between the estimated weight and the actual birthweight is 10–20% in ultrasound or external examination).
- A vaginal breech delivery can be contemplated if the estimated birthweight is between 2500 and 4000 g.
- Macrosomia and intrauterine growth restriction are contraindications for vaginal breech birth [LE B].
- Perform an internal pelvic examination.

  - Perform a cesarean section in case of abnormal findings.

- The best evidence of adequate fetopelvic relationships is a good labor and delivery progression.
- A mechanically difficult delivery in the medical history is a contraindication for vaginal breech birth [LE D].
- For a vaginal breech delivery, the presence of an experienced and competent gynecologist and well-trained assistant (for applying fundus pressure!) and the immediate availability of a pediatrician and an anesthesiologist are required [LE A1].

During the Delivery

- Perform an ultrasound and internal pelvic examination if these examinations were not performed recently.
- Insert an intravenous infusion.
- Provide CTG monitoring: external in case of unruptured membranes and internal in case of ruptured membranes, and continuous CTG monitoring starting at complete dilation [LE A1].
- Keep forceps at the ready in case the head does not follow and a forceps delivery of the aftercoming head is required.
- Ensure that an operating room and a surgical team and pediatrician are immediately available [LE A1].
- Avoid rupturing the membranes prematurely, unless there is an indication for this.
- When the membranes rupture spontaneously, do a vaginal examination to detect a possible prolapsed umbilical cord [LE D].
- Oxytocin may be administered in case of problematic contraction activity during the first and second stage [LE A2].
- In case of insufficient progress of dilation decide to perform a cesarean section [LE A2].
- An experienced gynecologist pronounces the "complete dilation" diagnosis [LE D].
- Encourage the woman to avoid active pushing (for at least 90 minutes with a good CTG) if on complete dilation the breech is not close to or on the pelvic floor yet. That allows time for the breech to engage [LE A1].
- Active pushing by the mother commences when the breech is on or near the pelvic floor. Decide to perform a cesarean section if the infant has not yet been born (with a good CTG) after 60 minutes [LE A2].
- Avoid a complete breech extraction in case of a non-progressing expulsion [LE B].
- Perform an episiotomy just before the crowning of the breech [LE B].
- Ensure proper documentation of the breech delivery.

References

1. Holmer AJM, Ten Berge BS, Van Bouwdijk Bastiaanse MA, et al (eds). Leerboek der Verloskunde. 3rd edition. Amsterdam: Van Holkema Warendorf, 1963.

2. Dudenhausen JW, Pschyrembel W. Praktische Geburtshilfe. Berlin/New York: Walter de Gruyter, 2000.

3. Cunningham G, Gant NF, Leveno KJ, et al (eds). Williams Obstetrics: Techniques for breech delivery. 21st edition. Stanford, Connecticut: Appleton & Lange, 2001, pp. 495–508.

4. Stoeckel W. Lehrbuch der Geburtshilfe. 7th edition. Jena: Fisher Verlag, 1943.

5. Gimovsky ML, McIlhargie CJ. Munro Kerr's operative obstetrics. London: Williams & Wilkins, 1995.

6. Martius H. Die geburtshilflichen Operationen. 8th edition. Stuttgart: Georg Thieme Verlag, 1958.

7. Hickock DE, Gordon DC, Milberg JA, et al. The frequency of breech presentation by gestational age at birth: a large population-based study Am J Obstet Gynecol. 1992;166:605–18.

8. Hsieh YY, Tsai FJ, Lin CC, et al. Breech deformation-complex in neonates. J Reprod Med. 2000;45:933–5.

9. Shipp TD, Bromley B, Benacerraf B. The prognostic significance of hyperextension of the fetal head detected antenatally with ultrasound. Ultrasound Obstet Gynecol. 2000;15:391–6.

10. Collea JV, Rabin SC, Weghorst GR, et al. The randomized management of term frank breech presentation. Vaginal delivery vs cesarean section. Am J Obstet Gynecol. 1978;131:186–95.

11. Krebs L, Langhoff-Roos J. Breech presentation at term: indications for secondary caesarean section. In: Künzel W (ed). Breech delivery, European practice in gynaecology and obstetrics. Paris: Éditions Scientifiques et Médicales/Elsevier SAS, 2002, pp. 129–37.

12. Fischl F, Janisch H, Wagner G. pH-Messungen nach Geburt aus Beckenendlage. Z Geburtshilfe Perinatol. 1979;58:183–7.

13. Zimmerman P, Zimmerman M, Dehnhard F. Noch eine Untersuchung zur Frage des optimalen Entbindungsmodus bei Beckenendlage. Z Geburtshilfe Perinatol. 1978;57:182–8.

14. Kubli F, Boos W, Rüttgers H. Caesarean section in the management of singleton breech presentation. In: Rooth G, Bratteby LE (eds). Perinatal medicine. 5th European Congress of Perinatal Medicine, Uppsala. Uppsala: Almqvist & Wiksell, 1976, pp. 69–75.

15. Kubli F. Geburtsleitung bei Beckenendlagen. Gynäkologe. 1975;8:48–57.

16. Flanagan TA, Mulchahey KM, Korenbrot CC, et al. Management of term breech presentation. Am J Obstet Gynecol. 1987;156:1492–9.

17. Society of Obstetricians & Gynaecologists of Canada. Vaginal delivery of breech presentation. Guideline Society of Obstetricians & Gynaecologists of Canada (www.sogc.org). J Obstet Gynaecol Can. 2009;31:557–66.

18. Verhoeven ATM, de Leeuw JP, Bruinse HW. Aterme stuitligging: onterechte keus voor de electieve keizersnede als standaardbehandeling vanwege te hoge risico's voor moeder en haar volgende kinderen. Ned Tijdschr Geneeskd. 2005;149:2007–10.

19. Rietberg C. Term breech delivery in the Netherlands. Unpublished Ph.D. thesis, University of Utrecht, 2006.

20. Goffinet F, Carayol M, Foidart JM, et al. Is planned vaginal delivery for breech presentation still an option? Results of an observational prospective survey in France and Belgium. Am J Obstet Gynecol. 2006;194:1002–11.

21. Verhoeven ATM. Tien jaar na de Term Breech Trial, een balans voor Nederland. Ned Tijdschr Obstet Gynaecol. 2011;124:143–7.

22. Dutch Society Obstetrics & Gynecology. Guideline Breech Position, 2008. www.nvog.nl.

23. Bergenhenegouwen LA, Meertens LJE, Schaaf J, et al. Vaginal delivery versus caesarean section in preterm delivery: a systematic review. Eur J Obstet Gynecol Reprod Biol. 2014;172:1–6.

24. Barrett JFR, Hannah ME, Hutton EK, et al. A randomized trial of planned cesarean or vaginal delivery for twin pregnancy. N Engl J Med. 2013;369:295–305.

25. Royal College of Obstetricians and Gynaecologists. The management of breech presentation. Guideline No 20b. London: RCOG, 2006.

26. Su M, McLeod L, Ross S, et al. Factors associated with adverse perinatal outcome in the Term Breech Trial. Am J Obstet Gynecol. 2003;189:740–5.

27. Mulder ME. Het ontwikkelen der armen en de extractie volgens A. Müller. Ph.D. thesis, University of Groningen, 1908.

28. Verhoeven ATM. Handgreep van Mauriceau (Levret-Smellie-Veit) – Eponiemen. Ned Tijdschr Obstet Gynaecol. 2010;123:86–92.

29. Bracht E. Vortrag: Zur Manualhilfe bei Beckenendlage. Z Geburtsh Gynäkol. 1936;112:271.

30. Bracht E. Zur Behandlung der Steisslage. Handelingen Internationaal Congres voor Verloskunde en Gynaecologie. Congresbericht II. Amsterdam: Brill, 1938, pp. 93–4.

31. Bracht E. Zur Beckenendlage-Behandlung. Geburtsh Frauenheilkd. 1965;25:635–7.

32. Verhoeven ATM. Methode van Bracht – 70 jaar – Eponiemen. Ned Tijdschr Obstet Gynaecol. 2006;119:8–12.

33. Verhoeven ATM, de Leeuw JP. De theorie van de methode van Bracht en de praktische gevolgen. Ned Tijdschr Obstet Gynaecol. 2008;**121**:58–60.

34. Løvset J. Schulterentwicklung ohne Armlösung bei natürlicher und künstlicher Beckenendlage. Arch Gynäkol. 1936;**161**:397–8.

35. Løvset J. Shoulder delivery by breech presentation. J Obstet Gynaecol Br Emp. 1937;**44**:696–704.

36. Løvset J. Vaginal operative delivery. Oslo: Scandinavian University Books, 1968.

37. Verhoeven ATM. Handgreep van Løvset – 70 jaar Eponiemen. Ned Tijdschr Obstet Gynaecol. 2007;**120**:21–3.

38. Verhoeven ATM. Dührssense incisies. Ned Tijdschr Obstet Gynaecol. 2010;**123**:61–3.

39. Verhoeven ATM. De handgreep van Wigand-Martin-Von Winckel – Eponiemen, Geschiedkundige ontwikkeling en betekenis voor de huidige praktijk. Ned Tijdschr Obstet Gynaecol. 2008;**121**:345–50.

40. van Loon AJ, Mantingh A, Serlier EK, et al. Randomised controlled trial of magnetic resonance pelvimetry in breech presentation at term. Lancet. 1997;**350**:1799–804.

41. de Leeuw JW de, Struijk PC, Vierhout ME, et al. Risk factors for third degree perineal ruptures during delivery. BJOG. 2001;**108**:383–7.

42. Kurz CS, Künzel W. Fetale Herzfrequenz, Dezelerationsfläche und Säure-Basen-Status bei Entbindung aus Beckenendlage-und Schädellage. Z Geburtshilfe Perinat. 1977;**181**:9–16.Ref in: Künzel W (ed). Breech delivery, European practice in gynaecology and obstetrics. Paris: Elsevier, 2002, p. 126.

43. de Leeuw JP. Breech presentation vaginal or abdominal delivery? A prospective longitudinal study. Ph.D. thesis, University of Maastricht, 1989.

44. Brady K, Duff P, Read JA, et al. Reliability of fetal buttock sampling in assessing the acid-base balance of the breech fetus. Obstet Gynecol. 1989;**74**:886–8.

45. Collea JV, Chein C, Quilligan EJ. The randomized management of term frank breech presentation: a study of 208 cases. Am J Obstet Gynecol. 1980;**137**:235–44.

46. Künzel W, Kirschbaum M. Management of vaginal delivery in breech presentation at term. In: Künzel W (ed). Breech delivery, European practice in gynaecology and obstetrics. Paris: Elsevier, 2002.

47. van Grinsven-Dmitrieva N, Verhoeven ATM. Stuitgeboorte volgens Bracht (1935) of Covjanov (1928). . . wie had de primeur? Ned Tijdschr Obstet Gynaecol. 2013;**126**:245–50.

48. Verhoeven ATM, De ontwikkeling van de armpjes bij stuitgeboorte volgens Müller – 110 jaar – Eponiemen. Ned Tijdschr Obstet Gynaecol. 2009;**122**:251–4.

49. von Mickulicz-Radecki F. Geburtshilfe des praktischen Ärztes. 3rd edition. Leipzig: Barth, 1943.

50. Verhoeven ATM, Methode volgens Sellheim. Ned Tijdschr Obstet Gynaecol. 2008;**121**:64–6.

51. Verhoeven ATM. Handgreep van De Snoo – Eponiemen. Ned Tijdschr Obstet Gynaecol. 2003;**116**:101–2.

52. de Snoo K. Leerboek der verloskunde. 4th edition. Groningen: Wolters, 1943.

53. Piper EB, Backman C. The prevention of fetal injuries in breech delivery. JAMA. 1929;**92**:217–21.

54. Gordon Douglas R, Stromme W. Operative obstetrics. 3rd edition. New York: Appleton Century Crofts, 1976.

55. Grady JP, Gimovsky M. Instrumental delivery: a lost art? In: Studd J (ed). Progress in obstetrics and gynecology. Vol **10**. Edinburgh: Churchill Livingstone, 1993.

56. Gabbe SG, Niebyl JR, Simpson JL, et al. Obstetrics, normal and problem pregnancies. 4th edition. Edinburgh: Churchill Livingstone, 2002.

57. Verhoeven ATM. De Piperforceps – 80 jaar – Eponiemen. Ned Tijdschr Obstet Gynaecol. 2009;**122**:180–5.

58. Verhoeven ATM. Handgreep van DeLee. In: Eponiemen en geschiedenis van de stuitgeboorte. Haarlem: DCHG, 2010, pp. 131–7.

59. Crowther CA. Caesarean delivery for the second twin. Cochrane Database Syst Rev. 2000;**2**:CD000047.

60. Ayres A, Johnson TR. Management of multiple pregnancy: labor and delivery. Obstet Gynecol Surv. 2005;**60**:550–6.

61. Rabinovici J, Barkai G, Reichman B, et al. Randomized management of the second nonvertex twin: vaginal delivery or caesarean section. Am J Obstet Gynecol. 1987;**156**:52–6.

62. Hofmeyr GJ, Kulier R. Expedited versus conservative approaches for vaginal delivery in breech presentation. Cochrane Database Syst Rev. 2000;**2**: CD000082.

63. Usta IM, Nassar AH, Awwad JT, et al. Comparison of the perinatal morbidity and mortality of the presenting twin and its co-twin. J Perinatol. 2002;**22**:391–6.

64. Caukwell S, Murphy DJ. The effect of mode of delivery and gestational age on neonatal outcome of the non-cephalic-presenting second twin. Am J Obstet Gynecol. 2002;**187**:1356–61.

Operative Vaginal Delivery (Vacuum and Forceps Extraction)

P.J. Dörr, G.G.M. Essed, and F.K. Lotgering

General Information

Introduction

To perform vacuum or forceps extraction requires knowledge of the indication, the instrumentation, and the procedure. Practitioners who perform assisted deliveries must be skilled in making the proper diagnosis and in carrying out the operative delivery.[1–3]

Definition

The operative vaginal deliveries discussed in this chapter relate to operative deliveries of infants in vertex presentation, for whom the second stage is accelerated through the use of vacuum or forceps extraction.

Incidence

The combined incidence of vacuum and forceps extraction varies all over the world and is between 3% and 13%.[3,4] In many countries, the percentage of forceps extractions has decreased and that of vacuum extractions has increased.[5] In the Netherlands, between 1990 and 2012, the percentage of forceps extractions decreased from 5.0% to 0.4% and that of vacuum extractions increased from 11.5% to 12.4%. In the United States the incidence of operative vaginal delivery continues to decline. In 2010 the incidence of vacuum and forceps delivery was 3.6%. The use of forceps declined from 6.6% in 1990 to 1% in 2010.[6]

Indications and Contraindications

The indications for a vaginal termination of a delivery may be decided on either fetal or maternal grounds; not infrequently there are combinations of factors that make intervention desirable. The following indications and contraindications are not absolute.

Indications

Indications for terminating a pregnancy with the aid of vacuum or forceps extraction are[2,3,7]:

- inadequate progress (of the bony part of the fetal skull) of the second stage:
  - in nulliparous women after 2 hours (with regional anesthesia after 3 hours);
  - in multiparous women after 1 hour (with regional anesthesia after 2 hours);
  - maternal fatigue/exhaustion;
- fetal: presumed fetal compromise (e.g., an abnormal fetal heart rate pattern on the cardiotocogram);
- maternal: contraindications to pushing (e.g., certain cardiac and neurological disorders).

Contraindications

Contraindications for assisted vaginal delivery are:

- fetal bleeding disorders, e.g., in fetal hemophilia (in a possibly male fetus) or thrombocytopenia: in general, the goal should be a non-traumatic delivery; an outlet forceps by an experienced gynecologist is not necessarily contraindicated [LE B][3,8];
- fetal demineralization (osteogenesis imperfecta) and connective tissue disease (Marfan and Ehlers–Danlos syndromes): the way of delivery and a possible contraindication for operative vaginal delivery depend on the kind of disorder and the accompanying risk factors for mother and child[3];
- face presentation: vacuum extraction is absolutely contraindicated in a face presentation.

There is a reported risk of cephalic hematomas and external bleeding in vacuum extraction following fetal scalp blood testing [LE C].[9,10]

Obstetric Interventions, ed. P. Joep Dörr, Vincent M. Khouw, Frank A. Chervenak, Amos Grunebaum, Yves Jacquemyn, and Jan G. Nijhuis. Published by Cambridge University Press. © Cambridge University Press 2017.

Classification of Vacuum and Forceps Deliveries[7]

Vacuum and forceps deliveries can be divided into:

- outlet vacuum or forceps:
  - the fetal skull has reached the pelvic floor (fourth plane of Hodge, H4, +5 station),
    - the sagittal suture is positioned at less than 45° relative to the midline, with the posterior fontanel anterior or posterior;
- low vacuum or forceps:
  - the fetal skull is engaged at ≥+2 station, which is ≥2 cm below the interspinal line (past the third plane of Hodge, which is indicated by H3[+]), but not yet at the pelvic floor, with the following subdivisions:
    - rotation <45° (the sagittal suture is positioned at less than 45° relative to the midline, with the posterior fontanel anterior or posterior);
    - rotation >45° (the sagittal suture is positioned at more than 45° relative to the midline, with the posterior fontanel anterior or posterior);
- midvacuum or midforceps:
  - the fetal skull is engaged (the largest skull circumference has passed the pelvic inlet), but not yet at 2 cm below the interspinal line);
- high vacuum or forceps:
  - the fetal skull has not yet engaged and is above the interspinal line (above 0 station, the third plane of Hodge).

Criteria for Vacuum or Forceps Delivery[11]

Criteria for performing a vacuum or forceps delivery are:
- information, explanation, and consent on the procedure;
- complete dilation;
- ruptured membranes;
- engaged head (the largest diameter of the fetal head has passed the pelvic inlet); in an infant in occiput presentation this generally means that the bony part of the head is at or below the interspinal line (0 station, H3);
- exact attitude and position of the head can be determined;

- empty bladder: remove any indwelling catheter;
- emergency plan: set a limit on the number of tractions and pop-offs beforehand, know what the next step has to be, and make sure that this step can be performed rapidly;
- anticipation of complications, such as shoulder dystocia and postpartum hemorrhage;
- availability of operating room and surgical team;
- availability of a pediatrician for neonatal resuscitation.

Important Points and Recommendations

- Consent: women should be informed about operative vaginal deliveries during the antenatal period. This information needs to be part of the birth plan of the mother. During delivery obtaining verbal consent is recommended.
- Macrosomia: the operative delivery of macrosomic infants (birthweight >4000 g) has a greater chance of failure and birth trauma after an operative vaginal delivery than after a natural delivery (relative risk factor [RR] 2.6) or an elective cesarean section (RR 4.2). An operative vaginal delivery, however, is not contraindicated, because it is hard to establish macrosomia before delivery and the absolute risk of persistent damage is small (0.3%). If an indication for operative vaginal delivery exists, between 50 and 99 cesarean sections are needed to prevent one infant from having permanent damage [LE B].[12]
- Prematurity: various guidelines recommend not to perform a vacuum extraction at a gestational age of less than 34 weeks because of increased risk of cephalohematoma, subgaleal and intracranial hemorrhage [LE D][3,11] Based on two cohort studies it appears that in prematurely born infants with a birthweight between 1500 and 2500 g there is no increased incidence of intracranial hemorrhage after vacuum extraction [LE B][13,14]
- Midpelvic rotation procedures and high vacuum extraction have higher failure rates than low pelvic procedures. Those who perform these operative deliveries must be skilled and consider the possibility of success to be high. In case of failure, an emergency cesarean must be possible. High forceps are no longer performed [LE D].[15]
- Ultrasound examination may be considered to establish the exact posture and position of the fetal head. Abdominal and transvaginal

ultrasound examination are superior to digital vaginal examination in establishing attitude and position of the fetal head [LE B].[16,17]

- In general, with an operative vaginal delivery, traction is applied during a contraction and while the woman is pushing [LE D].
- In the case of both vacuum and forceps extraction, the possibility of fetomaternal disproportion must be taken into account if there is no progression during successive tractions. There is an increased risk of birth trauma with an increased number of tractions (more than three pulls), the use of additional instruments (vacuum and forceps), and failure of an operative vaginal delivery (see Table 7.1) [LE B].[18] In this situation it should be decided to end the procedure and to switch to cesarean section [LE D].

Therefore, operative vaginal delivery should be abandoned following three pulls of a correctly applied instrument by an experienced operator.[3,10] If after three pulls delivery is clearly imminent, proceeding with instrumental delivery may be appropriate and less morbid than a cesarean delivery of an infant with its head on the perineum.

When deciding to do a forceps extraction after failed vacuum extraction, the increased risk of birth trauma in the infant must be weighed against the increased risk of a cesarean section in the mother. An easy to perform outlet forceps can be better in this situation than a surgically complicated cesarean section [LE D].

- Conclusive evidence that the routine use of episiotomy in operative vaginal delivery reduces anal sphincter injuries is lacking. Prospective and retrospective cohort studies show different results [LE B].[19–21] The only randomized controlled trial of routine versus restrictive use of episiotomy at operative vaginal delivery did not show differences in anal sphincter tears [LE A2].[22]
- It is recommended to perform a mediolateral episiotomy with vacuum and forceps delivery especially in primiparous women [LE D].
- Epidural analgesia in labor:
  - results in an increased risk of operative vaginal delivery compared with non-epidural or no analgesia (RR 1.42, 95% CI 1.28–1.57) [LE A1].[23]
  - results in a significant reduction in rotational or midcavity operative vaginal deliveries (RR 0.69, 95% CI 0.55–0.87) when pushing is

delayed for 1 or 2 hours or strong urge to push develops [LE A1].[24]

- Discontinuing epidural analgesia late in labor does not reduce the incidence of operative vaginal delivery [LE A1].[25]
- During the vacuum or forceps extraction the fetal condition should be monitored and documented. This can be done by means of continuous or intermittent internal or external recording.
- Proper documentation of a vacuum or forceps delivery is a requirement from a medical/legal point of view.

Choice Between Vacuum and Forceps Delivery

In the choice between vacuum or forceps extraction and the various types of these instruments, specific indications, knowledge of the complications for mother and child, and the personal experience of the person performing or supervising the operative delivery all play a role.

It is generally true that a vacuum cup is easier to apply than forceps, that with vacuum extraction the adaptations of the fetal head to the birth canal are more physiological (promoting synclitism and flexion) than with forceps extraction, and that with vacuum extraction there is an intrinsic limitation of the traction force, because the cup releases automatically in case of erroneous pulling direction or excessive traction force. Forceps is the only instrument of choice in case of indication for vaginal termination of a pregnancy with face presentation or aftercoming head in breech presentation (see Chapter 6 on breech delivery).

The results of a Cochrane Review of 10 RCTs on the advantages and disadvantages of vacuum and forceps extractions are shown in Table 7.2.[26]

Complications

Although the neonatal and maternal complications that may occur after an operative vaginal delivery are often the same as those after spontaneous vaginal delivery, the relative risks of operative vaginal deliveries are usually greater.

Neonatal Complications

Early neonatal complications of operative vaginal delivery generally occur within the first 10 hours after delivery [LE B].[27] The complications that may occur after vacuum or forceps extraction are caused

Table 7.1 Neonatal morbidity after different types of deliveries (figures per 10 000 deliveries)[28,29]

	Spontaneous	Vacuum	Forceps	Vacuum and forceps	Secondary cesarean section
Cephalic hematoma[a]	167.7	1116.6[b]	634.6[b]	1360.5[b]	
Subdural or intracerebral hemorrhage	2.9	8.0[b]	9.8[b]	21.3[b]	7.4
Intraventricular hemorrhage	1.1	1.5	2.6	3.7[b]	2.5[b]
Subarachnoidal hemorrhage	1.3	2.2	3.3	10.7[b]	1.2
Facial nerve lesion	3.3	4.6	45.4[b]	28.5[b]	3.1
Plexus-brachial lesion	7.7	17.6[b]	25.0[b]	46.4[b]	1.8[b]
Convulsions	6.4	11.7[b]	9.8[b]	24.9[b]	21.3[b]
Cerebral depression	3.1	9.2[b]	5.2	21.3[b]	9.6[b]
Feeding problems	68.5	72.1	74.6	60.7	117.2[b]
Artificial respiration	25.8	39.1[b]	45.4[b]	50.0[b]	103.2[b]

[a] From the study of Demissie et al.[28]; other data taken from the study of Towner et al.[29]
[b] Significantly different from spontaneous childbirth.

by compression and/or traction to the face, the scalp, and/or the skull, or traction in the wrong direction (i.e., against the pubic bone) and may consist of:

- lacerations and hematomas of the skin;
- lesions of the facial nerves;
- hemorrhages (Figure 7.1) of the retina, under the periosteum (cephalic hematoma), subgaleal and intracranial (subdural, subarachnoidal, intracerebral, and intraventricular);
- skull fractures.

The incidences of a number of the above-named complications are listed in Table 7.1 and are based on two extensive retrospective studies [LE B].[28,29]

Late neonatal complications are rare and can usually be considered to be late consequences of early complications (neuromuscular damage, hemorrhages). There are no indications that the cognitive development of children born after an operative vaginal delivery is different from that of spontaneously born infants [LE B].[30,31]

Infections

With operative vaginal deliveries there can be an increased chance of vertical transmission of various viral infections due to lacerations of the fetal scalp, which may occur with either vacuum or forceps extraction. Data are very limited on the risk of vertical transmission of viral infections with operative vaginal deliveries.

Until now there is no proof of an increased chance of vertical transmission of (asymptomatic) herpes simplex infection after vacuum extraction or hepatitis B viral infection (in case of immunization) after vacuum or forceps extraction [LE B].[32,33] No data are available in the literature on vertical transmission of HIV and hepatitis C infections with operative vaginal deliveries. The transmission risk probably depends primarily on the degree of viremia. In case of detectable viremia it seems prudent to avoid operative vaginal deliveries because of an increased chance of facial or scalp injuries [LE D].

Maternal Complications

Operative vaginal deliveries are associated with damage to the pelvic floor with symptoms of urinary and fecal incontinence and prolapse.

Urinary Incontinence

From patient–control studies it appears that:

- the prevalence of urinary incontinence 3 months after vaginal delivery is 29% and the urinary incontinence persists in three-quarters of these women;
- in the short term (<1 year) and the long term (1½ and 6 years), there are no differences in the occurrence of urinary incontinence after spontaneous delivery, vacuum, or forceps delivery [LE B].[34–36]

Table 7.2 Pros and cons of vacuum extractions (VE) and forceps extractions (FE)[26]

	Vacuum (%)	Forceps (%)	Odds ratio, 95% reliability interval	
Advantages of vacuum				
Vaginal and perineal ruptures	10	20	0.41	0.33–0.50
Pain during and after delivery	9	15	0.54	0.31–0.93
Advantages of forceps				
Failures	12	7	1.69	1.31–2.19
Cephalic hematoma	10	4	2.38	1.68–3.37
Retinal bleeding	49	33	1.99	1.35–2.96
Concern by the mother about her child	14	8	2.17	1.19–3.94
No difference between VE and FE				
C-section after VE or FE	2	3	0.56	0.31–1.02
Apgar score <7, 1 min	16	15	1.13	0.76–1.68
Apgar score <7, 5 min	5	3	1.67	0.99–2.81
Skin lesion	17	17	0.89	0.70–1.13
Phototherapy	4	4	1.08	0.66–1.77
Perinatal death	0.3	0.4	0.80	0.18–3.52

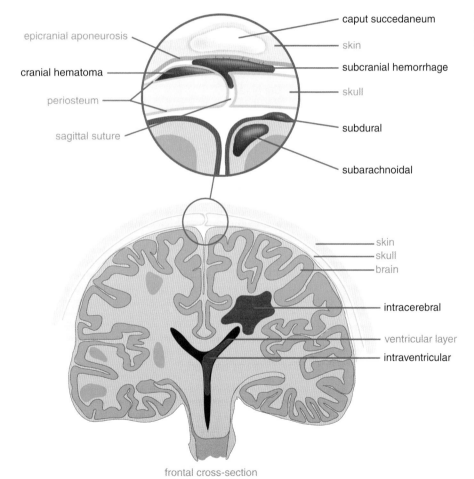

Figure 7.1 Anatomic overview of extra- and intracranial hemorrhages.

Table 7.3 Fecal incontinence after different types of childbirth

	Group 1: odds ratio (95% CI)	Group 2: odds ratio (95% CI)
Spontaneous delivery versus cesarean section	1.32 (1.04–1.68)[a]	1.86 (0.62–5.64)
FE versus spontaneous delivery	1.50 (1.19–1.89)[a]	1.52 (0.58–3.97)
VE versus spontaneous delivery	1.31 (0.97–1.77)	0.80 (0.29–2.18)
FE/VE versus spontaneous delivery	1.47 (1.22–1.78)[a]	1.91 (1.00–3.67)
FE versus VE	1.51 (1.07–2.13)[a]	1.63 (0.23–10.02)

[a] Significantly different.
FE = forceps extractions; VE = vacuum extractions.
Group 1: incontinence of loose stools, solid stools, or flatus;
Group 2: incontinence of solid stools.

Fecal Incontinence

A systematic review of patient–control studies shows that the prevalence of fecal incontinence, defined as incontinence of loose stools, solid stools, or flatus (Group 1), varies greatly and occurs in 3.8% to 39.5% of women within 1 year after childbirth. When the definition of fecal incontinence is limited to only loose and solid stools (Group 2), the prevalence lies between 0% and 4.9%. Table 7.3 shows fecal incontinence data from the review after different types of delivery.[37]

In one of the studies of this systematic review a 5-year follow-up study showed urinary incontinence of various severity in 47%, bowel urgency in 44%, and incidental or frequent loss of bowel control in 20%. There were no differences in urinary or fecal incontinence between forceps or vacuum deliveries.[31]

Prolapse

The literature is neither unanimous on the prevalence of prolapse during and after pregnancy, nor on the influence of operative vaginal delivery on that prevalence.[38]

One patient–control study suggests that vacuum or forceps extraction does not constitute a risk factor for the occurrence of prolapse symptoms.[39]

Forceps

Over the years more than 700 types of forceps have been developed. There is no systematic study in which different types of forceps are compared with each other. There is no particular forceps that is the best choice in all cases. It is recommended to develop and maintain the skills of forceps extraction with a limited number of different types of forceps.

This chapter discusses several forceps with different characteristics, i.e., the forceps of Naegele, Kielland, DeLee, Luikart, and Piper. The benefits and limitations attributed to these forceps will be discussed.[40] This knowledge can be beneficial when choosing the right instrument.

Description

Forceps consist of two parts, i.e., a left and a right branch, which close in a lock. The branches are named after the side of the pelvis into which they are introduced.

The branches are composed of (Figure 7.2):

- the blades;
- the shank or the neck;
- the lock;
- the handle.

The Blades

The blades of the forceps can have two curves (Figure 7.2), i.e.:

- a cephalic curve, which conforms to the shape of the head;
- a pelvic curve, which follows the pelvic axis.

Most forceps have both a cephalic and a pelvic curve. Kielland forceps have only a cephalic curve. The blades can be fenestrated (good grip on the head) or solid (easy to insert). The Luikart forceps has a solid blade and a raised edge on the inside of the blade.

The Shank or the Neck

The shanks contain the lock. The left branch usually contains the prominent part; the neck of the right branch fits into the prominent part. A modification of the shank forms the perineal curve.

The Lock

The Naegele forceps has a socket or English lock (firm grip around the head). A sliding lock (Figure 7.3), such as in the Kielland and Luikart forceps (Figure 7.4), has the advantage in synclitism,

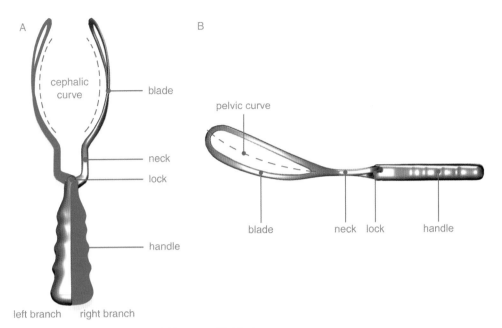

Figure 7.2 Forceps components. (A) Top view; (B) side view.

in that one branch can be inserted deeper than the other branch and slid into the other branch.

The Handles

There is little difference between the handles of the different types of forceps. Usually they are hollow to reduce their weight.

Characteristics of Different Forceps

The *Naegele* forceps (1854) was specifically developed as "midforceps" for application with a severely molded and stuck head to resolve relative cephalic-pelvic disproportion (Figure 7.4A). The specially developed socket lock makes it possible to firmly grasp the head and, if needed, adapt it to the pelvis.

Kielland left the pelvic curve out of the forceps named after him (1915, Figure 7.4B) and used the sliding lock developed by the Dutchman, Boerma (1907).

Owing to the lack of the pelvic curve, this forceps makes it possible to rotate more than 90° and by means of the sliding lock to use a forceps in case of asynclitism. The Kielland is not, by principle, a "pulling instrument," but was introduced as a "rotation instrument." The most popular modification to the classical Simpson forceps is the DeLee forceps (1920, Figure 7.4C). The difference with the prototype consists primarily of the lighter design. DeLee promoted his instrument for

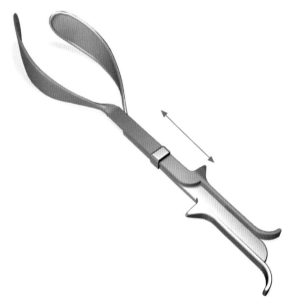

Figure 7.3 Sliding lock.

routine use as a protective cage around the (premature) head. In 1924, Piper introduced a special forceps (Figure 7.4D) with an extra curvature in the shank (perineal curve) to extract the aftercoming head in breech delivery. The idea of the perineal curve is to create room between the forceps and the infant's trunk. In 1937, Luikart designed a forceps

143

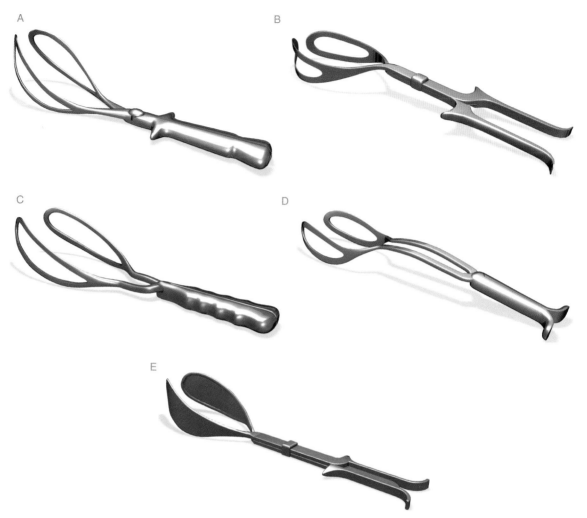

Figure 7.4 (A) Naegele forceps; (B) Kielland forceps; (C) DeLee forceps; (D) Piper forceps; (E) Luikart forceps.

(Figure 7.4E) with solid blades and raised edges. The degree of curvature of the Luikart forceps blades is midway between the forceps with a curve for a highly molded skull (Naegele forceps) and a forceps with a rounder skull curve for application to an unmolded skull (DeLee forceps) (Figure 7.5). The use of the sliding lock allows for adaptation to the position of the fetal skull.

Forceps Extraction Technique

Outlet or Low Forceps Extraction in Occiput Anterior Presentation (OA)[41]

See Animation 7.1.

After the indication has been made, the conditions for performing an operative vaginal delivery have been met and the proper instrument has been chosen, the steps in performing an outlet forceps on an OA infant are as follows:

- Explain the procedure.
- Ask and help the woman to place her legs in the stirrups.
- Perform vulvar cleaning.
- Catheterize if necessary and remove any indwelling catheter.
- Perform infiltration of the perineum or a pudendal block with local anesthetic.
- Carefully determine the engagement, attitude, and position of the fetal head (vaginal examination, ultrasound).
- Join the branches of the forceps together and hold out the forceps in the position to be used (Figure 7.6).

- Lubricate the blades.
- Insert the forceps (between contractions).
  - First insert the left branch, which is held with the thumb and index and middle fingers of the left hand (as in holding a pen) to prevent unwanted force from being exerted on the fetal and/or maternal tissues.
  - After the examining fingers of the right hand are inserted between the head and the vaginal wall, the left branch is introduced while being guided by the fingers and the thumb of the right hand in a smooth motion from the contralateral (right) groin (Figure 7.7).
  - In the same manner, the right branch is then introduced with the right hand from the left groin while guided with the inserted fingers of the left hand.
  - The right branch is then further inserted over the left branch, preferably while the left branch is held by an assistant (Figure 7.8).
  - The branches are locked together (Figure 7.9).
  - Check the proper position of the blades by holding the handles with one hand and check with the fingers of the other hand whether:

    - the sagittal suture runs from front to back and equally far between the blades;
    - the lock now points at the flexion point (see Figure 7.11).

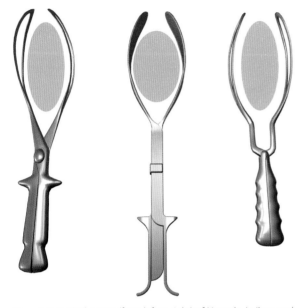

Figure 7.5 Skull curves (from left to right) of Naegele, Luikart, and DeLee forceps blades.

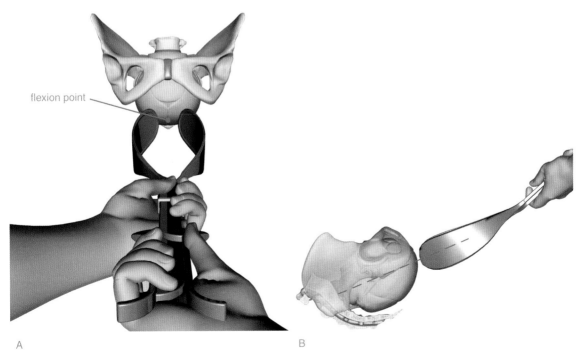

flexion point

A

B

Figure 7.6A–B Holding out the forceps.

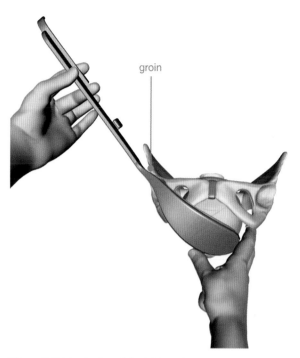

Figure 7.7 Introduction of the left branch.

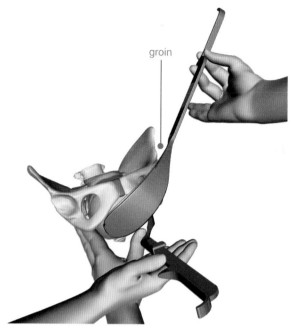

Figure 7.8 Introduction of the right branch.

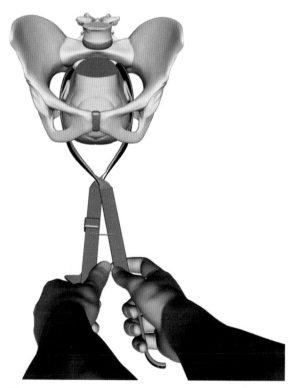

Figure 7.9 Locking of the branches.

- The branches are now situated "ideally around the head" (along the occipitomental circumference) and "ideally in the pelvis" (the left branch to the left and the right branch to the right in the pelvis);
- Traction is applied during a contraction and while the woman is pushing.
- Traction is applied with one hand (the pulling hand), while the other hand grasps the shank of the forceps to determine and adjust the – ever changing – traction direction (Figure 7.10A).
- With the so-called Pajot's maneuver, the direction of the traction can be "steered" by the combined traction of the "pulling hand" and downward pressure on the shank of the forceps by the other hand (Figure 7.10B).
- Traction is applied in the direction of the axis of the birth canal, thus first downward and then upward (Figure 7.10C).
- Make a mediolateral episiotomy when the perineum tightens.
- Move the handles further upward when the posterior hairline has passed under the symphysis and (gradually) deliver the head.
- After that, the branches may be disarticulated (first the right branch, then the left branch).

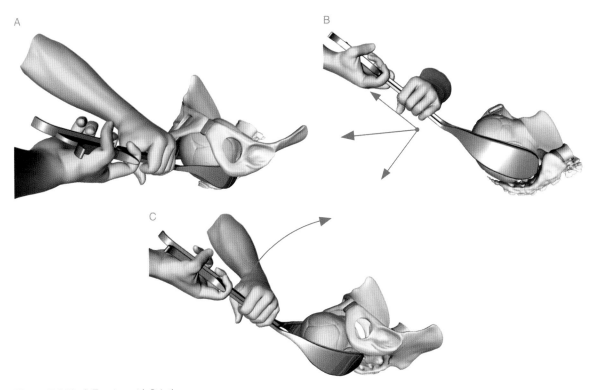

Figure 7.10A–C Traction with Pajot's maneuver.

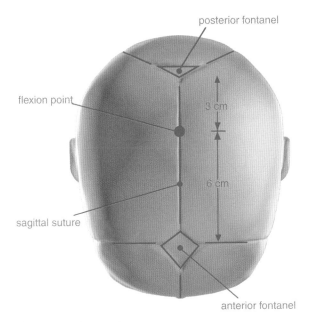

posterior fontanel

flexion point

3 cm

6 cm

sagittal suture

anterior fontanel

Figure 7.11 Flexion point.

- The delivery of the shoulders and trunk proceed as in normal delivery.

Comments

- The flexion point (Figure 7.11) refers to the part of the skull that – also in spontaneous deliveries with an occiput anterior position – is situated centrally in the birth canal axis. In a normally molded head the flexion point is situated in the midline on the sagittal suture, approximately 3 cm in front of the posterior fontanel and 6 cm behind the anterior fontanel.
- In general, the left branch is introduced first and then the right branch is slid over the top. This will allow the branches to be locked together without "crossing the branches" (crossing the branches may cause lacerations of the birth canal and the infant's scalp).
- If the branches do not close well, it must first be determined which branch is not situated properly and this branch must be repositioned while guided by the examining fingers.
- To prevent compression of the head while pulling, one finger of the pulling hand can be placed between the handles.

Outlet or Low Forceps Extraction in Occiput Presentation, Occiput Left Anterior (LOA) or Right Anterior (ROA)

See Animation 7.2.

Upon introducing the forceps, the head is encompassed biparietally, but the forceps will not lie ideally in the pelvis.

- *In the LOA position* the left branch is introduced in the left posterior pelvis from the middle between the right groin and the symphysis, while guided by the right hand. After insertion, the handle points to the left thigh (Figure 7.12).
- The right branch is crossed over into the right posterior pelvis starting from the left groin, guided by the left hand (Figure 7.13). After that, the right branch is made to "wander" to right anterior (Figure 7.14). After closing the lock both handles point to the left.
- Traction and rotation must be performed simultaneously.
- The rotation must be complete when the pelvic floor is reached.
- *In the ROA position* the same basic procedure is followed, but in that case you let the left branch wander.

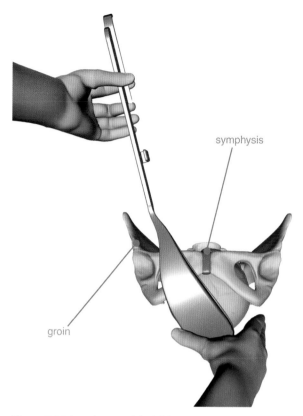

Figure 7.12 Introduction of the left branch with head in LOA.

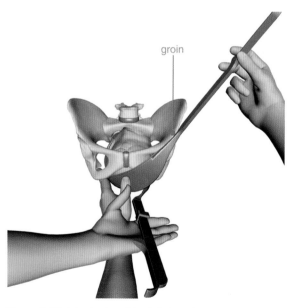

Figure 7.13 Introduction of the right branch.

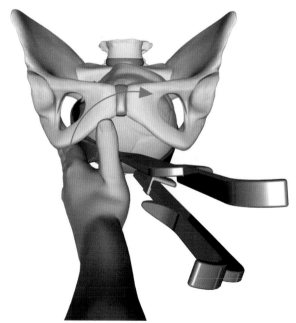

Figure 7.14 Wandering with the right branch.

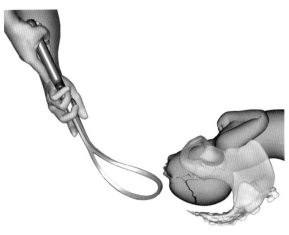

Figure 7.15 Positioning the forceps with head in MA presentation.

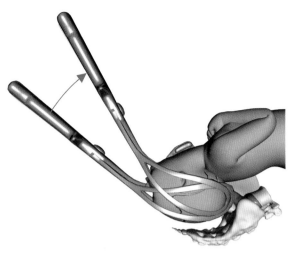

Figure 7.16 Move forceps ventrally before closing the branches.

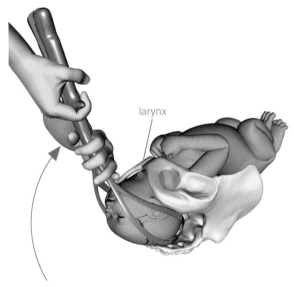

larynx

Figure 7.17 Traction applied in ventral direction after the larynx is exposed below the symphysis.

Forceps Extraction in Face Presentation

A forceps extraction with face presentation is only possible if the following conditions are met:

- head on the pelvic floor: only when at the pelvic floor the largest dimension of the head has passed the pelvic inlet;
- mentum anterior (MA) position; if the chin does not present right under the symphysis and the branches are introduced obliquely, there is a great chance of injuring the face. With the chin in posterior position, vaginal birth is impossible.

Technique

See Animations 7.3 and 7.4.

- In an MA position the forceps is placed ideally around the head and in the pelvis (Figure 7.15). The lock points to the chin. The branches lie along the mento-occipital circumference.

When closing the forceps, the handles of the not completely closed forceps are moved ventrally, so that the head is grasped alongside the aforementioned circumference and not over the forehead with the point of the branches in the neck (risk of plexus lesion!) (Figure 7.16).

- After the forceps is closed and the head is firmly grasped between the blades, traction is applied in a forward and dorsal direction, whereby the larynx can become a rotation point (hypomochlion) under the symphysis. Then the handles are moved in a ventral direction, whereby the forehead and then the occiput are born (Figure 7.17).

Comment

With an indication to terminate the delivery vaginally with the occiput in left or right transverse, left or right posterior, or posterior position, vacuum extraction is preferred. Ultimately, this facilitates "spontaneous" adaptation of the head to the birth canal and normal development of rotations [LE D].

Vacuum Extractor

The first clinically applicable obstetric vacuum extractor was invented in 1849 by James Young

Simpson. But vacuum extraction only became popular with the introduction of a mushroom-shaped cup designed by Malmström in 1957. This allowed for the same amount of negative pressure to provide greater traction than with the previously used clock-shaped cups. The advantage of this mushroom-shaped cup is lost, however, if the traction is not directly perpendicular to the surface of the cup, which causes the cup to tip to one side and pop off. Since the ideal direction of the traction follows the pelvic axis, and is therefore not always perpendicular to the cup, attempts have been made to remedy this disadvantage by either changing the technique (*Dreifingergriff* [three-finger grip]) or through adaptations to the instrument, such as with the O'Neil cup and the New Generation cup of Bird.

The Instrument

Different types of vacuum cups are available with differences in material, shape, and size.

Material

Currently used vacuum cups are made of metal or of flexible or hard plastic. Extractions made with soft cups fail more often than those made with metal cups (OR 1.65, 95% RI 1.19–2.29), but soft cups have the advantage of causing less injury to the fetal scalp (OR 0.45, 95% RI 0.34–0.60) [LE A].[42] Therefore, soft cups are an alternative for an outlet vacuum with OA position, while metal and hard plastic cups are preferred with other attitudes and positions of the fetal head (Figure 7.18).[43]

Shape

Metal cups usually have the shape of a mushroom, while soft cups are shaped like a clock. The pulling power of a mushroom-shaped vacuum cup is greater than that of a clock-shaped cup. Poor performance of the soft cup is probably more due to the clock shape than the material being employed.

The Kiwi OmniCup was introduced in 2001. This disposable ventouse is equipped with a plastic cup and, in contrast with other plastic cups, is mushroom shaped. The Kiwi OmniCup has a visual indicator, which allows the tractive force to be read. Little research has been done into the efficacy and safety of this cup.

Size

The size of the cup also determines the tractive force. With a vacuum pressure of 0.8 kg/cm^2 and a 5 cm diameter mushroom-shaped cup, a traction force of

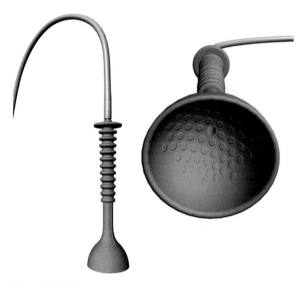

Figure 7.18 Soft cup.

15.7 kg is possible and 22.6 kg with a 6 cm cup. The most effective and safest cup size is not known. The same is true for tractive force.

Vacuum Pressure

In general, a vacuum pressure of 0.8 kg/cm^2 (= 600 mmHg) is recommended. At a lower pressure the chance of cup pop-offs increases and at a higher pressure the chances of fetal skin lacerations and cephalhematomas are increased.[44]

Creating continuous suction up to 0.8 kg/cm^2 is faster than and just as effective and safe as increasing the vacuum pressure in steps [LE A1].[45]

Characteristics of Different Vacuum Cups

Vacuum cups in current usage are all inspired by the *Malmström* cup and have the above-described mushroom shape. The suction tube is connected to a valve in the center of the cup. On the inside of the cup there is a metal plate to which a chain is attached. The chain runs through the exhaust tube to a handle. The Malmström cup is available in different sizes. The most used cup has a diameter of 50 mm (Figure 7.19). With this cup a maximum tractive force of more than 15 kg is only possible if the pull chain is directly perpendicular to the cup while traction is applied. As described with the extraction technique, traction is applied in the direction of the axis of the birth canal. When the direction of the traction is no longer perpendicular to the surface of the cup, even with a small deviation the tractive force will decrease considerably as a result of the tipping of the cup, which increases the chance of the cup popping off.

This drawback is remedied by the *O'Neil* cup (Figure 7.20). In this cup the connection point of the pull chain is flexibly attached to the top of the cup. This allows the connection point to follow the direction of the traction, with the result that no tipping or decreased tractive force occurs up to a deviation of 30° of the right angle (Figure 7.20). Thus, the cup maintains its tractive force also when, under traction, the axis of the birth canal is followed. The tube for supplying suction to the cup is located eccentrically on the top (anterior cup) or the side (posterior cup) of the cup and has therefore no relationship to the pull

chain. The O'Neil cup is available in diameters of 50 mm and 55 mm.

In the *Bird* cup the chain is in the center, without elevation, fastened to the surface of the cup, making the contact point of the tractive force closer to the surface of the fetal skull compared to the Malmström cup. This greatly decreases the tendency of the cup to tip when the direction of the traction is not perpendicular to the plane of the cup.

The suction tube of the regular OA cup – just as in the O'Neil cup – is located eccentrically on the cup (Figure 7.21A). The OA cup is recommended for use

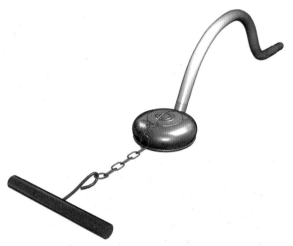

Figure 7.20 O'Neil cup

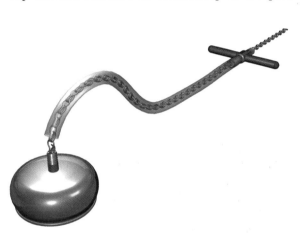

Figure 7.19 Malmström cup.

Figure 7.21 Bird cup: OA cup (A) and OP cup (B).

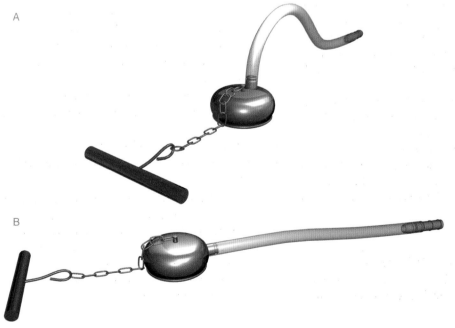

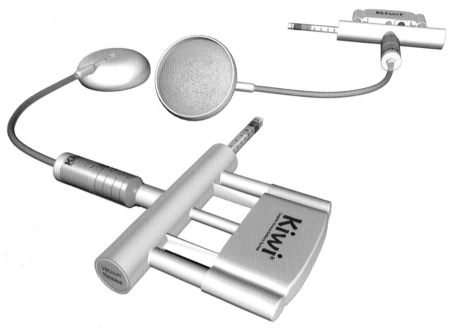

Figure 7.22 Kiwi OmniCup.

with OA position. In the occiput posterior (OP) cup the suction tube is located on the side of the cup (Figure 7.21B). This OP cup can be used to insert the cup deep toward the sacrum in case of an OP position. Cleaning the Bird cup and making it ready for use is easier than with the Malmström cup.

The *Kiwi OmniCup* is a plastic disposable cup that is fixed to a manual vacuum pump (Figure 7.22). In this cup the contact point of the pull cord lies considerably closer to the fetal skull surface than with the Malmström cup. The pull cord – as in the Malmström cup – runs through the vacuum suction tube. The suction tube has a small diameter (Figure 7.22).

As a result, the tube may easily become clogged at suction of even small amounts of amniotic fluid or blood, resulting in loss of vacuum.

The cup has a diameter of 50 mm.

The failure rate (not achieving a vaginal delivery) of the Kiwi OmniCup versus conventional cups shows heterogeneity of results. There are no differences in maternal or neonatal outcomes [LE A2].[45]

Vacuum Extraction Technique[41,43]

After the indication has been set, the conditions for performing an assisted vaginal delivery have been met,

and the proper instrument has been chosen, the steps in performing a vacuum extraction are as follows:

- Explain the procedure.
- Ask and help the woman to place her legs in stirrups.
- Perform vulvar cleaning.
- Catheterize if necessary and remove any indwelling catheter.
- Perform an infiltration of the perineum or a pudendal block with local anesthesia.
- Carefully determine the engagement, attitude, and position of the fetal head (vaginal examination, ultrasound).
- Connect the cup to the vacuum pump.
- Check whether the vacuum pump is functioning properly.
- Lubricate the outside of the cup.
- Introduce the cup beyond a contraction (Figure 7.23).

  – A metal or a hard plastic cup is inserted at an angle after spreading the labia; when the posterior side of the cup touches the fetal head the anterior side of the cup is pushed downwards till it lies on the fetal head.
  – A soft cup can be doubled and inserted after spreading the labia.

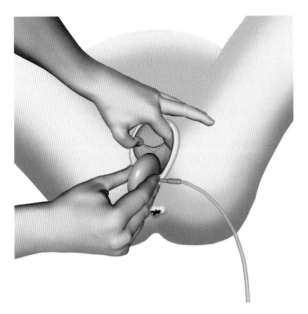

Figure 7.23 Inserting the cup.

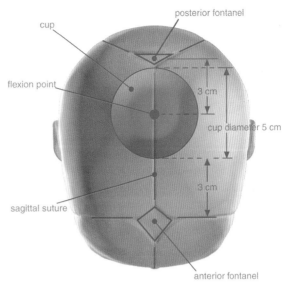

Figure 7.24 Location of cup on flexion point.

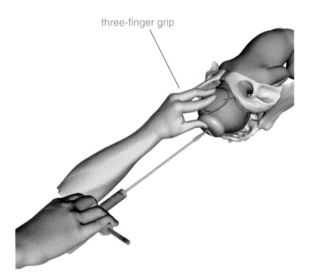

Figure 7.25 Traction with presenting head in OA.

- The center of the cup is placed at the flexion point of the fetal head (Figure 7.24); with a 5 or 6 cm cup, the center of the cup should be approximately 3 cm in front of the posterior fontanel, and the edge of the cup should be on the border of the posterior fontanel; the anterior fontanel forms the reference point after placing the cup, since the posterior fontanel is not readily palpable

after correct placement of the cup. Note: Placement of the cup on the flexion point promotes synclitism and flexion of the head and passage through the birth canal with the suboccipitofrontal circumference.

- After placing the cup, it must be carefully determined through palpation around the cup whether any part of the cervix or vaginal wall is stuck between the cup and the fetal scalp. If everything is clear, negative pressure is applied up to 0.1–0.2 kg/cm^2 and another check is performed by palpation for any possible entrapment of the cervix or vaginal wall (in case of entrapment the vacuum pressure is shut off and the cup is repositioned). Then negative pressure is applied up to 0.8 kg/cm^2.

- During the following contractions – and maternal expulsive efforts – tractions are performed.

  - The fingers of the dominant hand grasp the handle, while the fingers of the non-dominant hand are placed on the fetal head and on the cup (two fingers on the head and the thumb on the cup, the *Dreifingergriff* [three-finger grip], Figures 7.25 and 7.26) (see Animation 7.5), in order to determine the traction direction and to prevent premature pop off of the cup.

153

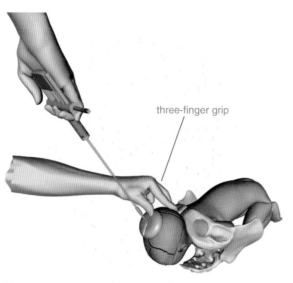

Figure 7.26 Traction with presenting head in OA.

three-finger grip

- The direction of the pulling must always follow the axis of the birth canal to prevent the head from getting stuck against the pubic symphysis. For that reason, the traction cannot always be perpendicular to the cup (Figure 7.27) (see Animation 7.6).

- If during the traction the pull chain is not perpendicular to the cup, a tilt moment occurs that must be corrected by digital pressure to the tilting side of the cup to prevent the cup from dislodging. Traction is gradually increased during a contraction. Jerking motions increase the chance of the cup popping off.

- During traction the head will rotate spontaneously if necessary as it descends. It should be avoided to make turning motions during the tractions – in order to promote rotation – as this increases the chance of scalp lesions.

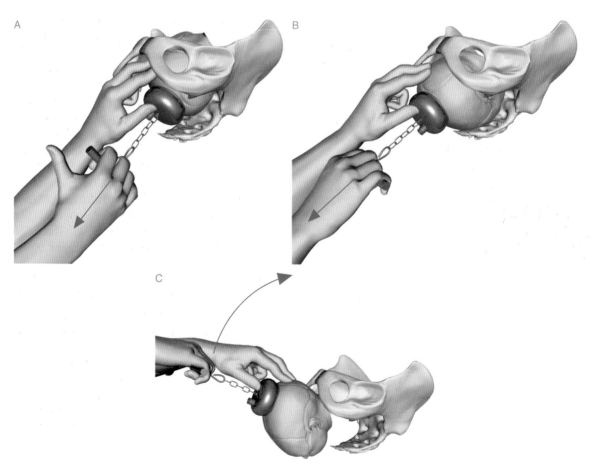

A

B

C

Figure 7.27A–C Traction with presenting head in LOA.

- It is recommended, at least in primiparous women, to perform a mediolateral episiotomy when the head crowns.
- When the head is born, the vacuum is shut off and the cup is removed.
- The delivery of the shoulders and trunk proceed as in normal delivery.

Reasons for Failure of Vacuum Extractions[43]

Failure of a vacuum extraction can be for various reasons, e.g.:

- fetomaternal disproportion;
- placement of the cup at a location other than the flexion point: this will result in a greater circumference of the head having to pass through the birth canal;
- incorrect traction direction: the chance of cup pop-offs increases when the pull chain does not follow the axis of the birth canal, such as when traction is applied upward before the head crowns;
- a large caput succedaneum.[46]

Important Points and Recommendations

- Prior to the vacuum or forceps extraction, carefully determine the engagement, posture, and position of the fetal head, if necessary with the aid of ultrasound [LE D].
- Establish an (emergency) plan when performing a vacuum or forceps extraction.
  - Determine the number of tractions and minutes, generally three or four tractions and 20 minutes [LE D].
  - Know what the next step has to be and make sure that this step can be carried out quickly [LE D].
  - Anticipate complications (shoulder dystocia, postpartum hemorrhage) [LE D].
- Ensure there is close observation of the neonate after a vacuum or forceps extraction. Early neonatal complications of assisted vaginal delivery generally occur within the first 10 hours after delivery [LE B].[27]
- Maintain the skills of forceps extraction by practicing on a dummy [LE D].

References

1 Essed GGM. Complicaties bij kunstverlossingen. In: Heineman MJ (ed.). Complicaties in obstetrie en gynaecologie. Bussum: Medicom Europe, 1994, pp. 19–30.

2 NVOG. Vaginale kunstverlossing (vacuümextractie, forcipale extractie). NVOG richtlijn, 2005.

3 Royal College of Obstetricians and Gynaecologists. Guideline No 26, Operative Vaginal Delivery, 2011.

4 Lumbiganon P, Laopaiboon M, Gülmezoglu M, et al. Method of delivery and pregnancy outcomes in Asia: the WHO global survey on maternal and perinatal health 2007–8. Lancet. 2010;**375**:490–9.

5 Goetzonger KR, Macones GA. Operative vaginal delivery: current trends in obstetrics. Womens Health (Lond Engl). 2008;**4**:281–90.

6 Births: Final data for 2010. Natl Vital Stat Rep. 2012;**61**:1–70.

7 ACOG. Operative vaginal delivery. ACOG Practice Bulletin No 17, 2000.

8 Meijer K, Bouman K, Sollie KM, et al. Begeleiding van de zwangerschap en de partus bij draagsters van hemofilie. Ned Tijdschr Geneeskd. 2008;**152**:1249–53.

9 Roberts IF, Stone M. Fetal hemorrhage: complication of vacuum extractor after fetal blood sampling. Am J Obstet Gynecol. 1978;**132**:109.

10 Thierry M. Fetal hemorrhage following blood sampling and use of vacuum extractor. Am J Obstet Gynecol. 1979;**134**:251

11 Wegner EK, Lockwood CJ, Baras VA. Operative vaginal delivery. UpToDate. 2013; April.

12 Kolderup LB, Laros RK Jr, Musci TJ. Incidence of persistent birth injury in macrosomic infant: association with mode of delivery. Am J Obstet Gynecol. 1997;**177**:37–41.

13 Morales R Adair CD, Sanchez-Ramos L, et al. Vacuum extraction of preterm infants with birthweights of 1500 to 2499 grams. J Reprod Med. 1995;**40**:127–30.

14 Castro MA, Hoey SD, Towner D. Controversies in the use of the vacuum extractor. Semin Perinatal 2003;**27**:46–53.

15 Hankins DV, Rowe TF. Operative vaginal delivery – Year 2000. Am J Obstet Gynecol. 1996;**175**:275–82.

16 Zahalka N, Sadan O, Malinger G, et al. Comparison of transvaginal sonography with digital examination and transabdominal sonography for the determination of fetal head position in the second stage of labor. Am J Obstet Gynecol. 2005;**193**:381–6.

17 Ramphul M, Kennelly M, Murphy DJ. Establishing the accuracy and acceptability of abdominal ultrasound to define the foetal head position in the second stage of labour: a validation study. Eur J Obstet Gynecol Reprod Biol. 2012;**164**:35–9.

18 Murphey DJ, Liebling RE, Patel R, et al. Cohort study of operative delivery in the second stage of labour and standard of obstetric care. Br J Obstet Gynaecol. 2003;**110**:610–15.

19 de Leeuw JW, de Wit C, Kuijken JPJA, et al. Mediolateral episiotomy reduces the risk for anal sphincter injury during operative vaginal delivery. Br J Obstet Gynaecol. 2008;**115**:104–8.

20 Räisänen SH, Vehviläinen-Julkunen K, Gissler M, et al. Lateral episiotomy protects primiparous women from obstetric anal sphincter rupture. Acta Obstet Gynecol Scand. 2009;**88**:1365–72.

21 Macleod M, Strachan B, Bahl R, et al. A prospective cohort study of maternal and neonatal morbidity in relation to use of episiotomy at operative vaginal delivery. Br J Obstet Gynaecol. 2008;**115**:1688–94.

22 Murphey DJ, Macleod M, Bahl R, et al. A randomized controlled trial of routine versus restrictive use of episiotomy at operative vaginal delivery: a multicenter pilot study. Br J Obstet Gynaecol. 2008;**115**:1695–702.

23 Anim-Somuah M, Smyth RM, Jones L. Epidural versus non-epidural or no analgesia in labour. Cochrane Database Syst Rev. 2011;**12**:CD000331. DOI: 10.1002/14651858.CD000331.pub3.

24 Roberts CL, Torvaldsen S, Camaron CA, et al. Delayed versus early pushing in women with epidural anesthesia: a systematic review and meta-analysis. BJOG. 2004;**111**:1333–40.

25 Torvaldsen S, Roberts CL, Bell JC, et al. Discontinuation of epidural analgesia late in labour for reducing adverse delivery outcomes associated with epidural analgesia. Cochrane Database Syst Rev. 2004;**4**:CD004457.

26 Johanson RB, Menon V. Vacuum extraction versus forceps for assisted delivery. Cochrane Database Syst Rev. 1999;**2**:CD000224. DOI: 10.1002/14651858.CD000224.

27 Smit-Wu MN, Moonen-Delarue DM, Benders MJ, et al. Onset of vacuum-related complaints in neonates. Eur J Pediatr. 2006;**165**:374–9.

28 Demissie K, Rhoads GC, Smulian JC, et al. Operative vaginal delivery and neonatal and infant adverse outcomes: population based retrospective analyses. BMJ. 2004;**329**:1–6.

29 Towner D, Castro MA, Eby-Wilkins BS, et al. Effect of mode of delivery in nulliparous women on neonatal intracranial delivery. N Engl J Med. 1999;**341**:1709–14.

30 Carmody F, Grant A, Mutch L, et al. Follow up of babies delivered in a randomized controlled comparison of vacuum extraction and forceps delivery. Acta Obstet Gynecol Scand. 1986;**65**:763–6.

31 Johanson RB, Heycock E, Carter J, et al. Maternal and child health after assisted vaginal delivery: five year follow of a randomized controlled study comparing forceps and ventouse. Br J Obstet Gynaecol. 1999;**106**:544–9.

32 Sedan O, Dishi M, Somekh E, et al. Vacuum extraction and herpes simplex virus infections. Int J Gynecol Obstet. 2005;**89**:242–6.

33 Wang J, Zhu O, Zhang X. Effect of delivery mode on maternal-infant transistor of hepatitis B virus by immunoprophylaxis. Chin Med J. 2002;**115**:1510–12.

34 MacArthur C, Glazener CM, Wilson PD, et al. Persistent urinary incontinence and delivery mode history: a six-year longitudinal study. BJOG. 2006;**113**:218–24.

35 Glazener CM, Herbison GP, MacArthur C, et al. New postnatal urinary incontinence: obstetric and other risk factors in primiparae. BJOG. 2006;**113**:208–17.

36 Gartland D, Donath S, MacArthur C, Brown SJ. The onset, recurrence and associated obstetric risk factors for urine incontinence in the first 18 months after a first birth: an Australian nulliparous cohort study. BJOG. 2012;**119**:1361–9.

37 Pretlove SJ, Thompson PJ, Toosz-Hobson PM, et al. Does the mode of delivery predispose women to anal incontinence in the first year postpartum? A comparative systematic review. BJOG. 2008;**115**:421–34.

38 Handa VL, Brubaker L, Flak S. Pelvic floor disorders associated with pregnancy. UpToDate. 2008;May.

39 Tegerstedt G, Miedel A, Maehle-Schmidt M, et al. Obstetric risk factors for symptomatic prolapse: a population-based approach. Am J Obstet Gynecol. 2006;**194**:75–81.

40 Essed GGM. Geschiedenis van de vaginale kunstverlossing. In: Merkus JMWM (ed.). Obstetrische interventies. Bussum: Medicom Europe, 1991, pp. 3–15.

41 O'Grady JP, McIlhargie CJ. Instrumental delivery. In: O'Grady JP, Gomovski ML, McIlhargie CJ (eds). Operative obstetrics. Baltimore: Williams & Wilkins, 1995.

42 Johanson R, Menon V. Soft versus rigid vacuum extractor cups for assisted vaginal delivery. Cochrane Database Syst Rev. 2000;**2**:CD000446. DOI: 10.1002/14651858.CD000446.

43 Greenberg J, Lockwood CJ, Barss V. Procedure for vacuum assisted operative vaginal delivery. UpToDate. 2013, March.

44 Suwannachat B, Lumbiganon P, Laopaiboon M. Rapid versus stepwise negative pressure application for vacuum extraction assisted vaginal delivery. Cochrane Database Syst Rev. 2012;**8**:CD006636. DOI:10.1002/14651858.CD006636.pub3.

45 O'Mahony F, Hofmeyr GJ, Menon V. Choice of instruments for assisted vaginal delivery. Cochrane Database Syst Rev. 2010;**11**:CD005455. DOI: 10.1002/14651858.CD005455.pub2.

46 Muise KL, Duchon MA, Brown RH. The effect of artificial caput on performance of vacuum extractors. Obstet Gynecol. 1993;**81**:170–3.

Shoulder Dystocia

P.P. van den Berg and S.G. Oei

General Information

Introduction

Shoulder dystocia constitutes an obstetric emergency due to the risk of morbidity to the infant, i.e., asphyxia and/or trauma, such as a brachial plexus injury.

Definition

Shoulder dystocia occurs during childbirth when the infant's anterior shoulder becomes impacted behind the symphysis of the mother after going through the customary steps. Since the definition of shoulder dystocia is rather subjective, the literature also speaks of a "head-to-trunk time interval" of more than 60 seconds. Another criterion for shoulder dystocia is the need for performing additional maneuvers to deliver the shoulders [LE D].[1]

Incidence

Shoulder dystocia occurs in 0.2–3% of vertex presentation deliveries.[2]

Risk Factors

There are different risk factors involved in the occurrence of shoulder dystocia:

- a previous delivery with shoulder dystocia;
- diabetes mellitus or gestational diabetes;
- obesity, post-term pregnancy;
- multiparity;
- high birthweight;
- pelvic disorders [LE C].[2,3]

Many of the risk factors are related to high birthweight. But the problem is that with the current methods, such as palpation and measuring the fundus height and ultrasound, fetal weight is difficult to estimate. The average margin of error between the estimated fetal weight and the actual birthweight is between 15% and 20%. Therefore, the predictive value of this risk factor is low [LE C].[2,3]

The risk of shoulder dystocia must be taken into account in the delivery of a fetus with a high estimated birthweight, as well as slow progress in dilatation and expulsion and operative vaginal delivery. Early symptoms of shoulder dystocia include the occurrence of *head bobbing* and the *turtle sign*. With head bobbing, the head shows in the perineum each time during pushing, but disappears again between contractions. With the turtle sign, the head is born slowly and pulled back against the perineum (Figure 8.1).

Indications

Prevention of the above-mentioned risk factors should provide the obstetrician with incentive to exercise extra care. A case of estimated high fetal weight and protracted dilatation or expulsion should trigger the notion of a possible shoulder dystocia.

In case of difficulty in delivering the anterior shoulder, be sure to:

- provide sufficient rest and room;
- do no more pushing, pulling, or turning the head;
- use a birthing bed with stirrups;
- have a plan of action, i.e., a series of maneuvers in a fixed order.

The indication to perform a certain maneuver in the event of a shoulder dystocia should be in an order from less to more stressful to the woman and the infant. The first maneuver to be performed should be the one that causes the least damage. If this does not solve the problem, the next step should be attempted.

Obstetric Interventions, ed. P. Joep Dörr, Vincent M. Khouw, Frank A. Chervenak, Amos Grunebaum, Yves Jacquemyn, and Jan G. Nijhuis. Published by Cambridge University Press. © Cambridge University Press 2017.

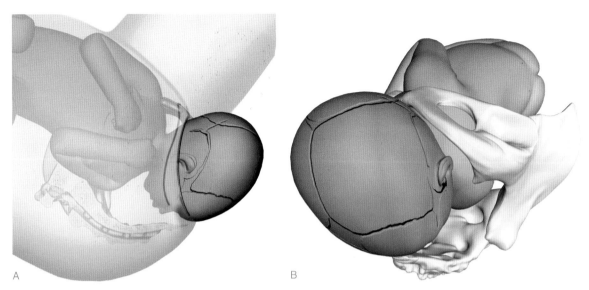

A   B

Figure 8.1 Turtle sign. (A) Side view; (B) perspective view.

Technique

The treatment of shoulder dystocia requires a series of successive actions that must be performed quickly and expertly by the obstetrics team. The order of the actions goes from less to more complicated, but may differ from clinic to clinic. It is important, however, that the obstetrics team in each clinic maintains a certain fixed order. One of the possibilities is the so-called *HELPERR* acronym, which is explained below [LE D][4,5]

Help

Call in extra help, from nursing to obstetrics personnel and a pediatrician. Start a time clock and record the actions performed. It is essential that each assistant is familiar with the protocol and his or her responsibility therein. This will prevent unnecessary time loss.

Episiotomy

Even though shoulder dystocia is a bony problem, an episiotomy should be contemplated when applying rotation maneuvers to create more room for the assistant and to prevent tissue injuries. Since the McRoberts maneuver together with suprapubic pressure provide a high success rate (40–50%), an episiotomy could be performed at a later stage.

Legs (McRoberts Maneuver)

Apply extreme flexion and abduction to the hips of the pregnant woman. This promotes pelvic rotation, which causes the symphysis to turn upward and the angle between the lumbar and the sacral spinal column to decrease (Figure 8.2) (see Animation 8.1). This allows the posterior shoulder to come down further and creates more room for the anterior shoulder.

Pressure Suprapubic

Through suprapubic pressure, applied laterally in the direction of the side of the fetal abdomen, an attempt is made to bring the anterior shoulder into an adduction position, so that it can slide under the symphysis (Figure 8.3) (see Animation 8.2). While applying suprapubic pressure, simultaneous dorsal traction is applied to the head (beware of brachial plexus injury). This maneuver can also be applied in combination with the McRoberts maneuver.

Enter Maneuvers (Internal Rotation)

The *enter maneuvers* concerns a number of rotation techniques, all leading to the goal of having the anterior shoulder to pass obliquely under the symphysis.

- In the Rubin method, pressure is applied with two fingers to the back of the scapula of the anterior shoulder to decrease the shoulder-to-shoulder distance through adduction (Figure 8.4) (see Animation 8.3).
- With the Woods maneuver, pressure is also applied to the front of the posterior shoulder toward the back of the infant, thereby initiating a "corkscrew-like" movement with both hands

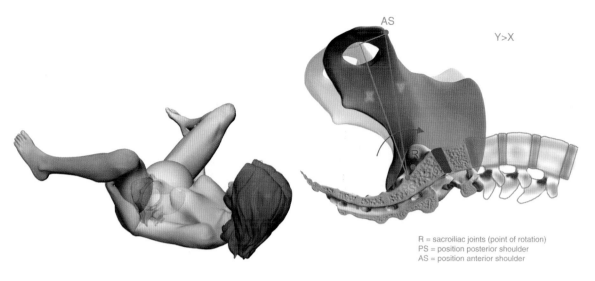

R = sacroiliac joints (point of rotation)
PS = position posterior shoulder
AS = position anterior shoulder

Figure 8.2 McRoberts maneuver.

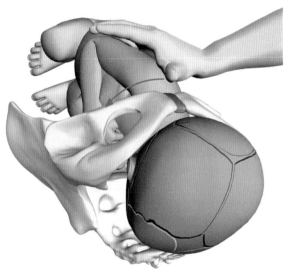

Figure 8.3 Pressure suprapubic.

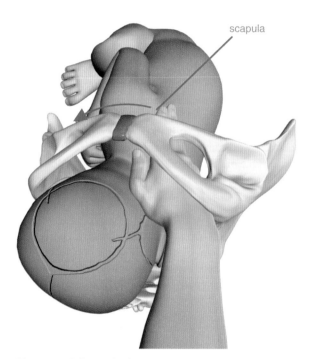

Figure 8.4 Rubin method.

(Figure 8.5) (see Animation 8.4). This causes a combination of adduction of the anterior shoulder and abduction of the posterior shoulder, which should dislodge the anterior shoulder that was wedged behind the symphysis. This maneuver could be continued for 180°, thereby making the posterior shoulder become the anterior shoulder.

Remove the Posterior Arm

The posterior arm of the fetus is extracted by reaching along the back of the curvature of the sacrum

with the hand that coincides with the abdominal side of the infant (thus, with the left hand if the abdomen is to the right and vice versa). The fingers follow the humerus up to the elbow. By applying pressure to the fold in the elbow the lower arm flexes, which allows it to be swept past the thorax and the face to the outside.

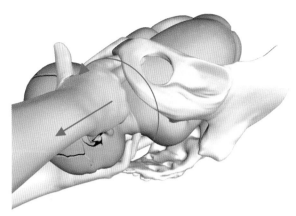

Figure 8.5 Woods method.

This maneuver decreases the biacromial width, whereby the fetus descends further into the sacral cavity and thereby resolves the impaction.

Grasping and pulling of the fetal arm must be avoided, as this can cause humerus fracture. When performing internal maneuvers, it is preferable to use the whole hand, including the thumb. Otherwise it is virtually impossible to reach high into the birth canal to dislodge the posterior arm (Figure 8.6) (see Animation 8.5).

Roll the Patient (All-fours Maneuver)[6–8]

Applying the *all-fours maneuver:* the patient rolls from a dorsal position to a knees and elbows position. By turning, the anterior shoulder often dislodges spontaneously. The posterior arm moves also toward the abdomen due to gravity, which produces extra sacral space and facilitates internal rotation procedures or sweeping of the posterior arm (Figure 8.7) (see Animation 8.6) [LE C/D].

It depends on the attending obstetric team whether they will first attempt to perform the R of *Remove* (sweeping the posterior arm down while the pregnant woman lies on her back) or whether the R of *Roll* (patient is placed in a knees and elbows position, after which an attempt is made to free the posterior arm) is applied first in the HELPERR acronym.

If the above-mentioned procedures did not lead to the infant's birth even after repeated efforts, there are still a number of other options.[4] However, you must always ask yourself whether a risky procedure would be the best choice, especially if the team lacks the experience. The options are as follows:

- The clavicle is broken on purpose.

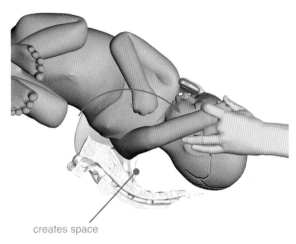

creates space

Figure 8.6 Remove the posterior arm.

- The Zavanelli maneuver: the head is replaced into the pelvis. After tocolysis, the head is returned to the original occiput anterior or occiput posterior position, flexed and pushed back into the vagina, followed by cesarean section.
- Symphysiotomy (Figure 8.8) (see Animation 8.7).
  - Two assistants must support the legs to prevent sudden abduction of the legs after the symphysiotomy (the angle between the legs may be no more than 60–80°).
  - Ensure infiltration of the skin and symphysis with lidocaine 2%.
  - Insert a transurethral catheter and keep the catheter away from the midline with the index and middle fingers.
  - Make an incision with a scalpel of the skin above the symphysis, followed by incision of the symphysis fibers until the pressure of the scalpel is felt by the index and middle fingers.
  - Remove the catheter after transecting the symphysis and allow the birth to take place.[9]

Complications

The occurrence of shoulder dystocia can have serious complications for the neonate. The morbidity reported in the literature is 8–20% [LE C].[2,10,11] Excessive traction to the head may cause a brachial plexus injury (C5–T1) due to avulsion or stretching of the corresponding nerve fibers. This leads to limited motion of the arm or hand. Moreover, the trauma resulting from the maneuvers can cause clavicular or humeral fracture.

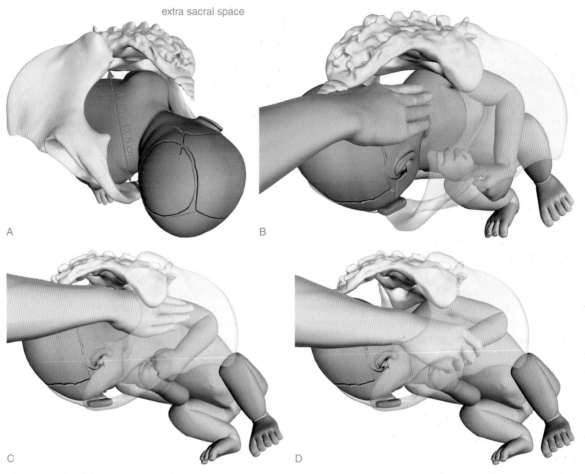

Figure 8.7 The all-fours maneuver and sweeping of the "posterior" arm. (A) Extrasacral space; (B and C) locating posterior arm; (D) sweeping posterior arm.

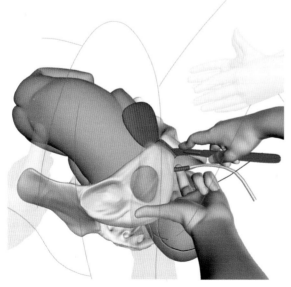

Figure 8.8 Symphysiotomy.

Insufficient oxygenation of the fetus due to poor perfusion can lead to permanent neurological damage and death. After the delivery of the head, the fetal pH can decrease by 0.04 for each minute the birth of the trunk is delayed. Therefore, a head-to-trunk time interval of less than 5 minutes must be pursued. The possibility of permanent fetal brain damage increases progressively with a time interval of 10 minutes.[9]

In pregnant women, serious shoulder dystocia and the corresponding maneuvers can lead to trauma to the birth canal (symphysiolysis) and hemorrhage. These complications can also occur if the corresponding maneuvers were performed adequately.

The social and medical/legal ramifications of the complications of a shoulder dystocia during parturition should be borne in mind. This is another reason why it is good to maintain proper medical reporting

[LE D].[12] The following checklist will be useful for this [LE D]:[8,12]

- date and time of delivery;
- caregivers present during the delivery;
- shoulder dystocia described as a complication;
- indication of the anterior shoulder;
- time between the birth of the head and that of the trunk;
- maneuvers applied and the order thereof;
- birthweight and Apgar scores;
- blood analysis results of the umbilical cord blood;
- pediatric examination, primarily for function limitations of the upper extremities and fractures;
- blood loss;
- condition of the perineum.

In addition, good communication between the obstetrician and the parents is essential in the event of morbidity in mother and/or child. Explain what happened and what was done to resolve the shoulder dystocia. Provide adequate advice, a clear plan of action, and any necessary referrals. In cases where a delivery was complicated by a shoulder dystocia, a subsequent prepregnancy consultation should discuss the possibility of an elective cesarean section for the next pregnancy, regardless of the occurrence of any neonatal morbidity.

Prevention

For patients with a history of risk factors, preventive measures could possibly lessen the occurrence of shoulder dystocia. The results of older randomized studies are disappointing [LE A1/2].[13,14] However in a recent RCT, induction of labor for suspected large-for-date fetuses was associated with a reduced risk of shoulder dystocia compared with expectant management [LE A2].[15] Stringent glucose control in pregestational diabetes mellitus type I and II but also in gestational diabetes has been shown to be effective in prevention of macrosomia and shoulder dystocia [LE A2].[16,17]

Considering the unpredictability of the occurrence of shoulder dystocia, the emergency nature of the event, and everyone's limited experience due to the low incidence, all personnel should be properly trained in resolving this complication. Training on a shoulder dystocia simulation model will improve the skills for resolving a case of shoulder dystocia [LE A2/C].[18,19] This is not only true for the obstetrician, but also for the entire delivery team. A protocol approach can provide support in this respect. In case of simulation training, we recommend that all caregivers involved become familiar with the protocol [LE B/D].[8,20–24]

Important Points and Recommendations

- The occurrence of shoulder dystocia is usually not predictable [LE C].
- A large time differential between the birth of the head and the trunk can result in serious hypoxia for the child, with a chance of permanent neurological damage [LE C].
- The risk, however, of a hasty approach is that the head will be pulled too much to be able to deliver the shoulders. Too much traction to the head can lead to permanent damage of the brachial plexus [LE C].
- There are certain procedures that can be performed as a team to safely resolve a shoulder dystocia [LE A2].
- A protocol approach with proper reporting and good communication with the parents is essential [LE D].
- In cases where a delivery was complicated by a shoulder dystocia, the possibility of an elective cesarean section in a subsequent pregnancy must be discussed, regardless of the occurrence of any neonatal morbidity [LE D].

References

1 Resnik R. Management of shoulder girdle dystocia. Clin Obstet Gynecol. 1980;**23**:559–64.

2 Dutch Society of Obstetrics and Gynaecology. Guideline Shoulder dystocia. September 2008.

3 Geary M, McParland P, Johnson H, et al. Shoulder dystocia – is it predictable? Eur J Obstet Gynecol Reprod Biol. 1995;**62**:15–18.

4 Gobbo R, Baxley EG. Shoulder dystocia. In: Leeman L (ed.). ALSO: advanced life support in obstetrics provider course syllabus. Leawood: American Academy of Family Physicians, 2000; p. 5.

5 Baxley EG, Gobbo RW. Shoulder dystocia. Am Fam Physician. 2004;**69**:1707–2014.

6 Gaskin IM. For the first time in history an obstetrical maneuver is named after a midwife. Birth Gaz. 1998;**14**:50.

7 Bruner JP, Drummond SB, Meenan AL, et al. All-fours maneuver for reducing shoulder dystocia during labor. J Reprod Med. 1998;**43**:439–43.

8 Coppus SFPJ, Langeveld J, Oei SG. Een onderschatte techniek voor het opheffen van schouderdystocie: baren op handen en knieën ('all-fours manoeuvre'). Ned Tijdschr Geneeskd. 2007;**151**:1493–7.

9 Grady K, Howell C, Cox C (eds). Shoulder dystocia. In: The MOET Course Manual, 2nd edition. London: RCOG Press, 2007; pp. 221–33.

10 Gherman RB, Ouzounian JG, Goodwin TM. Obstetric maneuvers for shoulder dystocia and associated fetal morbidity. Am J Obstet Gynecol. 1998;**178**:1126–30.

11 McFarland MB, Langer O, Piper JM, et al. Perinatal outcome and the type and number of maneuvers in shoulder dystocia. Int J Gynaecol Obstet. 1996;**55**:219–24.

12 Borell U, Femstrom I. A pelvimetric method for the assessment of pelvic mouldability. Acta Radiol. 1957;**47**:365–70.

13 Boulvain M, Stan C, Irion O. Elective delivery in diabetic pregnant women. Cochrane Database Syst Rev. 2001;**2**:CD001997.

14 Irion O, Boulvain M. Induction of labour for suspected fetal macrosomia. Cochrane Database Syst Rev. 2000;**2**: CD000938.

15 Boulvain M, Senat MV, Perrotin F, et al. Induction of labour versus expectant management for large-for-date fetuses: a randomised controlled trial. Lancet. 2015;**385**(9987):2600–5. DOI: 10.1016/ S0140-6736(14)61904-8.

16 Metzger BE; HAPO Study Cooperative Research Group. Hyperglycemia and adverse pregnancy outcomes. N Engl J Med. 2008;**358**:1991–2002.

17 Landon MB, Spong GY, Thom E, et al. A multicenter, randomized trial of treatment for mild gestational diabetes. N Engl J Med. 2009;**361**:1339–48.

18 Deering S, Poggi S, Macedonia C, et al. Improving resident competency in the management of shoulder dystocia with simulation. Obstet Gynecol. 2004;**103**: 1224–8.

19 Deering S, Poggi S, Hodor J, et al. Evaluation of residents' delivery notes after a simulated shoulder dystocia. Obstet Gynecol. 2004;**104**:667–70.

20 Draycott T, Sibanda T, Owen L, et al. Does training in obstetric emergencies improve neonatal outcome? BJOG. 2006;**113**:177–82.

21 Draycott TJ, Crofts JF, Ash JP, et al. Improving neonatal outcome through practical shoulder dystocia training. Obstet Gynecol. 2008;**112**:14–20.

22 Fransen AF, van de Ven J, Merién AE, et al. Effect of obstetric team training on team performance and medical technical skills: a randomised controlled trial. BJOG. 2012;**119**(11):1387–93.

23 Grobman WA, Miller D, Burke C, et al. Outcomes associated with introduction of a shoulder dystocia protocol. Am J Obstet Gynecol. 2011;**205**:513–17.

24 Grobman W. Shoulder dystocia. Obstet Gynecol Clin North Am. 2013;**40**:59–67.

Chapter 9

Retained Placenta

H.J. van Beekhuizen and J.H. Schagen van Leeuwen

General Information

Introduction

The third stage of labor refers to the period between the birth of the infant and the detachment and expulsion of the placenta and membranes. The "3rd stage of labor" may be managed either expectantly or actively. The latter is recommended by the WHO,[1] as it limits the average blood loss. Active management reduces the risk of severe bleeding (postpartum hemorrhage [PPH] >1000 ml) with a risk ratio of 0.34 (95% CI 0.14–0.87) [LE A1].[2] It does not, however, reduce the need for manual removal of the placenta (MRP) as compared to expectant management (RR 1.21, 95% CI 0.82–1.78) [LE A1].[2] Recently a large RCT on management of the third stage of labor in 4000 women showed a beneficial effect of controlled cord traction (CCT) on the incidence of retained placenta (RP): the incidence of RP was 4.2% in the CCT group versus 6.1% in the group that received only oxytocin (RR 0.69, 95% CI 0.53–0.90) [LE A2].[3] Of the three components of active management oxytocin administration is the most important[4] and recent recommendations advise delaying clamping of the cord for at least 2 to 3 minutes since delayed cord clamping does not increase the risk of PPH, but can be advantageous for the infant by improving iron status, which may be of clinical value particularly in infants where access to good nutrition is poor [LE A1].[5] Emptying the bladder in case of retained placenta may help to expel the placenta [LE D].

The normal length of the third stage of labor is not defined. The average duration of the third stage of labor in term births is 5 to 6 minutes [LE B].[6,7] Ninety percent of term placentas are delivered within 15 minutes and 97% are delivered within 30 minutes.[6] In preterm labor the duration of the third stage is usually longer.[7]

Professional societies in different countries have their own policies on when to perform MRP. Early MRP possibly reduces blood loss at the cost of too many interventions, while late MRP may lead to more blood loss. The timing of when to perform MRP depends not only on clinical factors, but also on the logistical restraints of the environment in which one is working. It should be borne in mind that underestimation of blood loss following delivery is a common problem. The diagnosis is usually made subjectively and many cases with clinically significant blood loss remain undetected. It is advisable to weigh or measure the blood loss [LE D]. A decision to perform MRP should not be unduly delayed.

Definition

A retained placenta is defined as a placenta that has not been delivered within 30 to 60 minutes after the birth of the infant [LE D][1] and is a frequent cause of PPH (WHO definition mild PPH >500 ml vaginal blood loss within 24 hours after the delivery; severe PPH >1000 ml/24 hours).

A (partially) retained placenta prevents normal contraction and retraction activity of the uterus and can therefore cause blood loss.

Incidence

Retained placenta affects approximately 0.5–3.3% of deliveries worldwide.[6–18] Review of observational studies showed that the median rate of RP at 30 minutes was higher in developed countries than in low-resource countries (2.67% vs 1.46%, p < 0.02), as was the rate of MRP (2.24% vs 0.45%, p < 0.001)[18] [LE C]. This may be explained in part by differences in the healthcare accessibility, i.e., high-risk women having a hospital delivery, (accuracy of) RP registration, reluctance to perform MRP in a low-resource setting, and definition and timing of MRP. In addition one may speculate that other factors, including ethnicity, parity, and previous cesarean section, may contribute to the differences.

Risk Factors

Risk factors are: history of retained placenta, cesarean section, and curettage as well as high maternal age, high parity, induction of labor, and preterm delivery. Gestational age is a risk factor that influences the length of the third stage of labor and the chance of a retained placenta. At less than 37 weeks, the chance of a prolonged third-stage labor as a result of a retained placenta is three times greater than in term birth [LE B].[6] This is also the case in second trimester pregnancy terminations. Recently a case–control study was published in which augmentation of labor with oxytocin was a risk factor with an OR of 2.00 (95% CI 1.20–3.34) for oxytocin augmentation of 195–415 minutes [LE B].[19]

Prevention of Retained Placenta

The effectiveness of strategies to prevent RP with interventions during the third stage of labor has been studied extensively, as shown in Table 9.1. Only CCT was significantly effective.[3] In prevention of MRP, ergometrine is apparently contra-productive (compared to oxytocin).[20]

Treatment of Retained Placenta

MRP is the standard of care in the treatment of RP. MRP is generally performed under anesthesia (general or regional), after disinfection of the vulva and vagina and application of a single dose of antibiotic. No data are available on the efficacy of antibiotics to prevent endometritis[26] or on the efficacy of MRP itself. It is known that MRP may be incomplete. Incomplete MRP requires re-intervention.

Medical drug treatment of RP with respectively nitroglycerin, intra-umbilical oxytocin, sulprostone, and misoprostol has been researched,[4,27–30] with MRP and excessive blood loss as endpoints. Only one study shows beneficial outcomes: intravenous 250 μg sulprostone (prostaglandin E2) administered

Table 9.1 Review of RCTs on the prevention of MRP during the third stage of labor

Intervention	Versus	Patients (number)	Relative risk	95% CI
Active management 3rd stage[2]	Expectant management	4 829	1.78	0.57–5.56
Active management 3rd stage[4]	Oxytocin 10 IU	18 831	0.97	0.68–1.37
Oxytocin[20]	Placebo	2 243	1.17	0.79–1.75
Ergometrine[21]	Placebo	2 429	3.75	0.14–99.7
Oral misoprostol 400 μg[22]	Placebo	900	0.43	0.06–2.89
Oxytocin[20]	**Ergometrine**	**2 800**	**0.57**	**0.41–0.79**
Oxytocin 5 IU plus ergometrine 0.5 mg[23]	Oxytocin 5 or 10 IU	9 932	1.03 (OR)	0.80–1.33
Oral misoprostol 600 μg[22]	Oxytocin/ergometrine	21 806	0.97	0.81–1.16
Prostaglandin $F_{2\alpha}$[22]	Oxytocin/ergometrine	231	1.09	0.31–3.81
Carbetocin 100 μg[24]	Oxytocin 5 IU plus ergometrine 0.5 mg	329	0.33	0.03–3.20
Drainage of umbilical cord plus CCT[25]	Expectant management	477	0.90	0.49–1.65
Active management with controlled cord traction[3]	**Active management without CCT**	4 000	**0.69**	**0.53–0.90**

OR, odds ratio; CCT, controlled cord traction.

when the placenta is retained 60 minutes after delivery of the infant decreases the number of manual placenta removals by 50% [LE A2].[28] Of course, before administering the drug the contraindications of sulprostone must be considered.

Indications

Indications for MRP are:

- more than 500–1000 ml blood loss due to retained placenta (depending on the national guidelines and the predelivery Hb level);
- retained placenta after 30 to 60 minutes postbirth of the infant;
- (suspicion of) a retained placental fragment;
- avulsion of the umbilical cord on controlled cord traction and lack of (spontaneous) expulsion [LE D].[31]

Anesthesia

A retained placenta is optimally removed in the operating room under adequate anesthesia, which could be regional when PPH is minimal and must be performed according to local protocol and in coordination with the anesthesiologist. As a minimum, the protocol must state that the patient has to have a properly running intravenous drip, that a blood sample was taken to determine the Hb count, as well as a cross-match for a possible blood transfusion, that the patient's bladder was emptied beforehand, and that before administering the anesthesia it was checked again whether the placenta dislodged by itself or through traction.

Technique of Manual Removal of the Placenta

An MRP is done under aseptic conditions and with gloves that reach to the elbows[27,31] and a sterile gown.

The technique of a manual placenta removal is as follows (see Animation 9.1).

- The external hand supports the fundus of the uterus.
- The other hand follows the umbilical cord and reaches the uterine cavity via the vagina and the cervix (Figure 9.1).
- It is important that the external hand continues to provide counterpressure to prevent ruptures and trauma to the birth canal.
- The margin of the placenta is then located and with the fingers pressed against each other the

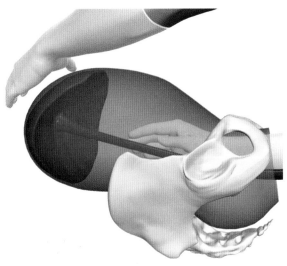

Figure 9.1 External hand supports the fundus, internal hand follows the umbilical cord.

dividing plane between the wall of the uterus and the placenta is located and the placenta is then peeled off the wall of the uterus. The cooperation of the internal hand (loosening of the placenta) and the external hand (supporting the uterus) is crucial in this procedure (Figure 9.2).

- After the placenta is completely separated, it is guided to the outside by the internal hand that remains in the uterus. Then the uterine cavity is palpated by the hand that remained inside the uterus to ensure that the placenta has been removed completely and that the uterine cavity has a normal shape (Figure 9.3).
- For women with a small area of placenta accreta, we suggest slow persistent finger dissection to create a plane of separation at the maternal–placental interface [LE D].
- *Unexpected placenta accreta.* Rarely, a placenta accreta is first recognized at the time of manual removal of the placenta. In these cases, there is no plane of dissection between the uterus and placenta and, almost invariably, attempts at manual removal lead to life-threatening hemorrhage. We suggest the following management in case the placenta does not separate.[32]

  . Administration of high-dose uterotonic drugs and preparation for hysterectomy. Hysterectomy is the definitive therapy of placenta accreta in patients who do not wish to preserve their fertility. It may be useful to perform a cystoscopy to

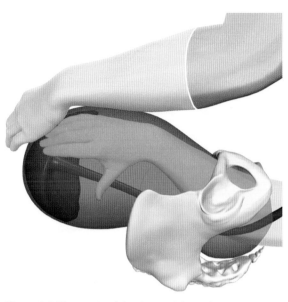

Figure 9.2 The margin of the placenta is located.

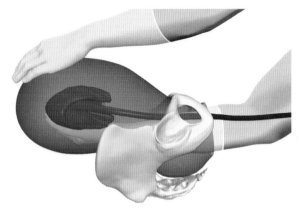

Figure 9.3 Placenta is dislodged and is brought to the outside.

assess for bladder invasion and to insert ureter catheters before hysterectomy.

- When there is a strong wish to preserve fertility in a patient who is willing to accept the risks of sudden bleeding, infection, and possible diffuse intravascular coagulation and when obvious hemorrhage is absent: leave placenta in place and administer antibiotics. Observe for spontaneous resorption of the placenta.
- If the placenta separates partially, deliver the separate parts and leave the adherent portions in place. This does not lead to postpartum hemorrhage as long as the uterus contracts well and there is no area of subinvolution at the site of the retained placental fragments. But one has to be careful: late postpartum hemorrhage may occur.

- The value of the prophylactic administration of antibiotics around MRP has not been proven [LE A1],[26] but can be included in a local protocol in consultation with the microbiologist.

Ultrasound scanning for complete removal of the placenta (fragments) is a simple procedure that can be performed after the intervention and could be useful, but its benefit has not been determined.[33]

After removal of the placenta, uterotonics are normally administered as a preventive measure and possible treatment of atonia of the uterus.

Complications

Inversion of the uterus is a rare complication of controlled cord traction and also of a manual removal of the placenta, in which the fundus of the uterus is pulled past the cervix and out of the uterus. In that case, immediate reposition is indicated after administering tocolytics as described in Chapter 11.

Manual removal of the placenta can lead to injury (through laceration or perforation) of the labia, introitus, vagina, cervix, or uterine cavity. In case of persistent blood loss after MRP these injuries should be excluded.

For diagnosis and treatment of placenta accreta and percreta we refer to Chapter 10.

In case of (suspected) retained placental fragments – either immediately after the delivery or later – it is not possible under certain circumstances to perform a manual placenta removal due to insufficient access to the uterus. In this situation curettage or hysteroscopic removal is indicated; the latter only if bleeding is not too profuse. Curettage can be done either with a vacuum instrument or with a blunt or sharp curette. It is recommended to perform postpartum curettage under ultrasound imaging to avoid perforation as much as possible and to ensure completeness of the placenta removal. Hysteroscopic removal is associated with less adhesions and higher pregnancy rate afterwards [LE C].[5]

Important Points and Recommendations

- Active management of labor does not reduce the risk for MRP [LE A1]; however it reduces the risk of severe PPH.

- Administering oxytocin and CCT are the most important components of active management of labor in case of RP [LE A1].
- Early cord clamping is no longer recommended by the WHO [LE A1].
- Use the definition of retained placenta if the placenta is not expelled within 30 minutes after delivery of the baby and start precautions to prevent and treat possible PPH such as putting up an IV drip and cross-match blood. If bleeding is heavy perform a MRP immediately. If blood loss is limited the MRP can be scheduled after 60 minutes. The 30 minutes between diagnosis of RP and treatment by MRP leaves ample time to study interventions that may help to expel the placenta and avoid MRP [LE D].
- In RP intravenous sulprostone 250 µg administration lessens the need for manual placenta removal [LE A2].
- MRP must be performed according to local protocol and in coordination with the anesthesiologist [LE D].

References

1. Mathai M, Gülmezoglu AM, Hill S. WHO Guidelines for the Management of Postpartum Haemorrhage and Retained Placenta. 2009. http://apps.who.int/iris/bit stream/10665/75411/1/9789241548502_eng.pdf?ua=1

2. Begley CM, Gyte GM, Murphy DJ, et al. Active versus expectant management for women in the third stage of labour. Cochrane Database Syst Rev. 2010;7:CD007412.

3. Deneux-Tharaux C, Sentilhes L, Maillard F, et al. Effect of routine controlled cord traction as part of the active management of the third stage of labour on postpartum haemorrhage: multicentre randomised controlled trial (TRACOR). BMJ. 2013;346:f1541. doi: 10.1136/bmj. f1541.

4. Gulmezoglu AM, Lumbiganon P, Landoulsi S, et al. Active management of the third stage of labour with and without controlled cord traction: a randomised, controlled, non-inferiority trial. Lancet. 2012;379 (9827):1721–7.

5. McDonald SJ, Middleton P. Effect of timing of umbilical cord clamping of term infants on maternal and neonatal outcomes. Cochrane Database Syst Rev. 2008;2: CD004074.

6. Combs CA, Laros RK, Jr. Prolonged third stage of labor: morbidity and risk factors. Obstet Gynecol. 1991;77(6):863–7.

7. Dombrowski MP, Bottoms SF, Saleh AA, Hurd WW, Romero R. Third stage of labor: analysis of duration and clinical practice. Am J Obstet Gynecol. 1995;172(4, Part 1):1279–84.

8. Adelusi B, Soltan MH, Chowdhury N, Kangave D. Risk of retained placenta: multivariate approach. Acta Obstet Gynecol Scand. 1997;76(5):414–18.

9. Bais JM, Eskes M, Pel M, Bonsel GJ, Bleker OP. Postpartum haemorrhage in nulliparous women: incidence and risk factors in low and high risk women. A Dutch population-based cohort study on standard (> or = 500 ml) and severe (> or = 1000 ml) postpartum haemorrhage. Eur J Obstet Gynecol Reprod Biol. 2004;115(2):166–72.

10. Chhabra S, Dhorey M. Retained placenta continues to be fatal but frequency can be reduced. J Obstet Gynaecol. 2002;22(6):630–3.

11. Owolabi AT, Dare FO, Fasubaa OB, et al. Risk factors for retained placenta in southwestern Nigeria. Singapore Med J. 2008;49(7):532–7.

12. Panprai P, Boriboonhirunsarn D. Risk factors of retained placenta in Siriraj Hospital. J Med Assoc Thai. 2007;90(7):1293–7.

13. Soltan MH, Khashoggi T. Retained placenta and associated risk factors. J Obstet Gynaecol. 1997;17(3):245–7.

14. Tandberg A, Albrechtsen S, Iversen OE. Manual removal of the placenta: incidence and clinical significance. Acta Obstet Gynecol Scand. 1999;78(1):33–6.

15. Titiz H, Wallace A, Voaklander DC. Manual removal of the placenta – a case control study. Aust N Z J Obstet Gynaecol. 2001;41(1):41–4.

16. Weeks AD. The retained placenta. Best Pract Res Clin Obstet Gynaecol. 2008;22(6):1103–17.

17. Onwudiegwu U, Makinde ON. Retained placenta: a cause of reproductive morbidity in Nigeria. J Obstet Gynaecol. 1999;19(4):355–9.

18. Cheung WM, Hawkes A, Ibish S, Weeks AD. The retained placenta: historical and geographical rate variations. J Obstet Gynaecol. 2011;31(1):37–42.

19. Endler M, Grunewald C, Saltvedt S. Epidemiology of retained placenta: oxytocin as an independent risk factor. Obstet Gynecol. 2012;119(4):801–9.

20. Westerhoff G, Cotter AM, Tolosa JE. Prophylactic oxytocin for the third stage of labour to prevent postpartum haemorrhage. Cochrane Database Syst Rev. 2013;10:CD001808. doi: 10.1002/14651858. CD001808.pub2.

21. Liabsuetrakul T, Choobun T, Peeyananjarassri K, Islam QM. Prophylactic use of ergot alkaloids in the third stage of labour. Cochrane Database Syst Rev. 2007;2:CD005456.

22. Gulmezoglu AM, Forna F, Villar J, Hofmeyr GJ. Prostaglandins for preventing postpartum

haemorrhage. Cochrane Database Syst Rev. 2007;**3**: CD000494.

23. McDonald S, Abbott JM, Higgins SP. Prophylactic ergometrine-oxytocin versus oxytocin for the third stage of labour. Cochrane Database Syst Rev. 2004;**1**:CD000201.

24. Leung SW, Ng PS, Wong WY, Cheung TH. A randomised trial of carbetocin versus syntometrine in the management of the third stage of labour. BJOG. 2006;**113**(12):1459–64.

25. Giacalone PL, Vignal J, Daures JP, Boulot P, Hedon B, Laffargue F. A randomised evaluation of two techniques of management of the third stage of labour in women at low risk of postpartum haemorrhage. BJOG. 2000;**107**(3):396–400.

26. Chongsomchai C, Lumbiganon P, Laopaiboon M. Prophylactic antibiotics for manual removal of retained placenta in vaginal birth. Cochrane Database Syst Rev. 2006;**2**:CD004904.

27. Weeks AD, Alia G, Vernon G, et al. Umbilical vein oxytocin for the treatment of retained placenta (Release Study): a double-blind, randomised controlled trial. Lancet. 2010;**375**(9709):141–7.

28. van Beekhuizen HJ, de Groot AN, De Boo T, et al. Sulprostone reduces the need for the manual removal of the placenta in patients with retained placenta: a randomized controlled trial. Am J Obstet Gynecol. 2006;**194**(2):446–50.

29. van Beekhuizen HJ, Tarimo V, Pembe AB, Fauteck H, Lotgering FK. Misoprostol is not beneficial in the treatment of retained placenta in a low-resource setting. Int J Gynaecol Obstet. 2013;**122**(3):234–7.

30. van Stralen G, Veenhof M, Holleboom C, van Roosmalen J. No reduction of manual removal after misoprostol for retained placenta: a double-blind, randomized trial. Acta Obstet Gynecol Scand. 2013;**92**(4):398–403.

31. Johanson R, Cox C, Grady K, Howell C, editors. Managing Obstetric Emergencies and Trauma: The MOET Course Manual. 2nd edition. London: RCOG Press; 2007.

32. Rao KP, Belogolovkin V, Yankowitz J, Spinnato JA. Abnormal placentation: evidence-based diagnosis and management of placenta previa, placenta accreta, and vasa previa. Obstet Gynecol Surv. 2012;**67**(8): 503–19.

33. Herman A. Complicated third stage of labor: time to switch on the scanner. Ultrasound Obstet Gynecol. 2000;**15**(2):89–95.

Chapter 10

Placenta Accreta, Increta, and Percreta

W. Mingelen, F.M. van Dunné, and P.J. Dörr

General Information

Introduction

In placenta accreta, increta, or percreta, the decidua of the endometrium is lacking, causing the placenta to partially or completely insert itself into the myometrium (placenta accreta; Figure 10.1A), invade the myometrium (placenta increta; Figure 10.1B), or grow through the myometrium into the surrounding structures and organs (placenta percreta; Figure 10.1C).[1]

The maternal mortality and morbidity are considerable and primarily the result of massive blood loss due to the abnormal insertion of the placenta, wherein the placenta does not release from the uterine wall after the child's birth.[2] The incidence of placenta accreta has risen during the past decades and is expected to continue to rise. This rise is related, among other things, to the increased incidence of cesarean sections.[3]

Definition

A placenta accreta, increta, or percreta is a placenta that completely or partially adheres abnormally to the uterine wall.

Incidence

Before 1980, a placenta accreta was rare, with an incidence of 1 in 4000 pregnancies. Currently, the incidence is 3 in 1000 to 1 in 530 pregnancies.[3,4] This increase runs practically parallel to the rise in the number of cesarean sections [LE B].[5,6]

Risk Factors

Risk factors for a placenta accreta are:
- maternal age above 35 years;
- placenta previa;
- previous cesarean section;
- procedures that can lead to damage to the endometrium or myometrium, such as a myoma enucleation, curettage, endometrial ablation, embolization of the uterine artery, or a submucosal myoma.[7-9]

The risk is highest in women with a placenta previa that lies partially on the anterior wall of the uterus and with a cesarean section in their prior medical history. This risk increases to 3%, 11%, 40%, 61%, and 67% after one, two, three, four, and five cesarean sections are performed, respectively, and whether or not the placenta is located on the anterior wall over the old scar.[10] Both a cesarean section in the medical history (adjusted odds ratio [AOR] 5; 95% CI 3.4–7.7) and a placenta previa (AOR 51; 95% CI 36–73) constitute independent risk factors [LE B].[11] An elective cesarean section has a higher risk of a placenta accreta in a subsequent pregnancy than a secondary cesarean section (OR 3.0; 95% CI 1.5–6.1) [LE B].[12]

Diagnosis

Prenatal diagnosis of a placenta accreta is essential for adequate treatment. Timely prenatal diagnosis allows a multidisciplinary plan of action to be developed, by means of which maternal and fetal mortality and morbidity can be prevented.

The placenta location relative to the cervix and any uterine scar must be examined by means of a structural ultrasound scan. A transvaginal ultrasound is more accurate in a low-lying placenta than an abdominal ultrasound [LE B].

Upon suspecting a placenta previa or a placenta over a cesarean section scar, an ultrasound must be repeated at the start of the third trimester. This way

Obstetric Interventions, ed. P. Joep Dörr, Vincent M. Khouw, Frank A. Chervenak, Amos Grunebaum, Yves Jacquemyn, and Jan G. Nijhuis. Published by Cambridge University Press. © Cambridge University Press 2017.

A   B   C

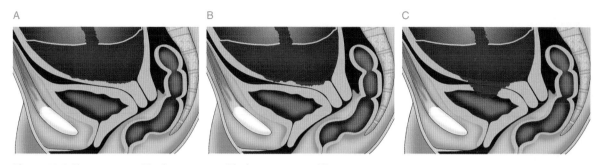

Figure 10.1 Placenta accreta (A), placenta increta (B), placenta percreta (C).

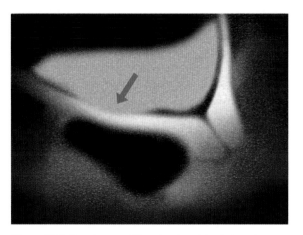

Figure 10.2 The absence of the retroplacental echolucent zone.

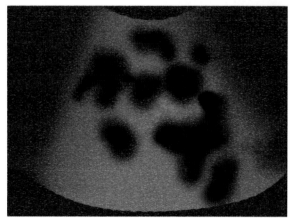

Figure 10.3 Multiple irregular placental lacunae.

there is sufficient time available to determine the multidisciplinary policy for the third trimester of the pregnancy.[13]

Ultrasound is a useful diagnostic tool (sensitivity: 91%; 95% CI 87–94; specificity: 97%; 95% CI 96–98; LR$^+$: 11; 95% CI 6–20; LR$^-$ 0.2: 95% CI 0.1–0.2 with a diagnostic OR of 99; 95% CI 49–199), but is never entirely conclusive.[14,15] The definitive diagnosis can only be made during a surgical procedure (cesarean section or manual placenta removal) [LE D].[13]

The ultrasound characteristics of a placenta inserting itself into the uterine wall are:

- the absence of the retroplacental echolucent zone (Figure 10.2);
- retroplacental myometrium thickness of less than 1 mm;
- multiple irregular placental lacunae (Figure 10.3);
- focal exophytic growth of the placenta invading the bladder.

The use of color Doppler ultrasound and three-dimensional (3D) power Doppler ultrasound does not increase the sensitivity or specificity as independent diagnostic tools, but may, in combination with conventional ultrasound, contribute to the diagnosis. Patients with a false-positive diagnosis are generally patients with one isolated ultrasound feature of a placenta accreta.[16]

Color Doppler ultrasound can be used to visualize a diffuse or focal lacunar flow, an increased amount of vascularization at the transition point from the uterus to the bladder (Figure 10.4), and dilated blood vessels in the peripheral subplacental zone as characteristics of a placenta accreta.[17,18]

Of the above-mentioned isolated ultrasound characteristics, the color Doppler differences are the most sensitive.[15]

In comparison with conventional ultrasound, MRI has produced comparable results.[19,20] MRI offers diagnostic possibilities when the ultrasound findings are not conclusive. MRI also offers added value in determining the infiltration depth in surrounding structures (the parametrium) and when suspecting a placenta accreta of the fundus and of the posterior wall of the uterus [LE B].[20]

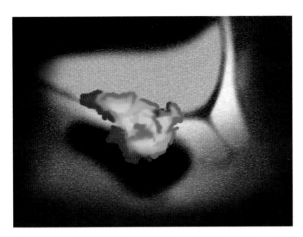

Figure 10.4 An increased amount of vascularization at the point of transition from the uterus to the bladder.

Policy

Women with a suspected placenta accreta should be instructed concerning the risks and potential complications of a placenta accreta. The main risks are massive blood loss and the need for a hysterectomy. In view of the blood loss, anemia must be prevented and treated prenatally, if necessary.[21]

The preferred mode of delivery in case of a suspected placenta accreta is a planned cesarean section. If there is no desire for additional children, the first choice of treatment in a placenta accreta is a hysterectomy following the cesarean section, while leaving the placenta in place.[22]

A scheduled cesarean section is preferable to an emergency cesarean section. An emergency cesarean section generally leads to more complications and blood loss than a planned cesarean section.

If the pregnancy progresses without complications, it is advisable to plan the cesarean section at 37 weeks' gestation [LE D]. The administration of corticosteroids to promote fetal lung maturation at this stage is still under discussion. Prenatal corticosteroids in an elective cesarean section appear to lower the risk of RDS (RR 0.46; 95% CI 0.23–0.93, p = 0.02) [LE B], but it is not clear whether the administration of prenatal corticosteroids after a gestation period of 36 weeks does not have adverse effects on the neonate.[23,24] In the event of blood loss during the second half of the pregnancy or in case of an increased risk of premature birth the performance of the cesarean section should be considered at 34 weeks' gestation or earlier if necessary [LE D], after the administration of corticosteroids for the fetal lung maturation [LE A2].[24,25]

To optimize the maternal and fetal outcomes, a multidisciplinary consultation should take place in the planning of the cesarean section, not only including an anesthesiologist, a perinatologist, a gynecologist with extensive surgical skills, and a neonatologist, but also with the intensivist, urologist, hematologist, intervention radiologist, and a general surgeon. In case of a suspected placenta percreta with invasion into the bladder, a preoperative cystoscopy should be performed.[26]

Treatment with Hysterectomy

The opinions regarding the performance of the procedure are as follows.

- Ultrasound testing immediately prior to the cesarean section for precise localization of the placenta. In case of doubt about the location, an ultrasound test can be performed during the operation.
- Lithotomy position related to controlling vaginal blood loss and a possible cystoscopy during the operation.
- Consider pre- or perioperative placement of ureteral catheters for easier localization of the ureters if a hysterectomy has to be performed.
- Consider preoperative placement of sheaths in both uterine arteries by the intervention radiologist for a possible balloon occlusion.
- The location of the placenta determines the place of the incision into the skin and the uterus. A median incision provides a better overview and makes it possible, if necessary, to open the uterus in the fundus or (after lifting the uterus out of the abdomen) in the posterior wall.
- The uterus should be opened at a distance from the placenta. An incision through the placenta involves a lot of blood loss and must therefore be avoided [LE B].
- After the child is born, it is checked whether the placenta releases spontaneously since the positive predictive value of the prenatal diagnosis of a placenta accreta is not 100%.
- If the placenta is not born spontaneously, it is left in place and a hysterectomy is performed immediately after the cesarean section.
- Attempting to remove a placenta accreta manually is not recommended, as this is related to high

maternal morbidity and mortality due to massive blood loss [LE B].[22]

- When suspecting a placenta percreta with invasion of the bladder, that part of the bladder must be removed together with the uterus.[27]
- General anesthesia is recommended due to the prolonged surgery time, but a combination of spinal and general anesthesia allows the patient to be awake for the birth of her child, after which a hysterectomy is performed under general anesthesia.[28]
- Standard prophylactic administration of antibiotics is indicated, with a repeated dose after a surgery time of 2 to 3 hours and after a blood loss of 1500 ml.[1]
- The transfusion laboratory should be informed of this risky surgical procedure. The current Dutch transfusion guidelines state that in case of massive blood loss multicomponent transfusions with fixed ratios between erythrocytes, plasma, and platelets (3:3:1) increase the survival by preventing or correcting a dilution coagulopathy. The optimal ratios among the three components are still unclear.[29]

In case of intensive vascularization of the pelvis, a hysterectomy may be considered at a later stage in a hemodynamically stable patient. Vascularization usually decreases with time. A hysterectomy at a later stage may also be considered in case experienced surgeons and/or adequate operating room and laboratory facilities are not available.[25]

Treatment with Conservation of the Uterus

Conservative treatment of women with a placenta accreta, with the purpose of preserving the uterus, is possible. This treatment leaves the placenta in place and closes the uterus after the child's birth. This option should only be considered if there is a strong desire to have more children in the future and in a hemodynamically stable patient with a normal coagulation status. Risks of this conservative treatment are blood loss, infection, diffuse intravascular coagulation, and the possibility of still having to perform a hysterectomy after the fact.

The available data in a group of 253 patients treated conservatively show a success rate (with the preservation of the uterus) of 80%.[30–32] The majority of these conservatively treated patients were additionally treated with arterial embolization, bilateral ligation of the hypogastric vessels, or methotrexate. The value of

the above-mentioned additional treatments is unclear due to the limited number of patient groups in which they are described. Methotrexate is the most described additional treatment option. There are indications that methotrexate decreases the vascularization of the placenta and therefore leads to necrosis and rapid involution of the placenta.[33] On the other hand, methotrexate has been proven effective only in rapidly dividing cells, such as in trophoblast proliferation, and it has a significant side-effect profile.[34]

There are insufficient data to make a reliable statement about a successful pregnancy after conservative treatment of a placenta accreta. The results of the largest study available appear to be positive. Of the 96 patients treated conservatively with success, ultimately only 27 patients desired to have more children. Twenty-four of the 27 women became pregnant.[35] The risk of renewed abnormal placentation in a subsequent pregnancy is significant; numbers range from 29% to 100% of the pregnancies.[30,31,35,36]

Important Points and Recommendations

- Prenatal discovery of a placenta accreta, increta, or percreta is essential to adequate multidisciplinary treatment.
- In a pregnant woman with this medical condition a planned cesarean section must be considered, wherein the placenta may be left in place and followed immediately by a hysterectomy.
- An attempt to manually remove (part of) the placenta is associated with a significant increase in massive blood loss.
- In the event of a significant future desire for more children and after due counseling of the patient with respect to the risks, it may be decided after the birth of the child by means of a planned cesarean section to close the uterus with the placenta left in place.

References

1. American College of Obstetricians and Gynecologists. Placenta accreta. ACOG. 2012;**529**:207–11.
2. O'Brien JM, Barton JR, Donaldson ES. The management of placenta percreta: conservative and operative strategies. Am J Obstet Gynecol. 1996;**175**:1632–8.
3. Wu S, Kocherginsky M, Hibbard JU. Abnormal placentation: twenty-year analysis. Am J Obstet Gynecol. 2005;**192**:1458–61.

4. Miller DA, Chollet JA, Goodwin TM. Clinical risk factors for placenta previa-placenta accreta. Am J Obstet Gynecol. 1997;**177**:210–14.

5. Higgins MF, Monteith C, Foley M, O'Herlihy C. Real increasing incidence of hysterectomy for placenta accreta following previous caesarean section. Eur J Obstet Gynecol Reprod Biol. 2013;**171**:54–6.

6. Morlando M, Sarno L, Napolitano R, et al. Placenta accreta: incidence and risk factors in an area with a particularly high rate of cesarean section. Acta Obstet Gynecol Scand. 2013;**92**:457–60.

7. Al-Serehi A, Mhoyan Q, Brown M, et al. Placenta accreta: an association with fibroids and Asherman syndrome. J Ultrasound Med. 2008;**27**:1623–8.

8. Hamar BD, Wolff EF, Kodaman PH, et al. Premature rupture of membranes, placenta increta and hysterectomy in a pregnancy following endometrial ablation. J Perinatol. 2006;**26**:135–7.

9. Pron G, Mocarski E, Bennet J, et al. Pregnancy after uterine artery embolization for leiomyomata: the Ontario multicenter trial. Obstet Gynecol. 2005;**26**:89–96.

10. Silver RM, Landon MB, Rouse DJ, et al. Maternal morbidity associated with multiple repeat cesarean deliveries. Obstet Gynecol. 2006;**107**:1226–32.

11. Eshkoli T, Weintraub AY, Sergienko R, Sheiner E. Placenta accreta: risk factors, perinatal outcomes, and consequences for subsequent births. Am J Obstet Gynecol. 2013;**208**:219.e1–7.

12. Kamara M, Henderson JJ, Doherty DA, et al. The risk of placenta accreta following primary elective caesarean delivery: a case-control study. BJOG. 2013;**120**:879–86.

13. Royal College of Obstetricians and Gynaecologists. RCOG Green-top Guideline No. 27: Placenta praevia, placenta praevia accreta and vasa praevia: diagnosis and management. London: RCOG, 2011.

14. Calì G, Giambanco L, Puccio G, Forlani F. Morbidly adherent placenta: evaluation of ultrasound diagnostic criteria and differentiation of placenta accreta from percreta. Ultrasound Obstet Gynecol. 2013;**41**:406–12.

15. D'Antonio F, Iacovella C, Bhide A. Prenatal identification of invasive placentation using ultrasound: systematic review and meta-analysis. Ultrasound Obstet Gynecol. 2013;**42**:509–17.

16. Shih JC, Palacios Jaraquemada JM, Su YN, et al. Role of three-dimensional power Doppler in the antenatal diagnosis of placenta accreta: comparison with gray-scale and color Doppler techniques. Ultrasound Obstet Gynecol. 2009;**33**:193–203.

17. Comstock CH. Antenatal diagnosis of placenta accreta: a review. Ultrasound Obstet Gynecol. 2005;**26**:89–96.

18. Warshak CR, Eskander R, Hull AD, et al. Accuracy of ultrasonography and magnetic resonance imaging in the diagnosis of placenta accreta. Obstet Gynecol. 2006;**108**:573–81.

19. Dwyer BK, Belogolovin V, Tran L, et al. Prenatal diagnosis of placenta accreta: sonography or magnetic resonance imaging? J Ultrasound Med. 2008;**27**:1275–81.

20. Masseli G, Brunelli R, Casciani E, et al. Magnetic resonance imaging in the evaluation of placental adhesive disorders: correlation with color Doppler ultrasound. Eur Radiol. 2008;**18**:1292–9.

21. American College of Obstetricians and Gynecologists. ACOG Practice Bulletin No. 95: anemia in pregnancy. Obstet Gynecol. 2008;**112**:201–7.

22. Eller AG, Porter TF, Soisson P, et al. Optimal management strategies for placenta accreta. BJOG. 2009;**116**:648–54.

23. Stutchfield P, Whitaker R, Russell I; Antenatal Steroids for Term Elective Caesarean Section (ASTECS) Research Team. Antenatal betamethasone and incidence of neonatal respiratory distress after elective caesarean section: pragmatic randomised trial. BMJ. 2005;**331**:662.

24. Royal College of Obstetricians and Gynaecologists. Green-top Guideline No. 7: Antenatal corticosteroids to reduce neonatal morbidity and mortality. London: RCOG, 2010.

25. Rao KP, Belogolovkin V, Yankowitz Y, et al. Abnormal placentation: evidence-based diagnosis and management of placenta previa, placenta accreta and vasa previa. Obstet Gynecol Surv. 2012;**67**:503–19.

26. Eller AG, Bennett MA, Sharshiner M, et al. Maternal morbidity in cases of placenta accreta managed by a multidisciplinary care team compared with standard obstetric care. Obstet Gynecol. 2011;**117**:331–7.

27. Hoffman MS, Karlnoski RA, Mangar D, et al. Morbidity associated with nonemergent hysterectomy for placenta accreta. Am J Obstet Gynecol. 2010;**202**:628.e1–5.

28. Kato R, Terui K, Yokota K, et al. Anesthetic management for cases of placenta accreta presented for cesarean section: a 7-year single-center experience [article in Japanese; English abstract]. Masui. 2008;**57**:1421–6.

29. Dutch Blood Transfusion Guideline, 2011. Core group: F.J.L.M. Haas, Prof. D.J. van Rhenen, Prof. R.R.P. de Vries, Mrs. M.A.M. Overbeeke, Dr V.M.J. Novotny, Dr Ch.P. Henny. http://www.sanquin.nl/repository/docu menten/en/prod-en-dienst/287294/blood-transfusion-guideline.pdf

30. Timmermans S, van Hof AC, Duvekot JJ. Conservative management of abnormally invasive placentation. Obstet Gynecol Surv. 2007;**62**:529–39.

31. Bretelle F, Courbiere B, Mazouni C, et al. Management of placenta accreta: morbidity and outcome. Eur J Obstet Gynecol Reprod Biol. 2007;**133**:34–9.

32. Sentilhes L, Ambroselli C, Kayem G, et al. Maternal outcome after conservative treatment of placenta accreta. Obstet Gynecol. 2010;**115**:526–34.

33. Arulkumaran S, Ng CS, Ingemarsson I, et al. Medical treatment of placenta accreta with methotrexate. Acta Obstet Gynecol Scand. 1986;**65**:285–6.

34. Winick M, Coscia A, Noble A. Cellular growth in human placenta: normal placental growth. Pediatrics. 1967;**39**:248–51.

35. Sentilhes L, Kayem G, Ambroselli C, et al. Fertility and pregnancy outcomes following conservative treatment for placenta accreta. Hum Reprod. 2010;**25**:2803–10.

36. Kayem G, Clement D, Goffinet F. Recurrence following conservative management of placenta accreta. Int J Gynecol Obstet. 2007;**99**:142–3.

Inversion of the Uterus

J.B. Derks and J. van Roosmalen

General Information

Introduction and Definition

Uterine inversion is a serious complication, in which – after delivery of the infant – the uterus protrudes completely or partially inside out through the cervix to the outside.

Classifications

There are several classifications:

- based on duration (acute <24 hours postpartum; subacute diagnosis >24 hours, but <4 weeks; chronic >4 weeks);
- based on severity (first degree: uterus in cervix; second degree: uterus passed through cervix; third degree: uterus reaches the perineum; total: the inverted uterus passes the perineum).

All recent cases of uterine inversion in the Netherlands were acute with different degrees of seriousness, whereby in some cases the inversion was only diagnosed upon internal examination prior to manual removal of the placenta.[1]

Incidence

Uterine inversion is a rare disorder. *Williams Obstetrics* cites an incidence of 1 in 6400 deliveries.[2] During the period from August 1, 2004 to August 1, 2006, 15 cases of uterine inversion were reported in the Netherlands out of a total of 358 874 deliveries, i.e., one uterine inversion in 23 925 deliveries.[1]

Causes

Causes of uterine inversion are:

- excessive traction on the umbilical cord when the placenta is implanted in the fundus, possibly in combination with a relaxed uterus and fundal pressure;
- placenta accreta, in which the placenta has invaded the myometrium.

Symptoms

The symptoms are:

- severe pain in the lower abdomen;
- life-threatening bleeding and often deep shock; the shock is often disproportional to the amount of blood loss due to a severe vagal reaction as a result of traction to the peritoneum.

All 15 Dutch patients presented with postpartum hemorrhage, for which they needed blood transfusions. Five of the 15 patients were in shock at the time of diagnosis and 4 presented with placenta accreta.[3]

Physical Examination

During physical examination the uterine fundus is not felt on abdominal palpation and upon vaginal examination the uterus may come out of the introitus inside out or be palpable in the vagina. Sometimes the inversion extends to the perineum. Often the placenta is still present.

Therapy

The therapy consists of:

- call for extra help (nursing staff, obstetric assistants, anesthesiologist);
- treatment of shock (oxygen, two functioning IVs, administration of crystalloids [0.9% NaCl], and if

Obstetric Interventions, ed. P. Joep Dörr, Vincent M. Khouw, Frank A. Chervenak, Amos Grunebaum, Yves Jacquemyn, and Jan G. Nijhuis. Published by Cambridge University Press. © Cambridge University Press 2017.

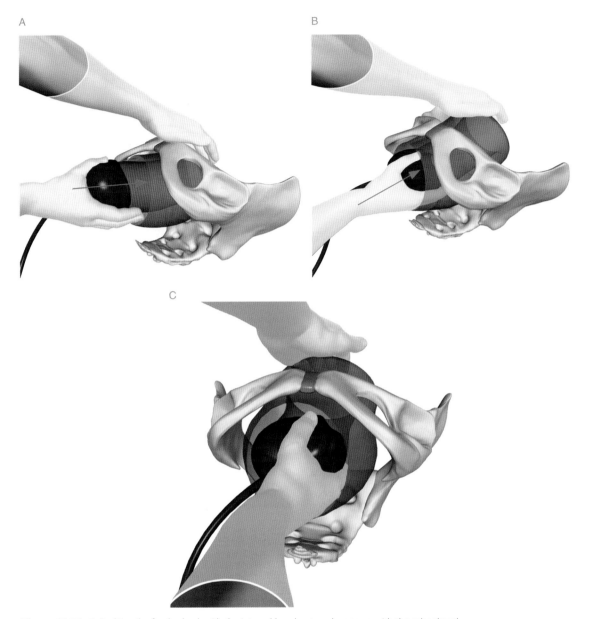

Figure 11.1A–C Pushing the fundus back with the internal hand; external pressure with the other hand.

necessary, administration of plasma expanders and blood products);
- repositioning of the uterus as soon as possible; the sooner this is done, the greater the chance of success.

Technique

Repositioning is done as follows (see Animations 11.1 and 11.2):

- Push the uterine fundus back through the cervix, while applying external pressure with the other hand (Johnson's maneuver, Figure 11.1).[3,4]
- Remove the placenta, if still present, only after reposition.
- Keep the hand in the uterus until the uterus, after administering an oxytocic agent, contracts to such a degree that there is no further fear of recurrence of the inversion (Figure 11.2).

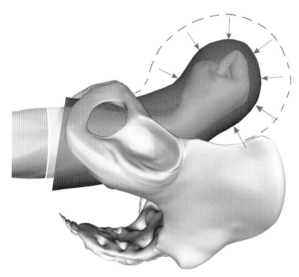

Figure 11.2 Internal hand stays inside until the uterus is properly contracted.

For all 15 patients, except 1, this was sufficient to treat the inversion.[3] One of the patients needed a Rusch balloon in the uterus to stop the hemorrhage and to prevent the inversion from recurring.[5]

Another possibility is to reposition the uterus with the help of hydrostatic pressure, by filling the vagina with warm saline solution and closing off the introitus with one hand or with a silicone cup (O'Sullivan's technique).[6]

If repositioning of the uterus is not immediately possible in the delivery room, the patient must be taken urgently to the operating room, where the procedure must be performed as soon as possible under general anesthesia. This was the case for all 15 patients. Sometimes it may be necessary to administer tocolytic drugs for uterine relaxation, such as intravenous ritodrine or atosiban or sublingual nitroglycerin spray.

When repositioning of the uterus under anesthesia is not possible, laparotomy will be needed. This is rarely necessary when the inversion is diagnosed soon enough after delivery. Earlier literature reports an incidence of three laparotomies on a total of 102 uterine inversions.[7] This procedure was not needed in any of the 15 recent cases in the Netherlands.[3]

During laparotomy, the uterine fundus can simultaneously be pulled from above, possibly with a traction suture, under vaginal pressure from below.

If repositioning is still not possible because of shrinkage of the constriction ring, the uterus can be incised posteriorly, after which repositioning should be possible. A careful inspection must be conducted of the internal organs after repositioning in order to treat any lacerations. Uterotonic agents (oxytocin or sulprostone) must be administered as soon as the uterus has been repositioned, to prevent recurrent inversion. If after reposition of the uterus there is a case of placenta accreta, it is sometimes necessary to perform a hysterectomy.

Prevention

Uterine inversion can be prevented through controlled cord traction during the third stage of labor only after the uterus has adequately contracted.

Important Points and Recommendations

- Uterine inversion is a rare, but potentially life-threatening, acute situation in which the uterus protrudes entirely or partially through the cervix to the outside. This is accompanied by severe abdominal pain, profuse bleeding, and symptoms of shock. The placenta may still be present, especially in the case of placenta accreta. Treatment is focused on alleviating shock and repositioning the uterus as soon as possible. If it is not possible to do this directly in the delivery room, repositioning should be done as soon as possible under general anesthesia [LE D].

References

1 Zwart JJ, Richters JM, Öry F, et al. Severe maternal morbidity during pregnancy, delivery and puerperium in the Netherlands: a nationwide population-based study of 371000 pregnancies. BJOG. 2008;**115**:842–50.

2 Cunningham FG, Gant NF, Leveno KJ, et al. *Williams obstetrics*. NewYork: McGraw-Hill, 2001.

3 Witteveen T, van Stralen G, Zwart J, van Roosmalen J. Puerperal uterine inversion in the Netherlands: a nationwide cohort study. *Acta Obstet Gynecol Scand*. 2013;**92**(3):334–7.

4 Kochenour NK. Diagnosis and management of uterine inversion. In: Hankins GDV, Clark SL, Cunningham FG, et al (eds). *Operative obstetrics*. Connecticut: Appleton & Lange, 1995: pp. 273–81.

5 Soleymani Majd H, Pilsniak A, Reginald PW. Recurrent uterine inversion: a novel treatment approach using SOS Bakri balloon. BJOG. 2009;**116**:999–1001.

6 Grady K, Howell C, Cox C. *Managing obstetric emergencies and trauma: The MOET course*

manual. Uterine inversion. London: RCOG Press, 2007: pp. 239–42.

7 Brar HS, Greenspoon JS, Platt LD, et al. Acute puerperal uterine inversion: New approaches to management. J Reprod Med. 1989;**34**:173–7.

Chapter 12

Technique for Cesarean Delivery

S.A. Scherjon, J.G. Nijhuis, and W.J.A. Gyselaers

General Information

Introduction

This chapter provides a description of the technique for performing cesarean sections. As in any other surgical procedure, the aim is a technique in which tissue damage is minimal, ischemia and infection are prevented where feasible, and the formation of adhesions is as slight as possible. Additionally, the goals are complete hemostasis with a precise approximation of the wound planes, which are sutured rather loosely, with the stitches at a reasonable distance and using the smallest amount of suturing material possible.

Present day cesarean sections are relatively safe procedures with low maternal morbidity and mortality. In one study there were no differences in maternal morbidity between delivery after an intended cesarean section and after an intended vaginal delivery: odds ratio (OR) 1.02 (95% CI: 0.77–1.34) [LE A1/C].[1,2] Potential risks of cesarean delivery included greater complications in subsequent pregnancies, such as uterine rupture, placenta previa, placenta accreta, bladder and bowel injuries, and the need for hysterectomy [LE C].[3] A Canadian study of primiparous women with singleton pregnancies showed an increased risk of postpartum cardiac arrest, wound hematoma, hysterectomy, major puerperal infection, anesthetic complications, venous thromboembolism, and hemorrhage that required hysterectomy in patients who had a planned primary cesarean delivery [LE C].[4]

Developments outside the realm of obstetrics, such as the availability of safe blood products and antibiotics, as well as improvements in anesthetics, have contributed to this [LE D].[5] If serious complications do arise, they are usually related to a deficiency in basic surgical skills, unexpected complications, and insufficient experience in resolving specific, cesarean-related, problems.

Incidence

Cesarean sections are the most practiced surgical procedure around the world. Recently, there has been a sharp increase in the incidence of cesarean sections. In 1977, the percentage was approximately 3–5%. For the United States, cesarean section rates were 5.5% in 1970, rising to a rate of 30.5% in 2007. Data from 119 countries between 1991 and 2003 on the median cesarean section rate showed a 100-fold difference in rate between countries of 0.4–40%. If categorized by income (low-, medium-, high-income countries), the median cesarean section incidence is (with interquartile ranges in parentheses) 4.0% (2.3–9.6%), 16.1% (13.6–21.9%), and 17.0% (15.0–21.3%), respectively. Cesarean section rates above 20% were found in respectively 3%, 36%, and 31% of these countries [LE C].[6]

Perioperative Phase

General

As in any other surgical procedure, it is important to evaluate and document the patient's medical history and the current status. In that way, the standard cesarean technique, as described in this chapter, can be individualized and potential problems can be anticipated.

Counseling

The decision to perform a cesarean section must always be based on appropriate indications and a balanced interaction between the physician in charge and the pregnant woman (and her partner). Aspects on counseling in general are described in

Obstetric Interventions, ed. P. Joep Dörr, Vincent M. Khouw, Frank A. Chervenak, Amos Grunebaum, Yves Jacquemyn, and Jan G. Nijhuis. Published by Cambridge University Press. © Cambridge University Press 2017.

more detail in Chapter 14. The pregnant woman and her partner must give their consent to the procedure. Even though an *informed consent* is not a universal rule yet, it is still recommended to make a note in the file that consent was obtained.

Preoperative Tests

Prior to performing a cesarean section it is good to know the recent hemoglobin (Hb) count, since in 4–8% of cesarean sections bleeding of >1000 ml occurs [LE A1].[7] In clinical situations with a potentially increased bleeding risk, such as placenta previa or abruption, it is recommended to perform the cesarean section where a 24-hour blood transfusion is available or to have cross-matched blood in stock before the surgery.

This specific measure is not indicated for a primary cesarean section after an uncomplicated pregnancy.

Antibiotics

Prophylactic administration of antibiotics for cesarean section reduces postpartum endometritis by more than 60% in both primary (RR 0.4; 95% CI 0.2–0.6) and secondary cesarean sections (RR 0.4; 95% CI 0.3–0.4). Additionally, this reduces wound infections by approximately 25% in primary (RR 0.7; 95% CI 0.5–0.99) and 65% in secondary cesarean sections (RR 0.4; 95% CI 0.3–0.5) [LE A1].[8] Also reductions in urinary tract infections are documented. The administration of antibiotics before the incision compared to after clamping the umbilical cord decreases the risk of endometritis (RR 0.5; 95% CI 0.3–0.9) and infections in general (RR 0.5; 95% CI 0.3–0.8), with a tendency toward less wound infections (RR 0.6; 95% CI 0.3–1.2). No differences have been observed in important neonatal results, such as suspected sepsis (RR 1.0; 95% CI 0.7–1.4), proven sepsis (RR 0.9; 95% CI 0.5–2.0), or admission to intensive care (RR 1.1; 95% CI 0.5–2.2) [LE A1/D].[9,10]

For cesarean section the use of cefazolin (1 g, single intravenous dose) and metronidazole (500 mg, single intravenous dose) as prophylaxis especially in secondary cesarean sections is recommended [LE C].[11] Cefazolin (a first generation broad-spectrum cephalosporin) is particularly effective against gram-positive cocci (*Ureaplasma* and *Mycoplasma*) and metronidazole against anaerobic bacteria. Besides this scheme, other antibiotics are also used for prophylaxis. Insufficient studies

have been conducted into the difference in efficacy between different prophylactic schemes.[10] Support for the use of azithromycin as a second-line broad-spectrum antibiotic (active against aerobes and anaerobes as well as *Ureaplasma* spp.) by preventing neonatal sepsis and chronic lung disease was suggested in several trials [LE C].[11] A definitive RCT has still to be performed (broad-range/preincision versus narrow-range/postincision). The importance of other measures to prevent postoperative wound infections, such as limiting the opening of the door of the operating room and keeping the patient's body temperature at a proper level, are often still overlooked.

Thrombosis Prophylaxis

Thrombosis prophylaxis is recommended for cesarean sections. Although the absolute risk is low, an increased risk of postoperative thromboembolic complications does exist and is an infrequent but potentially devastating contributor to maternal morbidity and mortality. The prophylactic method in all cesarean sections (e.g., use of compression hose, early mobilization, and short-term systematic administration of low-molecular-weight heparins [LMWH]) can be established by choice in local protocols, though recently protocols have been developed for routine use of low-dose heparin in all cesarean sections [LE C].[12] Compression hose are described as an additive effect along with simultaneous use of LMWH [LE A1].[13] With short-term use of LMWH in all cesarean sections there is a negligibly small risk of heparin-induced thrombopenia (HIT) and hemorrhage.

Prevention of Continued Bleeding

For the prevention of uterine atony and postpartum bleeding in cesarean sections the same recommendations are given as for the third stage in a vaginal delivery: 5 IU of oxytocin by slow IV, immediately after the infant has been delivered. However, oxytocin may be administered before clamping the infant's umbilical cord as this is beneficial for the autotransfusion of placental blood to the neonate.

For this indication – the prevention of an atony after a cesarean section under spinal or epidural anesthesia – carbetocin, a synthetic long-acting oxytocin analogue, has been registered. Four trials in women undergoing a cesarean section showed a decrease in the carbetocin-treated group (single dose of 100 µg by IV) versus oxytocin (different dosage schemes: from 5 HU [Howell unit] bolus to 32.5 HU in 16 hours) of the number of patients needing therapeutic uterotonics (RR 0.62; 95% CI 0.44–0.88), and the need for uterine massage (RR 0.54; 95% CI 0.37–0.79). There were no differences in terms of the risk for bleeding of 500 ml or more (RR 0.66; 95% CI 0.42–1.06), 1000 ml or more (RR 0.91; 95% CI 0.39–2.15), or mean blood loss (mean difference –29.00 ml; 95% CI –83–25 ml). No differences in adverse maternal effects were reported [LE A1].[14–16]

Maternal Positioning

It is customary to place the pregnant woman in a *left-tilt* position: a semi-prone left side lie by means of a wedge under the right flank or by tilting the OR table. This is an attempt to prevent vena caval compression due to the large uterine volume and thereby lessen the risk of maternal hypotension. The neonatal benefits still appear to be limited, with a trend to fewer low Apgar scores compared to supine position, without any difference in fetal pH values [LE A1].[7] At the moment there is no meta-analysis available.

Also in other positions – standing, half-sitting, and also with a 15° tilt – there is probably some aorta caval compression, which can be reinforced through (regional) anesthesia [LE C].[17]

Bladder Catheterization

Catheterization of the bladder, whether just one time or via an indwelling catheter, is customary in cesarean sections to prevent bladder lesions.

It has not been established whether one-time catheterization in cesarean sections is an advantage over an indwelling catheter [LE A1].[7] To prevent a bladder infection, especially if in an emergency cesarean section insufficient asepsis is (can be) observed, some recommend not to use catheterization [LE B].[18] It is also recommended after epidural anesthesia not to remove the bladder catheter until at least 12 hours after the last *top-up* and after the patient is mobile again [LE A1].[7]

Placental Localization

Placental localization may contribute to an increase in blood loss, and therefore it is good practice to know ahead of time where the placenta is located and whether you are dealing with an abnormal placentation such as a low-lying placenta, an anterior placenta that is located close to a prior uterine scar, or a placenta that lies over a prior myomectomy. If this is the case (regardless of the question whether the placenta lies against the anterior wall or the posterior wall) in a patient with a previous cesarean section, then the chance of having a placenta accreta is more than 20% [LE B].[19] This risk increases linearly up to 67% in the case of four prior cesarean sections [LE B/D].[20,21] The relative risk of placenta accreta, regardless of placental localization, is 8.7 (95% CI 3.5–21.2) in two or more prior cesarean sections [LE B].[22]

In a high-risk population, the indication of irregularly shaped lacunae in the placenta – a characteristic "cheese with holes image," with or without turbulent flow – has a high positive predictive value (PPV) of 93%. The combination of smallest sagittal myometrial thickness, lacunae, and bridging vessels, in addition to number of cesarean deliveries and placental location, yielded an area under the curve of 0.87 (95% CI 0.80–0.95) [LE C].[23]

Other characteristic disorders are a thin myometrium (<1 mm) and growth of the placenta into the bladder in cases of placenta percreta. The loss of the elongated clearing behind the placenta is less specific (PPV 6%) [LE D].[24] A high grade of suspicion should suggest next steps for further diagnostic evaluations such as imaging by means of an MRI or CT scan [LE D].[21] All patients with placenta previa and prior cesarean deliveries should be assumed to have a placenta accreta unless proven otherwise.

Anesthesia

Regional Anesthesia

Almost always, in more than 90% of all cases, the safest technique can be used: a form of *regional* anesthesia.

- *Efficacy*: the spinal and the epidural technique are equally effective in terms of relieving pain.
- *Contraindications* are:
  - coagulation disorders and (recent) anticoagulant use (coumarin derivatives and LMWH) (relative contraindication);
  - thrombocytopenia (commonly a marginal value of 50 × 109 thrombocytes/ml is used);
  - brain tumor (increased intracranial pressure) (relative contraindication) [LE C].[25]

Platelet aggregation inhibitors (acetylsalicylic acid) do not constitute a contraindication for both epidural and spinal techniques of regional anesthesia [LE C].[26]

Local protocols vary in the precise contraindications, depending on the LMWH dose used (low versus high prophylactic/therapeutic) and the technique – *single-shot* spinal anesthesia versus epidural anesthesia. The interval between the last moment of administration and the moment of regional anesthesia, preferably more than 10 hours, is an important factor [LE C].[26]

Comparison of Epidural and Spinal Technique

- The advantage of the epidural technique is that the decrease in blood pressure (and thereby the negative influence on the placenta perfusion) is less than in the spinal technique.
- The epidural pain relief can be continued successfully during the postoperative period with *patient-controlled analgesia* (PCA).
- The spinal technique is somewhat faster, but in order to prevent a blood pressure decrease the patient must first have an intravenous infusion with NaCl 0.9%.

Another method that is used is a combined spinal–epidural (SE) anesthesia technique [LE D].[27] In this method both techniques are combined and the dose needed for spinal analgesia can be decreased.

General Anesthesia

General anesthesia is considered the anesthesia of choice only for a few patients who have a cesarean section including those with the inability to have spinal or epidural anesthesia, for example because of prior back surgery or severe hematologic anomalies, or occasionally for emergent situations.

Comparison of General and Regional Anesthesia

- General anesthesia (GA) is less safe (complication risk is increased [OR 1.5; 95% CI 1.1–2.1]), because, among other things, of the increased chance of an aspiration and more blood loss (OR 2.0; 95% CI 1.5–2.7) [LE C].[28] A lower decrease in mean difference pre-postoperative hematocrit was found for regional anesthesia (RA) when compared to GA, both for epidural anesthesia (1.7%; 95% CI 0.5–2.9%) and spinal anesthesia (3.1%; 95% CI 1.7–4.5%). Also estimated maternal blood loss is lower with epidural anesthesia when compared to GA: –0.32 ml; 95% CI –0.59 to –0.07 ml [LE A1].[29]
- With GA there is no evidence that the infant is on average more depressed after birth: the mean adaptive score between GA and epidural anesthesia (EA) is not different (mean difference [MD] 2.17; 95% CI –1.1–5.5) and also no differences in Apgar score after 5 minutes were found (MD 0.2; 95% CI –0.2–0.6) [LE A1].[30] Also arterial and venous umbilical cord pH after GA is no different from that in epidural and spinal anesthesia [LE A1].[29]
- No difference in maternal death has been observed among the different techniques.
- It is doubtful whether GA, compared to regional techniques, leads to a faster operation in the case of an emergency cesarean section. Yet, compared to non-emergency cesarean sections, GA is used more often in emergency cesarean sections than in a control group in which there is no emergency factor (OR 18.5; 95% CI 6.0–64.0) [LE B].[31]
- One systematic review showed that women who had had a regional technique – compared to the general anesthesia group – have a lower preference of using the same technique again: epidural versus GA (RR 0.8; 95% CI 0.7–0.98) and spinal vs GA (RR 0.8; 95% CI 0.7–0.99) [LE A1].[29]
- No differences in adverse maternal outcome are evident if GA and RA are compared [LE A1].[29]

Local Anesthesia

Very rarely it may be preferred, for example where an intracranial space-occupying tumor in the mother increases the intracranial pressure, to employ a completely *local* technique. In this procedure, the abdominal wall is locally anesthetized with approximately 12 times 1–2 ml lidocaine (0.5–1%), with possible additional injections into the fascia and the peritoneum.

Obesity, Extra Risk Factor in Cesarean Sections?

The cesarean section percentage in obese patients has tripled (to 60%), in which the maternal weight has an independent association with the cesarean section percentage [LE B].[32–34] With obesity (BMI ≥30) there is a greater chance (42–74.4%) of a failed initial placement of an epidural catheter, compared to a population that is not overweight (6%) [LE B].[35]

General anesthesia presents greater problems concerning intubation (in approximately 33%) and aspiration [LE C].[36] Moreover, operative time is longer, there is more blood loss [LE C],[36] and there are more wound infections [LE C][37] and thromboembolic complications.

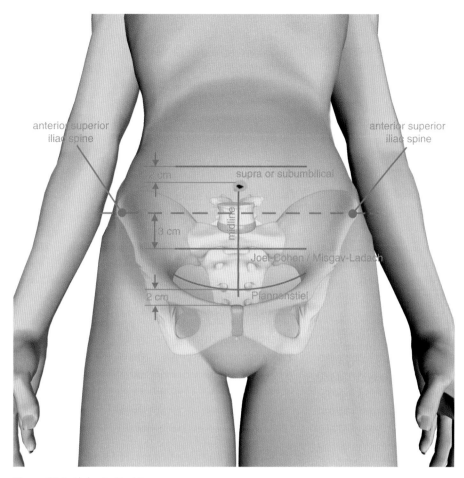

Figure 12.1 Abdominal incisions.

Surgical Aspects

Opening the Abdominal Wall

Five techniques are described for opening the abdominal wall in a cesarean section (Figure 12.1):

- the midline incision;
- the Pfannenstiel incision;
- the Joel-Cohen method;
  - the Misgav-Ladach method (Michael Stark Cesarean);
- the Maylard technique;
- the supra or subumbilical transverse incision.

General comments on abdominal incisions:

- To obtain a straight, symmetrical skin incision, the place of incision may be drawn on the skin before disinfection. This method is often applied in cosmetic surgery [LE C].[38]

- To prevent the skin incision from adhering to the fascia, some surgeons open the fascia slightly higher than the skin incision, which, after closing the skin, makes the subcutis automatically position itself between the skin and the fascia and the scars are therefore not superimposed on each other.

- It is not necessary to use a separate "skin scalpel" for all skin incisions and then switch to an "abdominal scalpel" [LE B].[39]

- The surgeon can follow his or her own preference for opening the abdomen, also of the skin, with a scalpel or with electrocautery.

  - Compared to other operative procedures, cesarean sections are prone to fluid spill. As such, the use of electrosurgery is theoretically at increased risk for misconduct of electrical current and subsequent burning wounds. Although this problem has not been investigated in randomized trials, surgeon's knowledge of safety measures for electrosurgery is highly recommended.[40]

185

- The use of a diathermal –midline– skin incision has clear advantages, such as a shorter operative time, less blood loss, and lower pain scores, and no drawbacks with regard to wound healing or infections [LE A2].[41]

- If a scar from a previous operation is particularly unsightly, it is customary to suggest excision of the old scar.

Midline Incision

Indications for a midline incision are:

- if additional exploration of the upper abdomen must also be performed;
- in case of specific obstetric complications, such as a neglected transverse lie, because of the longitudinal incision into the uterus in that case;
- if the patient had a previous midline lower abdominal laparotomy.

A midline incision is also preferred in emergency situations and if the need to limit blood loss was determined beforehand (in the event of thrombocytopenia, a patient who refused a blood transfusion [e.g., Jehovah's witness] or an operation under anticoagulant use). In both indications the benefit is doubtful because of wider experience with transverse incisions (therefore faster) and the use of blunt dissection techniques (less blood loss).

Disadvantages of midline incisions are:

- increased risk of bladder lesion and/or intestinal lesion (corrected OR 3.9 [CI 1.4–8.9] and 5.5, respectively [insignificant due to small numbers]). The risk (in midline as well as transverse incisions) of bladder lesions is (also) related to the number of cesarean sections in the patient's medical history [LE C].[42]
- greater risk (up to 3%) of wound dehiscence, which is almost 10 times higher than in a transverse incision (0.37%) [LE A1].[7]

Closure of Midline Incisions

For midline incisions there are sufficient data in the medical literature to justify a so-called continuous *mass-closure* with long-lasting absorbable material, in which the rectus muscle, fascia, and the parietal peritoneum are included in one continuous layer [LE A1].[7] This method has less risk of scar ruptures and dehiscence than closures in individual layers.

Pfannenstiel Incision

The most frequently used transverse incision is the "classical" Pfannenstiel method. With this method, all of the layers of the abdominal wall are incised sharply.

The following structures are opened in succession:

- The skin and the subcutaneous tissue are opened with a curvilinear incision of approximately 12 cm in length and two finger-widths above the pubis (Figure 12.2).

A

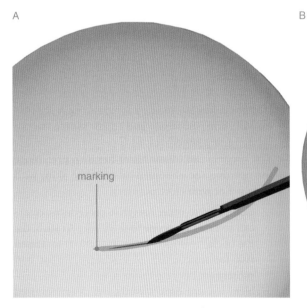

B

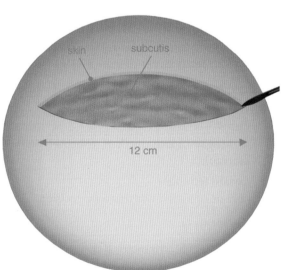

Figure 12.2 Skin incision (A) and situation after opening the skin (B).

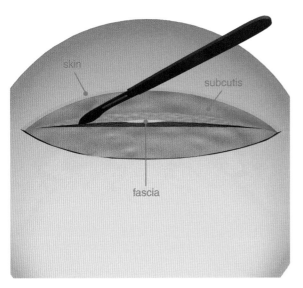

Figure 12.3 Incision of the subcutis.

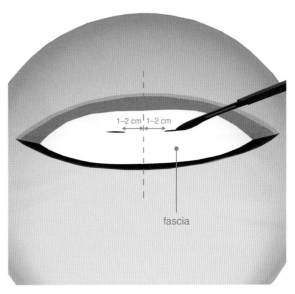

Figure 12.4 Incision of the fascia.

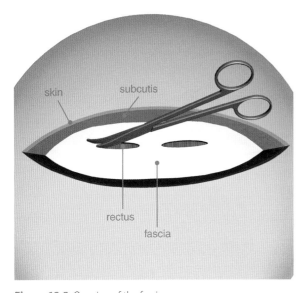

Figure 12.5 Opening of the fascia.

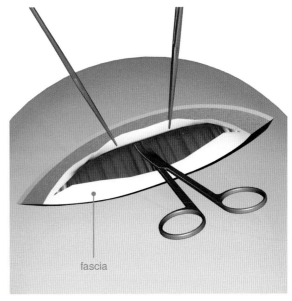

Figure 12.6 Dissecting the fascia.

- The subcutis is incised sharply over the entire length down to the fascia (Figure 12.3).
- The fascia is incised for 1–2 cm on each side next to the midline (Figure 12.4).
- The fascia is opened sharply with surgical scissors, e.g., curved Mayo scissors (Figure 12.5).

- The fascia is dissected sharply upward and downward off of both rectus muscles (Figure 12.6).
- The rectus muscles are separated sharply from each other in the midline (Figure 12.7) and then the rectus muscles are further opened by traction (Figure 12.8).

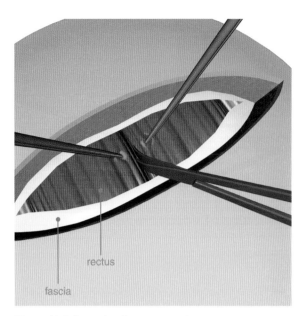

Figure 12.7 Separating the rectus muscles.

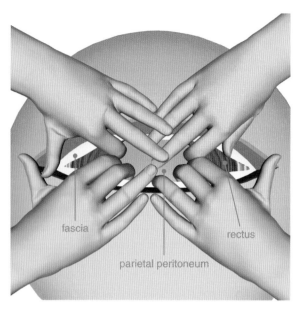

Figure 12.8 Separating the rectus muscles by digital traction.

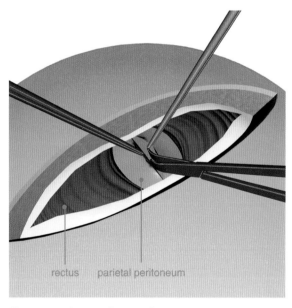

Figure 12.9 Opening the parietal peritoneum.

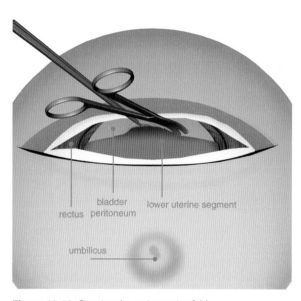

Figure 12.10 Opening the vesicouterine fold.

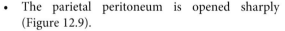

- The parietal peritoneum is opened sharply (Figure 12.9).
- The visceral peritoneum (the vesicouterine fold) is incised curvilinearly (Figure 12.10).
- The bladder is pushed caudally out of the way with a dabber (Figure 12.11).
- After placing a marking incision, the lower uterine segment is incised sharply in the center down to

the membranes (Figure 12.12), after which the incision is widened digitally in a transverse direction (Figure 12.13). In this way the arterial branches are not severed by sharp cleavage, but pushed aside and kept intact.
- Upon opening the uterus, the membranes may or may not be ruptured. If opening the uterus with ruptured membranes or in case of

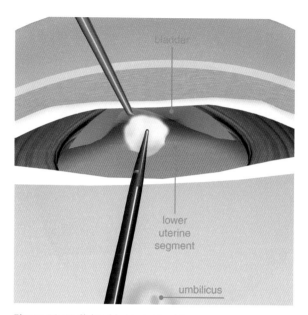

Figure 12.11 Sliding bladder to the side.

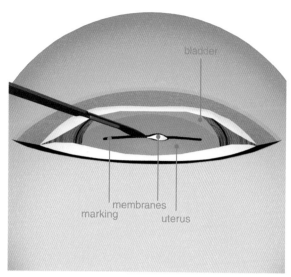

Figure 12.12 Marking incision and opening of the lower uterine segment.

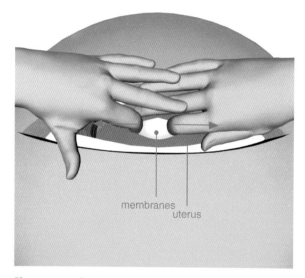

Figure 12.13 Digital widening of the incision.

oligohydramnios, it must be taken into account that the infant can be easily nicked with a scalpel, which could have serious consequences.

- After that, the infant is removed from the uterus.

After a Pfannenstiel incision moderate-to-severe chronic pain 2 years after the operation is reported in 7% of patients, while 9.8% of the respondents experience pain impairing their daily activities.

In 70% of the patients women experience the pain in the lateral portions of the scar. In half of the patients with moderate-to-severe pain the pain could be related to nerve entrapment of the iliohypogastric or ilioinguinal nerve [LE B].[43]

The Joel-Cohen Method

Joel-Cohen was particularly interested in shortening the time duration, although there is a bit more blood loss in the dissection of the subcutis than in a midline incision. In this "surgically minimalistic" variation of the Pfannenstiel cesarean section, no wound retractors are used, only the skin is incised sharply, and the subcutis is not separately "opened" sharply [LE B/D].[44–46]

The following structures are then opened in succession:

- Joel-Cohen's skin incision runs straight, approximately 3 cm below the line between both antero-superior iliac spines (Figure 12.14).
- A small section of the subcutis is incised sharply down to the fascia (Figure 12.15), after which it is opened further by blunt finger traction (Figure 12.16).
- The fascia is opened via two small incisions on each side of the midline (Figure 12.17) and then opened bluntly through bilateral traction above the rectus muscles (Figure 12.18).

189

A

B

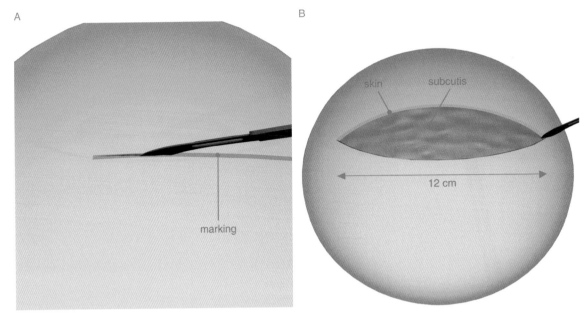

Figure 12.14 Skin incision (A) and situation after opening the skin (B).

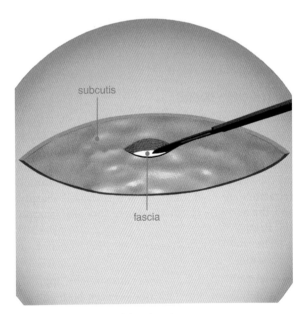

Figure 12.15 Incision of the subcutis.

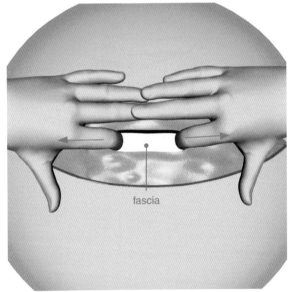

Figure 12.16 Digital opening of the subcutis.

- The rectus muscles are not dissected from the fascia, but are opened bluntly in the midline (Figure 12.19).
- The parietal peritoneum is opened digitally (Figure 12.20).
- The peritoneum, rectus muscle, and fascia are grasped completely on both sides with four fingers

and the abdomen is further opened by traction (Figure 12.21).
- The bladder peritoneum is not opened, which is a strategy that is also preferred according to more recent studies [LE A2/A2/C].[47–49] The omission of the bladder flap formation is associated with less fever and a significantly

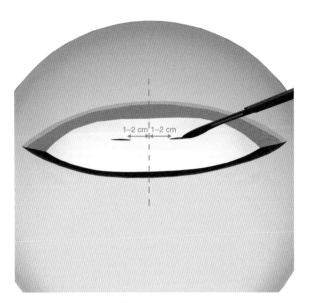

Figure 12.17 Incision of the fascia.

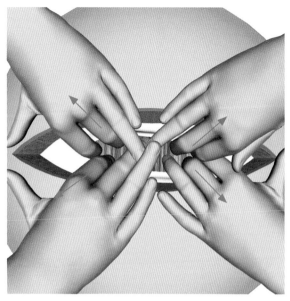

Figure 12.18 Digital opening of the fascia.

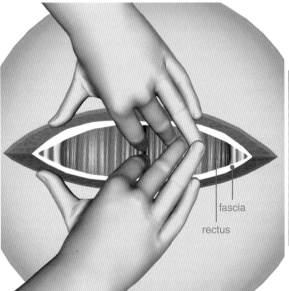

fascia

rectus

rectus

fascia peritoneum

Figure 12.19 Separating the rectus muscles.

decreased operation time, less blood loss, and improved patient outcome [LE C].[48] Because the incision is a little higher than in the Pfannenstiel incision, it is assumed that less damage occurs to the bladder.

- The lower uterus segment is incised sharply down to the membranes approximately 3 cm above the vesicouterine fold, after which the uterus is opened digitally (Figures 12.12 and 12.13).

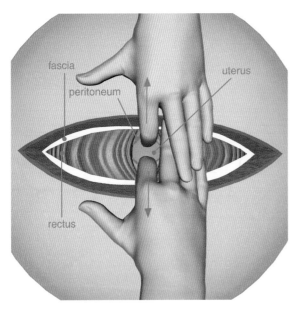

Figure 12.20 Digital opening of the parietal peritoneum.

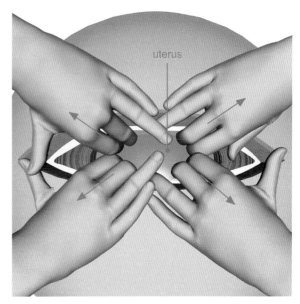

Figure 12.21 Opening the abdomen by traction.

Misgav-Ladach Method (Michael Stark Cesarean)

The method according to Misgav-Ladach (Michael Stark Cesarean), the modification named after a hospital in Jerusalem described in 1983 by Stark et al., does not differ in principle from the modification according to Joel-Cohen [LE D].[50,51] In this method the subcutis is also barely opened (approximately 2 cm down to the rectus sheath).

The following structures are then opened in succession:

- The skin and subcutis are opened as in the methods according to Joel-Cohen.
- After an incision in the midline of 2 cm (Figure 12.22A), the fascia is opened in a craniocaudal direction. This can be done with scissors or digitally (Figure 12.22B).
- The rectus muscles, the peritoneum, and the lower uterine segment are opened as in the method according to Joel-Cohen.

Dissection of the rectus sheath does not offer any advantages. Dissection of the (caudal) fascia seems to only result in negative consequences, such as more postoperative pain and lower postoperative Hb [LE A2].[52]

Of three steps originally described by the Misgav-Ladach method, i.e., carefully pushing the bladder out of the way, the standard procedure of a manual placenta removal (MPR), and the digital dilatation of the cervix, no advantages and even disadvantages have been reported. Closing the uterus outside the abdomen is possibly advantageous with respect to blood loss, because of a better view of the incision in the uterus. Also, the *locked* technique of uterine closure described in the Misgav-Ladach version is now discouraged. The subcutis is not closed and the skin is closed after approximation – by means of clamps – with only three sutures.

Maylard Method

In a Maylard incision both rectus muscles are severed crosswise with the aid of electrocoagulation. With this approach there are no advantages with respect to the amount of room over a midline incision and in terms of the muscle function analysis there may be disadvantages compared to the Pfannenstiel approach [LE A2].[53] Therefore, there seems to be no justification for the Maylard method in cesarean sections, except in the case of extreme obesity.

Supra or Subumbilical Transverse Incision

By using a skin incision 2 cm above the projection of the pubic symphyses, corresponding to a supra or subumbilical incision, in women with a voluminous panniculus a better approach to the lower uterine segment is realized. In the USA, 25% of the pregnant

A   B

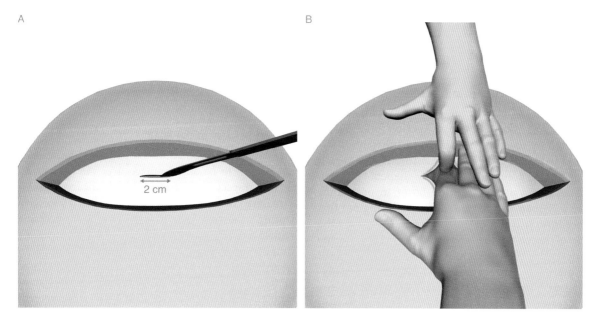

Figure 12.22 (A) Incision in the midline of 2 cm; (B) digital opening of the fascia.

population are obese. Obesity is defined as a BMI ≥30 kg/m² and morbid obesity as a BMI ≥40 kg/m². With this incision the panniculus is not moved and stays in the apron position [LE D].[54]

Uterine Incision

Corporeal Incision

A corporeal vertical incision of the uterus (a "classical cesarean section") is needed only rarely [LE D].[55]

The following are (relative) indications for a corporeal incision:

- extremely short gestational age (barely forming the lower uterine segment [LUS]);
- transverse lie, especially in case of preterm rupture of the membranes and with the back as presenting part ("back down"), so that the small extremities cannot be reached;
- large cervical myoma or serious adhesions in the true pelvis;
- placenta previa, in which large vessels run over the LUS. However, despite a presenting placenta, in an incision in the LUS, blood loss is still less than in a corporeal incision;
- cervical carcinoma during the pregnancy, in which a cesarean section is performed prior to the radical hysterectomy.

Incision of the Lower Uterine Segment

Digital Opening

To open the LUS, first a 2 cm sharp incision is made and then the uterus is further opened digitally. There is less blood loss with digital widening of the opening (843 ml versus 886 ml with a sharp incision: a difference of 43 ml; 95% CI –20 to –66 ml) and on sharp opening there is less need for transfusions (RR 0.22; 95% CI 0.1–1.01) [LE A1/2].[56,57] Blunt opening of the uterus is not associated with more endometritis [LE A1].[55] Extensions of the uterine incision are reported less often with blunt extension (RR 0.41; 95% CI 0.31–0.54) [LE A1].[56] Due to the frequent dextroposition of the uterus, a hemorrhage of the left parametric vessels or the left uterine artery may occur because of tearing of the left parametrium. As was shown in a non-blinded study, the use of an auto-suture technique suggests a clinically but not statistically significant decrease in blood loss (median –87 ml; 95% CI –175–1.1 ml) [LE A1].[56]

Transverse Versus Midline Opening of the LUS

A prospective randomized study showed that the digital opening of the uterus in both techniques (Pfannenstiel and Joel-Cohen) in the usual transverse direction compared to a craniocaudal technique results more frequently in lateral tearing (7.4% versus 3.4%: corrected OR 2.2; 95% CI 1.1–4.2) and also in more blood loss (>1500 ml: 0.2% versus 2.0%; corrected OR 8.4; 95% CI 4.2–18.5) [LE A2].[58]

Lengthening of the Transverse Incision in the LUS

Sometimes, for example in extreme growth restriction during the premature period, the space obtained by opening the LUS is insufficient and it is decided to "lengthen" the incision. In this case it is generally accepted that a "T-shaped" incision will lead to a uterine rupture faster in pregnancy than a "J-shaped" incision. Before carrying out this procedure, it is important to evaluate whether the lack of space in the uterus is due to a uterine contraction or contracture: simply waiting until the uterus relaxes again or administering a tocolytic agent (see Section: Tocolysis) may prevent any unnecessary iatrogenic trauma to the mother and the infant.

The "T-shaped" incision denotes a corporeal incision and the need for a primary cesarean section in a possible subsequent pregnancy. In a "J-shaped" incision this may not be the case, but it is something that needs to be considered. The indication for a primary cesarean section in a subsequent pregnancy must be indicated clearly by the surgeon, in both the surgical report and the discharge letter.

An extreme form of a surprise lie of the uterus is a uterine rotation of more than 180°, possibly resulting from a fixed retroflexion, in which an incision was made in the posterior wall of the uterus; which was only acknowledged after the delivery of the infant [LE D].[59] In inadequate progress of the second stage of delivery, the Bandl ring may have presented itself so high that the bladder is located much higher than expected. The bladder is then more easily damaged and is not infrequently opened iatrogenically.

In general and in order to prevent a skin lesion in the infant it is prudent to open the myometrium up to the chorion, in which the remaining fibers are pushed aside by blunt traction.

A randomized study has borne out the observation that the use of *stapling* during opening results in a (minimal) decrease in blood loss (–44 ml; 95% CI –66 to –20 ml) [LE A1][57] or no difference in blood loss [LE B],[60] in surgery of total equal duration [LE A1].[57]

Delivery

Delivery of the Head

The goal of the delivery is to have the infant's head flexed. This can usually be done with a flat hand. In an occiput or sinciput posterior presentation it is best to first turn the occiput to anterior.

Difficult Delivery of the Head

The standard use of instruments to deliver the head has not proven to be an advantage over the open hand. In this respect – in case of a non-engaged head – a (manual) vacuum cup (Kiwi) can be used if necessary. During a secondary cesarean after an unsuccessful vaginal attempt the fetal head can be deeply engaged – "impacted." Two techniques can then be used: the "push" technique, whereby the fetal head is displaced to the uterine cavity with manual pressure via the vagina and the reverse breech "pull" technique whereby there is a primary attempt to deliver first the breech (Figure 12.23). In small, non-randomized studies some advantages have been described for the "pull" technique. Less extension of the uterine incision is seen and also a "J-incision" is needed less frequently. Also less maternal fever and less urinary tract infections are reported, while neonatal outcomes are not different [LE C].[61,62]

Fundus Pressure

It has been hypothesized that the application of fundus pressure to assist extraction of the baby increases fetomaternal transfusion, and warrants careful preventive management of rhesus immunization in rhesus negative women. However, one randomized trial did not find any difference in transplacental microtransfusion between cesarean births with or without fundus pressure [LE A2].[63]

Tocolysis

In a difficult delivery of the infant some clinics use glyceryl trinitrate (= nitroglycerin). In a randomized study, a *routine* use of intravenous nitroglycerin (0.25 and 0.50 mg) or placebo showed no difference in the ease of the fetal extraction or in a decrease in uterine tone [LE A1].[64] A higher IV dose (100–250 μg) has been clinically applied, but not enough clinical trials have been done [LE A1/C].[65,66] Alternative forms of administration, such as sublingual (800 μg), have been described [LE D].[67] Until more evidence becomes

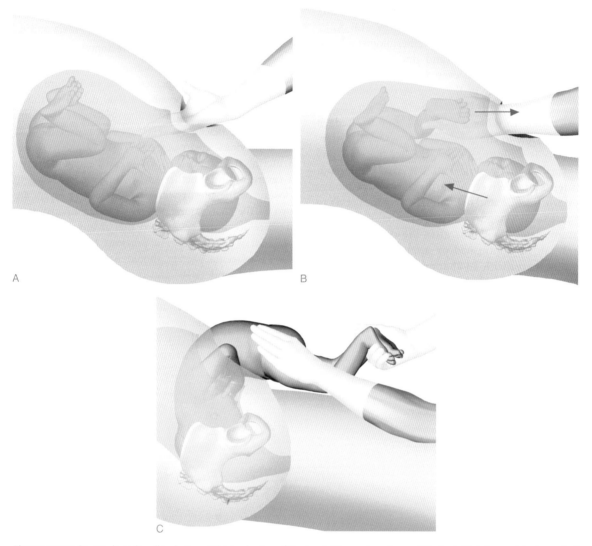

Figure 12.23 Reverse breech pull technique. (A) Introduction of the hand; (B) grasping of one of the feet; (C) delivery of the buttocks first, followed by the body and head.

available, as stated before, it is important that an operator demonstrates patience in allowing a contracting uterus to relax to prevent unnecessary surgical or medical harm to mother and child.

Delivery of the Placenta

A randomized study showed that a spontaneous placental delivery or with a lightly *controlled cord traction* has clear advantages over a manual removal of the placenta (MRP), i.e.:

- less blood loss, estimated 94 ml (95% CI 17–172 ml) [LE A1][68];
- higher Ht [LE A2][69] and Hb [LE A2].[70]

The performance of an MRP is associated with an increased risk of low Ht: –1.6 (95% CI –3.1–0.01) [LE A1][68];

- almost 40% lower risk of significant blood loss [LE A2].[71] The performance of an MPR is associated with an increased risk of blood loss of more than 1 l: 1.8 (95% CI 1.4–2.3) [LE A1].[68]

MRPs are also associated with a higher infection risk (endometritis) (OR 1.6; 95% CI 1.4–1.9), a tendency toward increased fetomaternal transfusion (OR 1.6; 95% CI 0.8–3.2) [LE A1/2],[68,69] and a longer hospital stay: 0.4 (95% CI 0.2–0.6) [LE A1].[68]

The administration of 5 IU of oxytocin (intravenous) [LE A1][7] or carbetocin 100 μg IV [LE A2][15] decreases the blood loss. The anesthesiologist administers the oxytocin by IV (and not in the uterus). Delaying cord clamping even for 3 minutes favors child outcome, even in the long term, and has no maternal drawbacks [LE D, A1].[72–74]

Although this has not been demonstrated, it seems sensible to check manually whether the uterine cavity is really empty and whether there are any abnormalities in the shape of the uterus. Wiping out the uterus after delivery of the placenta with a sponge is not worthwhile, and digitally opening the cervix to enhance the drainage from the uterus has no support in study data. Blood loss after the delivery of the infant can be diminished by applying pressure to the wound area with an abdominal gauze pad. This can also be consciously used to include a pause in the operation. The placement of (atraumatic) uterine clamps and the insertion of two hemostatic sutures at the corners of the incision may also decrease the blood loss.

Removal of the Placenta during the Cesarean Section in Case of a (Complete) Placenta Previa and/or Placenta Accreta (Cesarean Hysterectomy)

Placenta accreta is a morbid adherence of the placenta to the myometrium. The incidence was rare before 1950, but has increased to possibly 3/1000 deliveries; this is related to the increase in number of cesarean sections. Most of the placenta accreta are inserted at the scar of a previous cesarean section [LE C].[75] Whether a uterine dehiscence (niche) should be repaired after a cesarean, and whether such a finding is related to closure of the uterus with one versus two layers are two of the many questions that remain unanswered. It therefore must be realized that if any part of the placenta is located near a previous cesarean section scar, a placenta accreta should be considered. Both ultrasound and MRI are considered to be useful modalities in its diagnosis, although it can never be completely conclusive and the definitive diagnosis can only be made at surgery [LE D].[76] 3D power Doppler and MRI possibly have the same good test characteristics (sensitivity: 100%; specificity 85%;

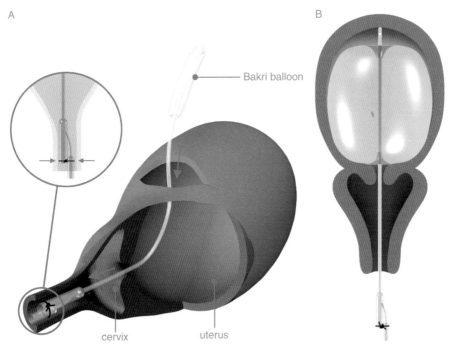

Figure 12.24 Bakri balloon tamponade. (A) Tip of Bakri balloon – the two "canals" fixed together with a suture thread – inserted via the uterine incision through the cervix; (B) the inflated Bakri balloon after closure of the uterine incision.

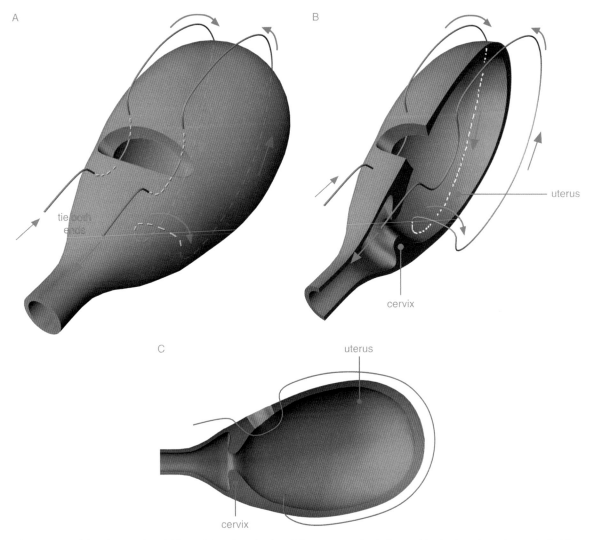

Figure 12.25 B-Lynch procedure. (A) Frontal view: introduction of the suture starting below and leaving just above the uterine incision. (B) Sagittal view: the suture is introduced and leaves at the dorsal side of the uterus, just above the cervix. (C) Sagital schematic view: the suture is tied at the frontal side of the uterus just above the cervix.

PPV 88%; risk 100%). Both placenta accreta and placenta previa increase the risk of severe postpartum hemorrrhage (PPH). As pharmacological treatment fails in general in these cases, massive hemorrhage occurring after removal of a placenta previa due to the poor contractility of the lower uterine segment is treated with different modalities by packing of the lower uterine segment with gauze, balloon tamponade (Figure 12.24) [LE C/D],[77,78] a stepwise ligation of the uterine vessels or of the internal iliac arteries, uterus compression with a (modified) B-Lynch procedure (Figure 12.25) [LE D],[79] and embolization or hysterectomy. The lower uterine segment full-thickness compression sutures, which are applied after anterior–posterior decompression of the LUS, have been shown to be successful in reducing blood loss. It consists of two fast absorbable sutures that are passed on both sides of the uterus, 2 cm from the edge of the uterus from anterior to posterior and then back, and then knotted (Figure 12.26) [LE D/C].[79,80] This seems a more rational choice for this complication than craniocaudal compression sutures (Hayman), which are primarily intended for treatment of uterine atony (Figure 12.27).

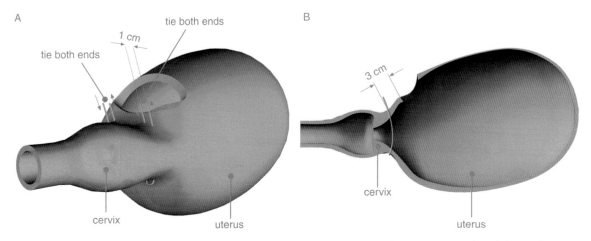

Figure 12.26 Full-thickness compression sutures. (A) An absorbable suture is introduced from the anterior side and then to the posterior side and back again. Both ends are 1 cm distant from each other and are tied in the frontal aspect of the uterus, above the cervix. (B) The compression sutures are introduced at the two sides: 3 cm under the uterine incision and 2 cm from the lateral uterine wall.

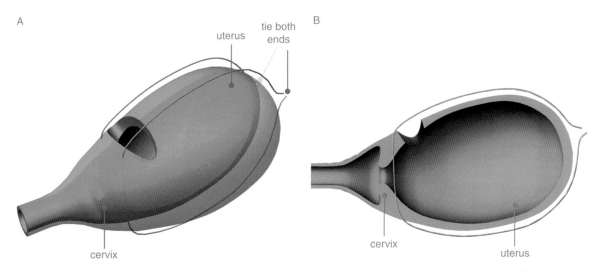

Figure 12.27 Hayman compression sutures. (A) Two separate sutures are introduced just below the uterine incision; (B) the sutures are tied at the fundal site of the uterus.

Extra-abdominal or Intra-abdominal Uterine Closure

It may be useful to *lift* the uterus out of the abdomen, as this improves the view of the uterine incision. Compared to the intra-abdominal closure of the uterus, this procedure is associated with a decrease in febrile periods of more than 3 days (RR 0.4; 95% CI 0.2–0.97), without a clear difference in other morbidity variables [LE A1].[81] More recent randomized studies indicate that the extra-abdominal closure of the uterus is done faster than the intra-abdominal closure [LE A2][82] and that intraoperative blood loss is less [LE A2],[83,84] but aside from that there is also an increase in perioperative nausea and tachycardia with spinal anesthesia [LE A2][85] and an increase in pain symptoms after 6 hours [LEA2][82] and during the first 2 postpartum days [LE A2].[86] It has also been reported that the intestinal function resumes more slowly after extra-abdominal closure [LE A2][79] and there is uncertainty on an increase (0.24 days; 95% CI 0.08–0.39) [LE A1][81] or decrease in the hospital stay (0.8 days) [LE A2].[87] However, a recent RCT does not confirm all these findings, suggesting that both methods can be valid options during surgery with a minor decrease in surgery time (3 minutes) and a minor difference (0.2 days) in hospital stay after intra-abdominal repair [LE A2].[87] A meta-analysis – including 11 RCTs published before 2008 – shows no differences in all these findings. There are no data on adhesion formation as a result of extra-abdominal closure of the uterus [LE C].[88]

Uterine Closure

The uterine incision is usually closed with a one- or two-layer, continuous, atraumatic (non-locking) stitch, using multifilament thread (e.g., with polyglactin 910–1). This produces a better tension distribution of the suture (compared to a locked technique and the knotted technique), which can spiral through the wound area in a shorter operative time: 7.4 minutes (95% CI −8.4–6.5) [LE A1],[57] with less blood loss: 70 ml (95% CI −102 to −39 ml) and less postoperative pain (RR 0.7; 95% CI 0.5–0.9) [LE A1/B].[57,60]

In the CAESAR trial no difference in maternal infectious morbidity was found after single- versus double-layer closure of the uterine incision (RR 1.0; 95% CI 0.9–1.2) [LE A2].[89]

Ultrasound testing performed regularly up to 6 weeks postpartum shows no difference between one-layer and two-layer closures in the decrease in thickness of the uterine scar [LE A2].[90]

There are no serious arguments against closing in two layers, although a minor study found that after closing the uterus in one layer there were radiologically fewer scar defects [LE B].[91] In patients who were randomized for one-layer or for two-layer closure, no difference was found in negative outcomes in a subsequent pregnancy for either the mother or the child (interpregnancy interval, vaginal delivery, preterm delivery, placental abruption, uterine dehiscence). However, the groups were small, including only 18% of the original cohort [LE B].[92] A retrospective study found more uterine ruptures after one-layer closure (OR 4.0; 95% CI 1.4–11.5). In this study, the uterus was closed in one layer with chromic catgut suture and a locked closure, two factors which contribute to additional necrosis of the uterine scar and therefore a poorer healing of the scar [LE B].[93] In a recent meta-analysis of eight observational studies and an RCT (n = 5810 pregnancies) the risk of uterine rupture and uterine dehiscence in a trial of labor in the next pregnancy was not different between single- versus double-layer closure (OR 1.7; 95% CI 0.7–4.4). Interestingly, confirming the former study, this risk is compared to double-layer closure, increased after a locked single-layer closure

(OR 5.0; 95% CI 2.6–9.5) and not after an unlocked single-layer closer (OR 0.5; 95% CI 0.2–1.2) [LE C].[94] The ever-continuing discussion led to setting up the previously mentioned randomized study ("CAESAR") into the different surgical techniques of a cesarean section (National Perinatal Epidemiology Unit: www.npeu.ox.ac.uk/caesar).[89] In addition to one-layer or two-layer closings, this study also looked into the effects of whether or not to close the parietal peritoneum. Long-term outcomes, especially on uterine rupture in a next pregnancy, await elucidation.

The thickness of the uterine wall for suturing has not been studied sufficiently, just as whether or not to include the serosa and/or the decidua in the suturing (inverted "endometrium-sparing" suturing). At this time, no valuable recommendations can be formulated on these aspects [LE A1].[95] The use of a large abdominal sponge after the infant's birth for applying pressure to the wound area results in a shorter operative time.

Inspection of the Adnexa and Sterilization

It is good practice to inspect (and possibly palpate) the adnexa after closing the uterus in order to rule out any adnexal pathology. No studies have been done on the usefulness of this procedure.

If the partners made a request for sterilization during the weeks prior to the cesarean section, this can be done during this phase of the intervention. The most frequently used method is the Pomeroy technique, in which a bilateral 2–3 cm portion of fallopian tube is resected at the isthmus level after prior distal and proximal ligation. Traditionally, for reasons of a greater inflammatory response, catgut was used for this procedure. By analogy with tubal ligation in general, the *lifetime* risk of a failing tubal ligation during a cesarean section is estimated at 1:200, but specific studies on this have not been published [LE A1].[7] Sterilizations are also done with a Falope Ring or a Filshie clip. It is assumed that by using one of these two techniques the chance of pregnancy is more successful after a possible refertilization. An observational study (2–15 years) showed no differences in pregnancy rate between a Pomeroy technique (0/203) and Filshie clips application (1/85) [LE C].[96] The Filshie clip application is quicker and is simpler. Intraoperative sterilization during a cesarean is a practical and safe method and has as a second advantage that less negative effects were found on ovarian reserve [LE C].[97] Also the placement of an intrauterine device (IUD) through the incision at the time of cesarean birth is a possibility [LE D].[98]

Peritoneal Closure

Despite the fact that since the 1926 article by Kerr it has been standard practice to close the visceral and parietal peritoneum to prevent adhesions, this method has been losing popularity in recent years. It appeared that when suturing the peritoneum there was a slower postoperative recovery.

The advantages of not closing the peritoneum compared to closing it are as follows:

- Owing to a possible diminished ischemia because of suturing and a decreased fibrinolysis shown in animal experiments it is now generally believed that closing the peritoneum actually causes more adhesion formation [LE A2/B].[45,99] The percentage of serious adhesions increases with each cesarean section. The percentage is 0.2% for the first cesarean section, while 11.5% of serious adhesions are encountered in the second cesarean, and this increases to 44.5% in the fourth cesarean [LE C].[100] In one follow-up study of an RCT comparing the Pfannenstiel cesarean with a modified (Joel-Cohen) cesarean technique (with without bladder formation and with non-closure of the peritoneum; 62 patients in each group), the number of adhesions seen at repeat cesarean (the primary outcome) was higher with a Pfannenstiel cesarean (RR 3.1; 95% CI 1.5–6.8). In the classic Pfannenstiel technique there was also more fibrosis of the anterior abdominal wall and the bladder was found adherent to the uterus more often [LE A2].[101] With the repeat cesarean, operation time, blood loss, time to mobilization, and postoperative hospital stay all favored the modified technique. In an RCT where closure and non-closure of both the visceral and parietal peritoneum were compared, the proportion of patients with adhesions at repeat cesarean was the same in both groups (60% in the closure and 51% in the non-closure group; p = 0.31), with comparable mean adhesion scores [LE A2].[102]
- This debate is still ongoing as a meta-analysis (33 observational studies) provided strong evidence for closure of the peritoneum. Two groups – with and without closure of the peritoneum – were compared using the Stark technique. More adhesions were found when the peritoneum was left open compared to when it was closed (OR 4.7; 95% CI 3.3–6.6) [LE A1].[103]

- A randomized study showed that there is less chance of ileus when the peritoneum is left open. Not closing both peritoneal layers is not linked to more wound dehiscence and it also shortens the surgical duration (7.3 minutes; 95% CI 8.4–6.4 minutes) [LE A1/2/B].[99,104–106]
- Fewer infections occur and there is a decrease in febrile duration (OR 0.62; 95% CI 0.41–0.94) [LE A1/2].[99,104] This finding was confirmed in the CAESAR trial where no difference in maternal infectious morbidity was found after closure versus non-closure of the pelvic peritoneum (RR 0.9; 95% CI 0.8–1.1) [LE A2].[89]
- The need for pain medication is lessened [LE A2].[105] All of this results in a decrease in hospitalization stay by less than 1 day (–0.4; 95% CI –0.5 to –0.3) [LE A1][104] making the cesarean section less expensive.

The problem with these data is that they are primarily based on short-term results. In contrast to the Stark study [LE B],[46] two recent prospective studies found that the number of adhesions increases in the long term [LE B].[106,107] In a group of patients who underwent a primary cesarean section after a prior cesarean in which the peritoneal layers were closed, there were clearly less adhesions (OR 0.20; 95% CI 0.08–0.49) compared to a group in which the peritoneal layers were not closed [LE B].[107] This was confirmed in a randomized study in which closure or non-closure of the peritoneal layers was observed in a second cesarean. More adhesions were observed in the non-closure group (RR 3.2; 95% CI 1.0–10.2) [LE B].[106] Although the evidence points in the direction of not closing the peritoneum, the results of the CAESAR trial should shed more light on this matter (National Perinatal Epidemiology Unit; www.npeu.ox.ac.uk/caesar).[89]

Fascia Closure

No study data are available on the short- and long-term results of methods and materials for closing the fascia [LE A1].[94] In most cases one continuous (non-locked) suture is used [LE A1],[108] either with a monofilament suture, e.g., polydioxanone (PDS) 0, or absorbable, twisted synthetic suture, such as polyglactin 910–1. For this, the 10–10 rule or the 20–10 rule can be used: the distance between the sutures, 10 or 20 mm, and the distance to the fascial edge, 10 mm. The advantage of a continuous suture is that the spiraling closure of fascia results in a more even pressure distribution on the fascial edges. This continuous suture may be fixed on both sides to separately placed corner stitches.

There are no study results on the benefits or adverse effects of approximating the rectus muscles over the midline. There is a general consensus that this intervention has potentially more disadvantages than advantages [LE A1].[94]

Subcutis Closure

The theoretical advantages and disadvantages of closing the subcutaneous fat layer are interpreted differently, depending on the thickness of the subcutis [LE A1].[108] As a theoretical advantage, closing the subcutaneous layer has better wound healing because of a lesser chance of hematomas and seromas. The value of the study is doubtful due to the subjectivity in the assessment of the endpoints of the study. In a randomized, non-blinded study no advantage was found in subcutis closure after 4 months, with respect to wound healing and patient satisfaction [LE B][109] Furthermore, the conclusion of most studies advise against subcutis closure. The meta-analysis of the whole group did not demonstrate any advantages in terms of wound infections, operational duration, and average blood loss. Nevertheless, there are indications that less hematoma and seroma formation occurs when the subcutis has been closed (RR 0.5; 95% CI 0.3–0.8) [LE A1].[108]

Thin Subcutis

In case of a very thin subcutis, it seems prudent to close it in order to prevent skin adhesions to the fascia. Also, the subcutis contains a very fine connective tissue net that, if approximated, decreases traction on the skin.

Thick Subcutis

If the subcutis is thicker (>2–3 cm), it is a good idea to close it, e.g., with polyglycolic acid 3.0 or Rapide polyglactin 910. This has a favorable effect on decreasing the amount of hematomas and seromas (RR 0.42; 95% CI 0.24–0.75) and infections [LE A1].[95]

It is recommended to close or drain a subcutaneous layer with a thickness of at least 2–3 cm. If, however, a subcutis of 2–3 cm or more is not closed, again fewer wound complications are reported with the placement of a 24-hour wound drain [LE A1].[95] There are no comparative studies on suturing versus draining, or on a combination of both.

In the CAESAR trial no difference in maternal infectious morbidity was found after liberal versus restricted use of a subrectus sheath drain (RR 0.9; 95% CI 0.8–1.1) [LE A2].[89]

Skin Closure

There is no general consensus on the method for closing the skin after a cesarean section.

The skin can be closed with a continuous, intracutaneous absorbable suture that does not have to be removed (e.g., Rapide polyglactin 910 or polyglactin 910 4-0). Using staples is a faster method (5–10 minutes) [LE A1],[110,111] but in one study more pain symptoms were reported [LE A1][110]; however, a more recent RCT shows significantly less pain 6 weeks postoperatively [LE A1/A2].[110,112] The results for incision appearance are comparable ([LE B][109] and [LE A2][112]), especially where the neat wound edges are not lost as a result of the (unnecessary) gain in speed. A meta-analysis, however, showed more wound separation (OR 4.0; 95% CI 2.1–8.0) and more wound complications (OR 2.1; 95% CI 1.3–3.5) [LE A1],[111] suggesting a possible benefit in using subcuticular stitches for closure of a cesarean section.

Conclusions

In summary, there appears to be an advantage to replacing several sharp incision steps in the cesarean section technique with digital steps [LE A1/2/C].[113–115] Two modifications, the Misgav-Ladach or the Joel-Cohen modification, have shown a number of advantages compared to the Pfannenstiel technique, whereby a reduction of 65% has been found in reported postoperative morbidity in general (RR 0.4; 95% CI 0.1–0.9). More specifically this concerns (except for adhesions) only the following short-term results:

- a shorter operation time: 11 minutes (95% CI –6 to –17 minutes);
- less blood loss: 58 ml (95% CI –8 to –109 ml);
- less fever (RR 0.35; 95% CI 0.1–0.9), and decreased antibiotics use (RR 0.5; 95% CI 0.3–0.8);
- less suturing material [LE C];[113]
- shorter duration of postoperative pain: 14.2 hours (95% CI –10.0 to –18.3 hours), less use of injections for pain relief: –0.9 injections (95% CI –0.6 to –1.2), and less use of analgesics (RR 0.6; 95% CI 0.4–0.8);
- shorter hospitalization time: 1.5 days (95% CI –0.8 to –2.2 days);
- tendency for a 6.7-hour (95% CI –15.3–1.8 hours) [LE A1][115] faster recovery of intestinal function [LE C];[113]

Table 12.1 Comparison between complication rates after cesarean and vaginal deliveries

	Absolute risk (%)		Relative risk (RR)		Evidence (LE)
	Cesarean section	Vaginal	Cesarean section versus vaginal	95% CI	Degree
Maternal effects					
Peripartum					
Perineal pain	2	5	0.3	0.2–0.6	A2
Abdominal pain	9	5	1.9	1.3–2.8	A2
Bladder or intestinal lesion	0.1	0.001	25.2–36.6	2.6–243.5	C
Re-intervention	0.5	0.03	17.58	9.4–32.1	B
Hysterectomy	0.7–0.8	0.01–0.02	44.0–95.5	22.5–136.9	B
Intensive care admission	0.9	0.1	9	7.2–11.2	C
Thromboembolism	General = 0.04–0.16		3.8	2.0–4.9	B
Hospitalization stay extension	3–4 days	1–2 days			A2
Readmission after discharge	5.3	2.2	3.8	2.0–4.9	B
Maternal death	0.008	0.002	4.9	3.0–8.0	C
Hemorrhage >1000 ml	0.5	0.7	0.8	0.4–4.4	A1
Infection	6.4	4.9	1.3	1.0–1.7	A1
Trauma of the genital tract	0.6	0.8	1.2	0.4–3.4	A1
Long term					
Urinary incontinence (3 months)	4.5	7.3	0.6	0.4–0.9	A2
Urethrocystocele	General = 5		0.6	0.5–0.9	C
Fecal incontinence	0.8	1.5	0.5	0.2–1.6	A2
Back pain	11.3	12.2	0.9	0.7–1.2	A2
Postnatal depression	10.1	10.8	0.9	0.7–1.2	A2
Dyspareunia	17	18.7	0.9	0.7–1.1	A2
Effect on next pregnancy					
No next pregnancy	42	29	1.5	1.1–2.0	B
Placenta previa	0.4–0.8	0.2–0.5	1.3–1.6	1.0–2.0	B
Scar rupture	0.4	0.01	42.2	31.5–57.2	B
Neonatal effects					
Intrauterine death	0.4	0.2	1.6	1.2–2.3	B
Respiratory morbidity after elective cesarean section	3.5	0.5	6.8	5.2–8.9	C
Neonatal death (excluding breech)	0.1	0.1	1.1	0.1–8.4	B
Intracranial bleeding	0.008–0.04	0.01–0.03	0.6	0.1–2.5	B
Brachial plexus lesion	General = 0.05		0.5	0.1–1.9	C
Cerebral palsy	General = 0.2				C

Source: NICE guidelines, 2004, pages 22–3.[7]

- less time before oral intake can begin: 3.9 hours (95% CI −0.7 to −7.1 hours);
- fewer adhesions in a second cesarean section [LE B];[45,107,116]
- no difference in the number of wound infections (RR 1.4; 95% CI 0.5–3.9);
- no difference in wound dehiscences (RR 0.9; 95% CI 0.4–2.1);
- no difference in Apgar scores <7 (RR 0.2; 95% CI 0.01–3.7 hours).

Complications

Maternal Complications

Complications in cesarean sections are not that rare and they must always be weighed against the possible complications of a vaginal delivery. A comparison between maternal and neonatal complications in a cesarean versus a vaginal delivery is shown in Table 12.1 [LE A1].[7] It is important to identify these complications correctly and communicate them to the pregnant woman during the informational discussion prior to the procedure. From a recent Norwegian study it appears that one or more apparent maternal complications occur in 21% of all cesarean sections, and have been coded as such by the surgeon [LE C].[28]

In the following circumstances the chance of maternal complications is increased:

- In an advanced (>9 cm or more) dilatation the risk of complication is 33%, compared to 17% in the case of no dilatation (OR 2.4; 95% CI 1.8–3.2). As the dilatation advances, a higher number of emergency cesarean sections take place and the percentage of GA – which carries a higher maternal risk – also increases drastically [LE C].[28] In emergency cesarean sections no increase has been found in blood loss and bladder or intestinal lesions [LE B].[31]
- Unplanned cesarean sections carry a higher risk of complications (24%) than planned ones (16%; OR 1.6; 95% CI 1.3–2.0) [LE B].[28]
- The risks are greater in case of insufficient supervision and insufficient experience. Experience can be improved by practicing in a *skills lab.*
- There is a greater risk with cesarean sections in the preterm period (<30 weeks): RR 1.0 (95% CI 1.1–3.1).
- There is a greater risk with ruptured membranes.
- There is a greater risk with a fully engaged head.
- A macrosomic infant increases the risk for the mother.
- "Haste" appears to be an independent risk factor (RR 1.7) [LE C].[28]
- Maternal obesity (BMI >30 kg/m^2) is an independent risk factor in the occurrence of complications after cesarean sections. As a result of obesity, surgeons not only find more technical difficulties that can lengthen the operational duration, but also there is more blood loss, as well as a greater chance of postoperative wound infections and thromboembolic complications [LE C].[37]
- Prior pelvic surgery also increases the chance of complications.

Re-closing of a dehiscent cesarean scar of the skin is associated with faster healing of the wound and fewer postoperative visits to the outpatient clinic than with secondary wound healing [LE A1].[117] Not enough study data are available regarding the moment and the technique of the re-intervention and the benefit of antibiotics [LE A1].[95]

Neonatal Complications

In a cesarean section respiratory complications, such as tachypnea (*wet lung syndrome* and *respiratory distress syndrome* [RDS] type II), RDS, and pulmonary hypertension, become elevated, possibly because in a cesarean section less amniotic fluid is removed from the lungs [LE C].[118] The literature describes greatly divergent ORs in this respect: for tachypnea (OR 1.2–2.8); RDS (OR 1.3–7.1); persistent pulmonary hypertension (OR 4.6; 95% CI 1.9–11).

The risk of neonatal complications is influenced by the following factors.

- *Contraction activity:* a protective effect is found in having had contractions (OR 1.9; 95% CI 1.2–2.9). Without contraction activity the OR is 2.6 (95% CI 1.3–2.8) [LE B].[119] In a cesarean section between 34 and 37 weeks (without prior contraction activity) there is an occurrence of neonatal intensive care hospitalization due to serious RDS in 28% of neonates; in 30%, admission is needed due to mild RDS.
- *Gestational age:* this is the most important risk factor (a cesarean section before 36 weeks has an OR of 2.1; 95% CI 1.0–4.4 of serious RDS). In addition, singleton pregnancies (OR 3.2; 95% CI 1.5–6.7) and a fetal indication of a cesarean section (OR 2.7; 95% CI 1.2–5.7) have a risk elevation effect, while early rupturing of the membranes has a protective action (OR 0.2; 95% CI 0.1–0.8) against contracting serious RDS [LE C].[120] In a group of children born after an elective cesarean section from the 37th week it appeared that between 5.1% and 6.2% of the children had contracted respiratory complications [LE B/C].[121,122] Prevention is highly dependent on the gestational age: at 37 weeks the incidence is 73.8/1000 and it decreases to 17.8 at 39 weeks [LE B].[118] See Table 12.2 [LE B/D].[120,123,124]

Table 12.2 Neonatal complications related to gestational age

Gestational age in weeks	Neonatal respiratory complications after elective cesarean section (range in %)	OR to respiratory morbidity [LE B][124]
37 0/7–37 6/7	7.4–11	3.9 (95% CI 2.4–6.5)
38 0/7–38 6/7	4.2–8.4	3.0 (95% CI 2.1–4.3)
39 0/7–40 0/7	0.8–2.1	1.9 (95% CI 1.2–3.0)

In the entire group of term pregnancies, after a planned cesarean section the number of pulmonary complications is low at 1.6% (but twice as much, however, compared to a planned vaginal delivery: RR 2.1; 95% CI 1.2–3.7) and there are also nearly twice the amount of admissions to the neonatal intensive care unit at 10% (RR 1.7; 95% CI 1.4–2.2) [LE B].[125]

For infants born at a gestational age of >39 weeks, no difference is encountered in pulmonary complications [LE B/D].[121,125] This is the decisive argument for planning an elective cesarean section as early as week 39 0/7 or to wait for spontaneous contraction activity and then perform a cesarean section [LE A2].[126] To decrease the number of emergency cesarean sections it can locally be agreed, in principle, to only perform primary cesarean sections from week 38 0/7.

Follow-up Care after Cesarean Sections

The following can be noted with regard to after-care for cesarean sections [LE A1].[7] Just as after a vaginal delivery, early direct skin contact between mother and child has a positive influence on the mother/child relationship, as well as the success rate of breastfeeding. It is therefore recommended to stimulate the mother/child contact as early as possible after the cesarean section [LE D].[127]

Besides continuing the epidural analgesic, opiates are indicated for perioperative and immediate postoperative pain relief, while in the later postpartum period preference is given to non-steroidal anti-inflammatory medication. During an uncomplicated postpartum development after a cesarean section, the woman may commence eating and drinking on request and an early discharge is not contraindicated.

Long-term Complications

After a previous cesarean section, the risk of serious complications is increased in a subsequent pregnancy.

- There is a greater chance of a cesarean section in a subsequent pregnancy. It is assumed that approximately 50% of cesarean sections concern a previous cesarean section in the medical history.
- The OR of a placenta previa is 1.9 (95% CI 1.7–2.2) to 2.7 (95% CI 2.3–3.2) [LE A1].[128] The risk of a placenta previa (or other serious maternal morbidity) increases with the number of cesarean sections in the medical history and the parity [LE B].[128,129] A para 2 with one cesarean section

in the history already has an increased risk of placenta previa (OR 1.4; 95% CI 1.1–1.8). This risk increases even more with the parity and the number of cesarean sections: para 3 with three prior cesarean sections (OR 4.1; 95% CI 1.5–11.0) [LE B].[130]

- Placenta accreta is found especially in a patient with a placenta previa and prior cesarean section. In a second cesarean section this percentage is 11%; in a third cesarean section it is as much as 40% [LE B].[130] In the absence of placenta previa, the OR for a placenta accreta is 2.4 (95% CI 1.3–4.3) in a third cesarean section. After a fourth cesarean section, the OR for a hysterectomy is 3.8 (2.4–6.0) [LE B].[130]
- There is an increased risk of a uterine rupture in a subsequent vaginal delivery of 3.9 per 1000 deliveries compared to 1.6 per 1000 in an elective subsequent cesarean section (OR 2.1; 95% CI 1.5–3.1) [LE A1].[131]
- Prenatal death beyond 39 weeks of a subsequent pregnancy is slightly increased: 1.1/1000 compared to 0.5/1000 in a pregnancy without cesarean section, in which the relative risk after 34 weeks is already increased: RR 2.7 (95% CI 1.7–4.3) [LE B].[132] This association is only found in the African American population (OR 1.4; 95% CI 1.1–1.7) [LE B].[133]
- There is more perinatal death in attempted vaginal delivery than in elective cesarean sections: RR 11.6 (95% CI 1.6–86.7) [LE B].[134]
- Maternal death remains rare, although many other forms of surgical morbidity, such as bladder and intestinal lesions, necessity of a blood transfusion, artificial respiration, and intensive care hospitalization, increase with the number of cesarean sections in the medical history.
- Subfertility is slightly increased after a term primary cesarean section (RR 1.2; 95% CI 1.1–1.2) [LE C].[135]

Pregnancy and Delivery after Cesarean Section

After a cesarean section for a non-repetitive indication, and in the absence of contraindications during the next pregnancy, a vaginal delivery can be pursued. It is not known whether this advice is also true after (two or) three cesarean sections in the medical history. The literature reports a variable chance of successful vaginal delivery after a cesarean section, varying between 21% and 86% [LE A1].[7] The choice of a delivery method after prior cesarean section is once again a joint decision between the physician and the pregnant woman and her partner, who must be sufficiently informed. The potential pros and cons of both delivery methods must be considered in this decision, as well as the potential risks of scar rupture and perinatal mortality/morbidity.

The chance of a vaginal delivery after a prior cesarean section increases if a vaginal delivery was already performed before that, and decreases if the woman has already had more than one cesarean section [LE A1].[7] Pregnant women with a cesarean scar are recommended to give birth in a setting with an availability of continuous electronic fetal monitoring and a possibility for emergency cesarean section under safe circumstances.

Perimortem Cesarean

After a maternal cardiac arrest and a non-immediate successful resuscitation, it is recommended to perform a cesarean section within 4 minutes, in order to increase the chance of survival of the infant as well as a chance of a successful cardiopulmonary resuscitation. Although the data are far from optimal, the neonatal results do not appear unfavorable, and there is a clear improvement of the cardiac output after the cesarean section [LE C].[136]

Important Points and Recommendations

Preoperative Aspects

- Regional anesthesia for cesarean section is safer than GA [LE A1].
- Positioning of the mother in a semi-prone sideways lie on the left side reduces the chance of maternal hypotension [LE D].

Operative Aspects

- To prevent neonatal respiratory morbidity, it is best to plan an elective cesarean section during the last week of the pregnancy (>39 weeks) [LE A1].
- Opening the abdominal wall according to the Joel-Cohen technique reduces the total operational time and the postoperative febrile morbidity [LE A1].

- It is advisable not to routinely slide the bladder out of the way and open the lower uterine segment above the vesicouterine fold [LE A1].
- Opening the lower uterine segment by digital extension of the scar reduces the blood loss and the need for postpartum transfusion [LE A1].
- A single RCT shows that digitally opening the lower uterine segment in a craniocaudal direction is preferred [LE A2].
- The one-time administration of antibiotics before making the skin incision reduces the chance of postpartum endometritis and wound infections [LE A1].
- The administration of oxytocin agonists (oxytocin or carbetocin) is desirable to prevent significant blood loss after a cesarean section [LE D].[137]
- Waiting for spontaneous expulsion of the placenta, with or without slight umbilical cord traction, reduces the risk of postpartum endometritis and blood loss [LE A1].
- Extra-abdominal placement of the uterus before closing the uterine incision reduces postpartum fever and blood loss [LE A1].
- Not suturing the peritoneum (both visceral and parietal) reduces the risk of postoperative fever, the total operational time, and hospitalization duration [LE A1].
- The closing of a midline abdominal wall incision with a continuous *mass closure* with slowly absorbable suture material reduces the risk of scar rupture [LE A1].
- Not closing a subcutis of less than 2–3 cm in thickness reduces the risk of wound infection or bleeding [LE A1].
- Closing a subcutis of greater than 2–3 cm in thickness reduces the risk of wound infection or bleeding [LEA1].
- The routine use of subcutaneous drains has no advantages [LE D].
- Placing a wound drain in a non-sutured subcutis between 2 and 3 cm in thickness reduces the risk of wound complications [LE A1].

Postoperative Aspects

- Immediate skin contact between mother and child as soon as possible after the cesarean section stimulates the mother/child bonding and increases breastfeeding success [LE A1].

- Opiates are the analgesics of choice during the early postpartum period after cesarean section, while during the late postpartum period non-steroidal anti-inflammatory agents are preferred [LE A1].
- During the uncomplicated postpartum period after cesarean section the patient may commence eating and drinking as desired [LE A1].

References

1   Leith CR, Walker JJ. The rise in caesarean section rate: the same indications but a lower threshold. Br J Obstet Gynaecol. 1989;**105**:621–6.

2   Wax JR. Maternal request cesarean versus planned spontaneous vaginal delivery: maternal morbidity and short term outcomes. Semin Perinatol. 2006;**30**:247–52.

3   American College of Obstetricians and Gynecologists. ACOG committee opinion no. 559: Cesarean delivery on maternal request. Obstet Gynecol. 2013;**121**:904–7.

4   Liu S, Liston RM, Joseph KS, et al. Maternal mortality and severe morbidity associated with low-risk planned cesarean delivery versus planned vaginal delivery at term. Maternal Health Study Group of the Canadian Perinatal Surveillance System. CMAJ. 2007;**176**:455–60.

5   Ecker JL, Frigoletto FD. Cesarean delivery and the risk–benefit calculus. N Engl J Med. 2007;**356**:885–8.

6   Althabe F, Sosa C, Belizan JM, et al. Cesarean section rates and maternal and neonatal mortality in low-, medium-, and high-income countries: an ecological study. Birth. 2006;**33**:270–7.

7   National Collaborating Centre for Women's and Children's Health. NICE Clinical Guideline. Caesarean section. Commissioned by the National Institute for Clinical Excellence. London: RCOG Press, 2004. http://www.nice.org.uk/pdf/CG013fullguideline.pdf

8   Hofmeyr GJ, Smaill FM. Antibiotic prophylaxis for caesarean section. Cochrane Database Syst Rev. 2002;**3**:CD000933. DOI: 10.1002/14651858.CD000933, 2002.

9   Costantine MM, Rahman M, Ghulmiyah L, et al. Timing of perioperative antibiotics for cesarean delivery: a metaanalysis. Am J Obstet Gynecol. 2008;**199**:301.e1–6.

10 Tita AT, Rouse DJ, Blackwell S, et al. Emerging concepts in antibiotic prophylaxis for cesarean delivery: a systematic review. Obstet Gynecol. 2009;**113**:675–82.

11 Lamont RF, Sobel JD, Kusanovic JP, et al. Current debate on the use of antibiotic prophylaxis for caesarean section. BJOG. 2011;**118**:193–201.

12 Anderson SB, Lin SN, Reiss J, Skupski D, Grunebaum A. Peripartum thromboprophylaxis before and after implementation of a uniform heparin protocol. J Perinat Med. 2014;**42**:219–23.

13 Quiñones JN, James DN, Stamilio DM, et al. Thromboprophylaxis after cesarean delivery: a decision analysis. Obstet Gynecol. 2005;**106**:733–40.

14 Su LL, Chong YS, Samuel M. Carbetocin for preventing postpartum haemorrhage. Cochrane Database Syst Rev. 2012;**4**:CD005457.

15 Borruto F, Treiser A, Comparetto C. Utilization of carbetocin for prevention of postpartum hemorrhage after caesarean section: a randomized clinical trial. Arch Gynecol Obstet. 2009;**280**(5):707–12. DOI 10.1007/S00404-009-0973-8.

16 Peters NCJ, Duvekot JJ. Carbetocin for the prevention of postpartum hemorrhage. A systematic review. Obstet Gynecol Surv. 2009;**64**:129–35.

17 Cluver C, Novikova N, Hofmeyr GJ, et al. Maternal position during caesarean section for preventing maternal and neonatal complications. Cochrane Database Syst Rev. 2009;**1**:CD007623. DOI: 10.1002/14651858.CD007623.

18 Senanayake H. Elective cesarean section without urethral catheterization. J Obstet Gynaecol. 2005;**31**:32–7.

19 Usta IM, Hobeika EM, Musa AA, et al. Placenta previa-accreta: risk factors and complications. Am J Obstet Gynecol. 2005;**193**:1045–9.

20 Clark SL, Koonings PP, Phelan JP. Placenta previa/accreta and prior cesarean section. Obstet Gynecol. 1985;**66**:89–92.

21 Mazouni C, Gorincour G, Juhan V, et al. Placenta accreta: a review of current advances in prenatal diagnosis. Placenta. 2007;**28**:599–603.

22 Wu S, Kocherginsky M, Hibbard JU. Abnormal placentation: twenty-year analysis. Am J Obstet Gynecol. 2005;**192**:1458–61.

23 Rac MW, Dashe JS, Wells CE, et al. Ultrasound predictors of placental invasion: the Placenta Accreta Index. Am J Obstet Gynecol. 2015;**212**:343.e1–7.

24 Comstock CH. Antenatal diagnosis of placenta accreta: a review. Ultrasound Obstet Gynecol. 2005;**26**:89–96.

25 Su TM, Lan CM, Yang LC, et al. Brain tumor presenting with fatal herniation following delivery under epidural anesthesia. Anesthesiology. 2002;**96**:508–9.

26 Butwick AJ, Carvalho B. Neuraxial anesthesia in obstetric patients receiving anticoagulant and antithrombotic drugs. Int J Obstet Anesth. 2010;**19**:193–201.

27 Jenkins JG, Khan MM. Anaesthesia for caesarean section: a survey in a UK region from 1992 to 2002. Anaesthesia. 2003;**58**:1114–18.

28 Hager RME, Daltveit AK, Hofoss D, et al. Complications of cesarean deliveries: rates and risk factors. Am J Obstet Gynecol. 2004;**109**:428–32.

29 Afolabi BB, Lesio FEA. Regional versus general anaesthesia for caesarean section. Cochrane Database Syst Rev. 2012;**10**:CD004350.

30 Ong BY, Cohen MM, Palahniuk RJ. Anesthesia for cesarean section – effects on neonates. Anesth Analg. 1989;**100**:50–4.

31 Lagrew DC, Bush MC, McKeown AM, et al. Emergent (crash) cesarean delivery indications and outcomes. Am J Obstet Gynecol. 2006;**194**:1638–43.

32 Abrams B, Parker J. Overweight and pregnancy complications. Int J Obes. 1988;**12**:293–303.

33 Soens MA, Birnbach DJ, Ranasinghe JS, et al. Obstetric anesthesia for the obese and morbidly obese patient: an ounce of prevention is worth more than a pound of treatment. Acta Anaesthesiol Scand. 2008;**52**:6–19.

34 Hood DD, Dewan DM. Anesthetic and obstetric outcome in morbidly obese patients. Anesthesiology. 1993;**79**:1210–18.

35 Munnur U, de Boisblanc B, Suresh MS. Airway problems in pregnancy. Crit Care Med. 2005;**33**(suppl 10):S259–68.

36 Jordan H, Perlow MD, Mark A, et al. Massive maternal obesity and perioperative caesarean morbidity. Am J Obstet Gynecol. 1994;**170**:560–5.

37 Rothrock RA, Kabiru W, Kelbick N, et al. Maternal obesity and postcesarean infectious morbidity. Obstet Gynecol. 2006;**107**:675.

38 Terris DJ, Seybt MW, Elchoufi M, et al. Cosmetic thyroid surgery: defining the essential principles. Laryngoscope. 2007;**117**:1169–72.

39 Hasselgren PO, Hagberg E, Malmer H, et al. One instead of two knives for surgical incision. Does it increase the risk of postoperative wound infection? Arch Surg. 1984;**119**:917–20.

40 Lipscomb GH, Givens VM. Preventing electrosurgical energy-related injuries. Obstet Gynecol Clin North Am. 2010;**37**:369–77.

41 Kearns SR, Connolly EM, McNally S, et al. Randomized clinical trial of diathermy versus scalpel incision in elective midline laparotomy Br J Surg. 2001;**88**:41–4.

42 Makoha FW, Fathuddien MA, Felimban HM. Choice of abdominal incision and risk of trauma to the uterine bladder and bowel in multiple cesarean sections. Eur J Obstet Gynecol Reprod Biol. 2006;**125**:50–3.

43 Loos MJ, Scheltinga MR, Mulders LG, Roumen RM. The Pfannenstiel incision as a source of chronic pain. Obstet Gynecol. 2008;**111**:839–46.

44 Joel-Cohen S. Abdominal and vaginal hysterectomies. New techniques based on time and motion studies. London: W Heinemann Books, 1972, p.170.

45 Stark M. Clinical evidence that suturing the peritoneum after laparotomy is unnecessary. World J Surg. 1993;**17**:419.

46 Stark M, Finkel AR. Comparison between the Joel-Cohen and Pfannenstiel incisions in caesarean section. Eur J Obstet Gynecol Reprod Biol. 1994;**53**:121–2.

47 Hohlagschwandter M, Ruecklinger E, Husslein P, et al. Is the formation of a bladder flap at cesarean necessary? A randomised trial. Obstet Gynecol. 2001;**98**:1089–92.

48 Mahajan NN. Justifying formation of bladder flap at cesarean section? Arch Gynecol Obstet. 2009;**279**: 853–5.

49 Tuuli MG, Odibo AO, Fogertey P, et al. Utility of the bladder flap at cesarean delivery: a randomized controlled trial. Obstet Gynecol. 2012;**119**:815–21.

50 Stark M, Chavkin Y, Kupfersztain C, et al. Evaluation of combinations of procedures in cesarean section. Int J Gynecol Obstet. 1993;**48**:273–6.

51 Holmgren G, Sjoholm L, Stark M. The Misgav-Ladach method for cesarean section: method description. Acta Obstet Gynecol Scand. 1999;**78**:615–21.

52 Kadir RA, Khan A, Wilcock F, Chapman L. Is inferior dissection of the rectus sheath necessary during pfannenstiel incision for lower segment caesarean section? A randomised controlled trial. Eur J Obstet Gynecol Reprod Biol. 2006;**128**:262–6.

53 Giacalone PL, Daures JP, Vignal J, et al. Pfannenstiel verus Maylard incision for cesarean delivery: a randomized controlled trial. Am J Obstet Gynecol. 2002;**99**:745–50.

54 Tixier H, Thouvenot S, Coulange L, et al. Cesarean section in morbidly obese women: supra or subumbilical transverse incision? Acta Obstet Gynecol Scand. 2009;**88**:1049–52.

55 Hema KR, Johanson R. Techniques for performing caesarean section. Best Pract Res Clin Obstet Gynaecol. 2001;**15**:17–47.

56 Magann EF, Chauhan SP, Bufkin L, et al. Intra-operative haemorrhage by blunt versus sharp expansion of the uterine incision at caesarean delivery a randomised clinical study. BJOG. 2002;**109**:448–52.

57 Dodd JM, Anderson ER, Gates S. Surgical techniques for uterine incision and uterine closure at the time of caesarean section. Cochrane Database Syst Rev. 2012;**8**:CD004732. DOI: 10.1002/14651858.CD004732.pub2.

58 Cromi A, Ghezzi F, Di Naro E, et al. Blunt expansion of the low transverse uterine incision at caesarean delivery a randomised comparison of 2 techniques. Am J Obstet Gynecol. 2008;**199**:292.e1–6.

59 Picone O, Fubini A, Doumere S, et al. Cesarean delivery by posterior hysterotomy due to torsion of the pregnant uterus. Obstet Gynecol. 2006;**107**:533–5.

60 Gilson GJ, Kephart WH, Izquierdo LA, et al. Comparison of absorbable uterine staples and

traditional hysterotomy during cesarean delivery. Obstet Gynecol. 1996;**87**:384–8.

61 Levy R, Chernomoretz T, Appelman Z, et al. Head pushing versus reverse breech extraction in cases of impacted head during Cesarean section Eur J Obstet Gynecol Reprod Biol. 2005;**121**:24–6.

62 Bastani P, Pourabolghasem S, Abbasalizadeh F, Motvalli L. Comparison of neonatal and maternal outcomes associated with head-pushing and head-pulling for impacted fetal head extraction during cesarean delivery. Int J Gynaecol Obstet. 2012;**118**:1–3. Erratum in Int J Gynaecol Obstet. 2012;**119**:292.

63 Owens M, Bhullar A, Carlan SJ, O'Brien WF, Hirano K. Effect of fundal pressure on maternal to fetal microtransfusion at the time of cesarean delivery. J Obstet Gynaecol Res. 2003;**29**:152–6.

64 David M, Halle H, Lichtenegger W, et al. Nitroglycerin to facilitate fetal extraction during cesarean delivery. Obstet Gynecol. 1998;**91**:119–24.

65 Dodd JM, Reid K. Tocolysis for assisting delivery at caesarean section. Cochrane Database Syst Rev. 2006;**2**:CD004944. DOI: 10.1002/14651858.CD004944.

66 Smith GN, Brien JF. Use of nitroglycerin for uterine relaxation. Obstet Gynecol Surv. 1998;**53**:559–65.

67 Clift K, Clift J. Uterine relaxation during caesarean section under regional anaesthesia: a survey of UK obstetric anaesthetists. Int J Obstet Anesth. 2008;**17**: 374–5.

68 Anorlu RI, Maholwana B, Hofmeyr GJ. Methods of delivering the placenta at caesarean section. Cochrane Database Syst Rev. 2008;**3**:CD004737. DOI: 10.1002/14651858.CD004737.pub2.

69 Hidar S, Jennane TM, Bouguizane S, et al. The effect of placental removal method at caesarean section delivery on preoperative hemorrhage: a randomized clinical trial ISRCTN 49779257. Eur J Obstet Gynecol Reprod Biol. 2004;**117**:179–82.

70 Dehbashi S, Honarvar M, Fardi FH. Manual removal or spontaneous placental delivery and postcesarean endometritis and bleeding. Int J Gynaecol Obstet. 2004;**86**:12–15.

71 Morales M, Ceysens G, Jastrow N, et al. Spontaneous delivery or manual removal of the placenta during caesarean section: a randomized controlled trial. BJOG. 2004;**111**:908–12.

72 van Rheenen P. Delayed cord clamping and improved infant outcomes. BMJ. 2011;**343**:d7127.

73 Andersson O, Hellström-Westas L, Andersson D, Clausen J, Domellöf M. Effects of delayed compared with early umbilical cord clamping on maternal postpartum hemorrhage and cord blood gas sampling: a randomized trial. Acta Obstet Gynecol Scand. 2013;**92**(5):567–74. DOI: 10.1111/j.1600-0412.2012.01530.

74 Andersson O, Hellström-Westas L, Andersson D, Domellöf M. Effect of delayed versus early umbilical cord clamping on neonatal outcomes and iron status at 4 months: a randomised controlled trial. BMJ. 2011;**343**:d7157.

75 Timor-Tritsch IE, Monteagudo A. Unforeseen consequences of the increasing rate of cesarean deliveries: early placenta accreta and cesarean scar pregnancy. A review. Am J Obstet Gynecol. 2012;**207**:14–29.

76 RCOG. Guideline no. 27: Placenta praevia, placenta praevia accreta and vasa praevia: diagnosis and management, 2011. https://www.rcog.org.uk/en/guide lines-research-services/guidelines/gtg27

77 Vrachnis N, Iavazzo C, Salakos N, et al. Uterine tamponade balloon for the management of massive hemorrhage during cesarean section due to placenta previa/increta. Clin Exp Obstet Gynecol. 2012;**39**: 255–7.

78 Ishii T, Sawada K, Koyama S, et al. Balloon tamponade during cesarean section is useful for severe post-partum hemorrhage due to placenta previa. J Obstet Gynaecol Res. 2012;**38**:102–7.

79 Penotti M, Vercellini P, Bolis G, Fedele L. Compressive suture of the lower uterine segment for the treatment of postpartum hemorrhage due to complete placenta previa: a preliminary study. Gynecol Obstet Invest. 2012;**73**:314–20.

80 Amorim-Costa C, Mota R, Rebelo C, Silva PT. Uterine compression sutures for postpartum hemorrhage: is routine postoperative cavity evaluation needed? Acta Obstet Gynecol Scand. 2011;**90**:701–6.

81 Jacobs-Jokhan D, Hofmeyr GJ. Extra-abdominal versus intra-abdominal repair of the uterine incision at caesarean section. Cochrane Database Syst Rev. 2004;**4**: CD000085. DOI: 10.1002Z14651858.CD000085.pub2.

82 Coutinho IC, Ramos de Amorim MM, Katz L, et al. Uterine exteriorization compared with in situ repair at cesarean delivery: a randomized controlled trial. Obstet Gynecol. 2008;**111**:639–47.

83 Orji EO, Olaleye AO, Loto OM, Ogunniyi SO. A randomised controlled trial of uterine exteriorisation and non-exteriorisation at caesarean section. Aust N Z J Obstet Gynaecol. 2008;**48**:570–4.

84 Wahab MA, Karantis P, Eccersley PS, et al. A randomised, controlled study of uterine exteriorisation and repair at caesarean section. Br J Obstet Gynaecol. 1999;**106**:913–16.

85 Siddiqui M, Goldszmidt E, Fallah S, et al. Complications of exteriorized compared with in situ repair at cesarean delivery under spinal anesthesia: a randomized controlled trial. Obstet Gynecol. 2007;**110**:570–5.

86 Nafisi S. Influence of uterine exteriorization versus in situ repair on post-cesarean maternal pain: a randomized trial. Int J Obstet Anesth. 2007;**16**:135–8.

87 Ozbay K. Exteriorized versus in-situ repair of the uterine incision at cesarean delivery: a randomized controlled trial. Clin Exp Obstet Gynecol. 2011;**38**: 155–8.

88 Kearns SR, Connolly EM, McNally S, et al. Infection rates after cesarean delivery with exteriorized versus intraperitoneal uterine closure. Obstet Gynecol. 2006;**107**:68–95.

89 CAESAR Study Collaborative Group. Caesarean section surgical techniques: a randomised factorial trial (CAESAR). BJOG. 2010;**117**:1366–76.

90 Hamar BD, Saber SB, Cackovic M, et al. Ultrasound evaluation of the uterine scar after cesarean delivery: a randomized controlled trial of one- and two-layer closure. Obstet Gynecol. 2007;**110**:808–13.

91 Lal K, Tomso K. Comparative study of single and conventional closure of uterine incision in cesarean section. Int J Obstet Gynecol. 1988;**27**:349–52.

92 Chapman SJ, Owen J, Hauth JC. One- versus two-layer closure of a low transverse cesarean: the next pregnancy. Obstet Gynecol. 1997;**89**:16–18.

93 Bujold E, Bujold C, Hamilton EF, et al. The impact of a single-layer or double-layer closure on uterine rupture. Am J Obstet Gynecol. 2002;**186**:1326–30.Discussion: Am J Obstet Gynecol. 2002;**189**:895–6.

94 Roberge S, Chaillet N, Boutin A, et al. Single- versus double-layer closure of the hysterotomy incision during cesarean delivery and risk of uterine rupture. Int J Gynaecol Obstet. 2011;**115**:5–10.

95 Berghella V, Baxter JK, Chauhun SP. Evidence-based surgery for cesarean delivery. Am J Obstet Gynecol. 2005;**193**:1607–17.

96 Oligbo N, Revicky V, Udeh R. Pomeroy technique or Filshie clips for postpartum sterilisation? Retrospective study on comparison between Pomeroy procedure and Filshie clips for a tubal occlusion at the time of Caesarean section. Arch Gynecol Obstet. 2010;**28**:1073–5.

97 Ozyer S, Moraloğlu O, Gülerman C, et al. Tubal sterilization during cesarean section or as an elective procedure? Effect on the ovarian reserve. Contraception. 2012;**86**:488–93.

98 Nelson AL, Chen S, Eden R. Intraoperative placement of the Copper T-380 intrauterine devices in women undergoing elective cesarean delivery: a pilot study. Contraception. 2009;**80**:81–3.

99 Grundsell HS, Rizk DEE, Kumar MR. Randomized study of non-closure of peritoneum in lower segment cesarean section. Acta Obstet Gynecol Scand. 1998;**77**: 110–15.

100 Makoha FW, Felimban HM, Fathuddien MA, et al. Multiple cesarean section morbidity. Int J Gynecol Obstet. 2004;**68**:227–32.

101 Nabhan AF. Long-term outcomes of two different surgical techniques for cesarean. Int J Gynaecol Obstet. 2008;**100**:69–75.

102 Kapustian V, Anteby EY, Gdalevich M, et al. Effect of closure versus nonclosure of peritoneum at cesarean section on adhesions: a prospective randomized study. Am J Obstet Gynecol. 2012;**206**:56.e1–4.

103 Shi Z, Ma L, Yang Y, et al. Adhesion formation after previous caesarean section–a meta-analysis and systematic review. BJOG. 2011;**118**:410–22.

104 Bamigboje AA, Hofmeyr GJ. Closure versus non-closure of the peritoneum at cesarean section. Cochrane Database Syst Rev. 2003;**4**:CD000163. DOI: 10.1002/14651858.CD000163.

105 Rafique Z, Shibli KU, Russell LF, et al. A randomised controlled trial of the closure or non-closure of peritoneum at caesarean section: effect on post-operative pain. BJOG. 2002;**109**:694–8.

106 Zareian Z, Zareian P. Non-closure versus closure of peritoneum during caesarean section: a randomized study. Eur J Obstet Gynecol Reprod Biol. 2006;**128**: 267–9.

107 Lyell DJ, Caughy AB, Hu E, et al. Peritoneal closure at primary cesarean delivery and adhesions. Obstet Gynecol. 2005;**106**:275–80.

108 Anderson ER, Gates S. Techniques and materials for closure of the abdominal wall in caesarean section. Cochrane Database Syst Rev. 2004;**4**:CD004663. DOI: 10.1002/14651858.CD004663.pub2.

109 Gaertner I, Burkhardt T, Beinder E. Scar appearance of different skin and subcutaneous tissue closure techniques in caesarean section: a randomized study. Eur J Obstet Gynecol Reprod Biol. 2008;**138**:29–33.

110 Alderdice F, McKenna D, Dorman J. Techniques and materials for skin closure in caesarean section (Cochrane Review). In: The Cochrane Library Issue 2. Chichester, UK: John Wiley & Sons, Ltd, 2004.

111 Clay FSH, Walsh CA, Walsh SR. Staples vs subcuticular sutures for skin closure at cesarean delivery: a metaanalysis of randomized controlled trials. Am J Obstet Gynecol. 2011;**202**:378–83.

112 Rousseau J-A, Girard K, Turcot-Lemay L, Thomas N. A randomized study comparing skin closure in cesarean sections: staples vs subcuticular sutures. Am J Obstet Gynecol. 2009;**200**:265.e1–4.

113 Ferrari AG, Frigero LG, Candotti G, et al. Can Joel-Cohen incision and single layer reconstruction reduce cesarean section morbidity? Int J Obstet Gynecol. 2001;**72**:135–43.

114 Mathai M, Hofmeyr GJ. Abdominal surgical incisions for caesarean section. Cochrane Database Syst Rev. 2007;**1**:CD004453. DOI: 10.1002/14651858. CD004453.pub2.

115 Hofmeyr GJ, Mathai M, Shah AN, et al. Techniques for caesarean section. Cochrane Database Syst Rev. 2008;**1**:CD004662. DOI: 10.1002Z14651858. CD004662.pub2.

116 Joura EA, Nather A, Husslein P. Non-closure of peritoneum and adhesions: the repeat caesarean section (letter). Acta Obstet Gynecol Scand. 2001;**80**;286.

117 Wechter ME, Pearlman MD, Hartmann KE. Reclosure of the disrupted laparotomy wound: a systematic review. Obstet Gynecol. 2005;**106**:376–83.

118 Hansen AK, Wisborg K, Uldbjerg N, et al. Elective caesarean section and respiratory morbidity in the term and near-term neonate. Acta Obstet Gynecol Scand. 2007;**86**:389–94.

119 Gerten KA, Coonrod DV, Bay RC, et al. Cesarean delivery and respiratory distress syndrome: does labor make a difference? Am J Obstet Gynecol. 2005;**193**:1061–4.

120 LeRay C, Boithias C, Castaigne-Meary V, et al. Caesarean before labour between 34 and 37 weeks: what are the risk factors of severe neonatal repiratory distress? Eur J Obstet Gynecol Reprod Biol. 2006;**127**:56–60.

121 van den Berg A, van Elburg RM, van Geijn HP, et al. Neonatal respiratory morbidity following elective caesarean section in term infants: a 5-year retrospective study and a review of the literature. Eur J Obstet Gynecol Reprod Biol. 2001;**98**:9–13.

122 Jain L, Dudell GG. Respiratory transition in infants delivered by cesarean section. Semin Perinatol. 2006;**30**:296–304.

123 Morrison JJ, Rennie JM, Milton PJ. Neonatal respiratory failure after elective repeat cesarean delivery: a potential preventable condition leading to extracorporal membrane oxygenation. Br J Obstet Gynaecol. 1995;**102**:101–6.

124 Hansen AK, Wisborg K, Uldbjerg N, et al. Risk of respiratory morbidity in term infants delivered by elective caesarean section: cohort study. BMJ. 2008;**236**:85–7.

125 Kolas T, Saugstad OD, Daltveit AK, et al. Planned cesarean versus planned vaginal delivery at term: comparison of newborn infant outcomes. Am J Obstet Gynecol. 2006;**195**:1538–43.

126 Stutchfield P, Whitaker R, Russell I. Antenatal betamethasone and incidence of neonatal respiratory distress after elective caesarean section: pragmatic randomized trial. BMJ. 2005;**331**:662.

127 Smith J, Plaat F, Fisk NM. The natural caesarean: a women-centered technique. BJOG. 2008;**115**:1037–42.

128 Faiz AS, Annath CV. Etiology and risk factors for placenta previa: an overview and meta-analysis of observational studies. J Matern Fetal Neonatal Med. 2003;**13**:175–90.

129 Gilliam M, Rosenberg D, Davis F. The likelihood of placenta previa with greater number of cesarean deliveries and higher parity. Obstet Gynecol. 2002;**99**:976–80.

130 Silver RM, Landon MB, Rouse RJ, et al, for the National Institute of Child Health and Human Development Maternal-Fetal Medicine Units Network. Maternal morbidity associated with multiple repeat cesarean deliveries. Am J Obstet Gynecol. 2006;**107**:1126–32.

131 Mozurkewich EL, Hutton EK. Elective repeat cesarean delivery versus trial of labor: a meta-analysis of the literature from 1989 to 1999. Am J Obstet Gynecol. 2000;**183**:1187–97.

132 Smith GCS, Peil JP, Dobbie R. Caesarean section and risk of unexplained stillbirth in subsequent pregnancy. *Lancet*. 2003;**362**:1779–84.

133 Salihu MH, Sharma PP, Kristensen S, et al. Risk of stillbirth following a cesarean delivery. Obstet Gynecol. 2006;**107**:383–90.

134 Smith GC, Peil JP, Cameron AD, et al. Risk of perinatal death associated with labor after previous cesarean delivery in uncomplicated term pregnancies. J Am Med Assoc. 2002;**287**:2684–90.

135 Smith GCS, Wood AM, Peil JP, et al. First cesarean birth and subsequent fertility. Fertil Steril. 2006;**85**: 90–5.

136 Katz V, Balderston K, DeFreest M. Perimortem cesarean delivery: were our assumptions correct? Am J Obstet Gynecol. 2005;**192**:1916–21.

137 Su LL, Chong YS, Samuel M. Oxytocin agonists for preventing postpartum hemorrhage. Cochrane Database Syst Rev. 2007;**3**:CD005457. DOI: 10.1002/14651858.CD005457.

Chapter

13

Sphincter Injury

M. Weemhoff, C. Willekes, and M.E. Vierhout

General Information

Introduction

It is very important to properly diagnose and repair sphincter injuries, as there is a significant chance of long-term morbidity. After a sphincter injury, women often suffer from emotional, physical, and/or sexual problems. Even after optimal (peri)operative care there are still many residual symptoms and complications. The care for this patient group is therefore of great importance, not only immediately after the childbirth, but also in the long term and when counseling towards a new pregnancy. The goal of this chapter is to provide the information that is essential to achieve this care.

Definition

Sphincter injury (synonyms: third- or fourth-degree tears, complete tear) is defined as a tear involving the anal sphincters.

Prevalence

The prevalence of sphincter injuries was 2% in a Dutch study analyzing 284 783 deliveries in a national database [LE B].[1] However, recent studies show a much higher percentage. In a 2006 study, 251 postpartum primiparas were examined by the person who supervised the delivery and by an expert. In 24.5% of the deliveries a sphincter injury was diagnosed. There was a large difference between the physical examination performed by the person who had supervised the delivery (11%), and the expert (24.5%) [LE B].[2] This study shows the importance of good training in diagnosing sphincter injuries. Sphincter injuries will only heal properly if the injury is recognized and acknowledged in a timely manner.

Anatomy and Function

Anatomy

The anal sphincter complex consists of the external anal sphincter (EAS) and the internal anal sphincter (IAS) (Figure 13.1). These two sphincter components are separated from each other by a thin fibromuscular longitudinal layer, which is an extension of the longitudinal smooth muscle of the rectum and the internal transverse muscle fibers of the anal levator muscle. The internal anal sphincter is a widened extension of the circular smooth muscle layer of the intestine. Macroscopically, the internal anal sphincter has a pale aspect and can be distinguished from the red external anal sphincter. The difference in color can be described as the color of chicken meat versus the color of red beefsteak.

Alongside the sphincter there is ischioanal fat, which can serve as a marker to confirm that the structure is part of the sphincter. The external anal sphincter has a length of approximately 2 cm. In women, the external anal sphincter is thinner on the ventral side than on the dorsal side. On the anterior side, the muscle fibers of the anal sphincter are connected to the muscle fibers of the bulbospongiosus muscle and to the coccyx on the posterior side.

Besides the anal sphincter complex, the puborectal muscle is also important in maintaining continence (see Figure 13.3). The puborectal muscle is the most caudal part of the anal levator muscle. The puborectal fibers run from the rear of the pubic bone and from the tendinous arch in a loop around the rectum and are responsible for the formation of the anorectal angle.

Innervation

Since the involuntary internal anal sphincter is a continuation of the circular muscle fibers of the rectum, it has the same innervation from the cranial

Obstetric Interventions, ed. P. Joep Dörr, Vincent M. Khouw, Frank A. Chervenak, Amos Grunebaum, Yves Jacquemyn, and Jan G. Nijhuis. Published by Cambridge University Press. © Cambridge University Press 2017.

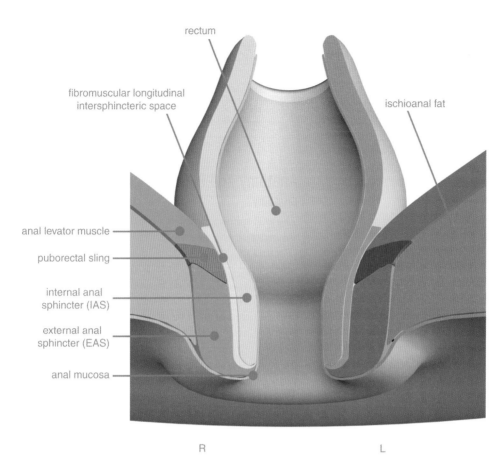

rectum

fibromuscular longitudinal
intersphincteric space

ischioanal fat

anal levator muscle

puborectal sling

internal anal
sphincter (IAS)

external anal
sphincter (EAS)

anal mucosa

R   L

Figure 13.1 Cross-section of the anal sphincter complex.

direction through sympathetic nerves of the pelvic plexus and parasympathetically from level S2–S4 via the splanchnic pelvic nerves. The voluntary external anal sphincter (striated muscle tissue) is innervated from the lateral side through rectal and sacral branches of the pudendal nerve, which comes from S2–S4. The puborectal muscle has a dual innervation through the anal levator nerve (S3–S4) on the inside and the pudendal nerve from the outside of the pelvic floor (Figure 13.2).

Continence

Stool continence takes more than a properly functioning sphincter complex. Many structures play a role in the continence mechanism. Incontinence can be a consequence of myogenic and neurogenic factors. The internal anal sphincter is in a continuous tonic contraction and determines 50–85% of the resting tonus of the anal sphincter. Injury to the internal

anal sphincter is associated with incontinence for flatus and *soiling* (unexpected leakage of small quantities of liquid stools). The external anal sphincter is also in a continuous state of tonic contraction. The external anal sphincter contributes 30% of the instinctive resting tonus through a reflex arch at the level of the cauda equina. Injury of the pudendal nerve can lead directly to incontinence problems. The puborectal sling forms the anorectal angle of almost 90°, which through contraction forms a type of functional valve action and consequently plays a role in the continence mechanism (Figure 13.3).

Risk Factors and Sphincter Injury Prevention

The most important risk factors for the occurrence of third- or fourth-degree tears are instrumental vaginal delivery, the first vaginal delivery, a large infant,

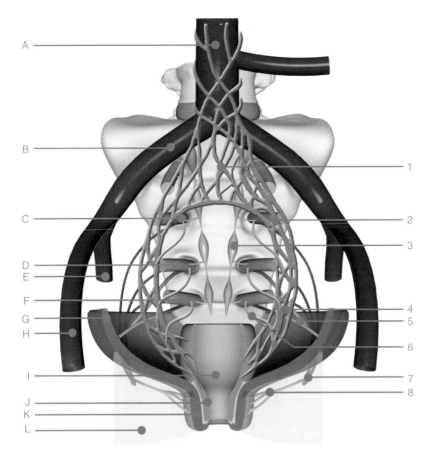

A. aorta
B. a. iliaca communis
C. S2
D. S3
E. a. iliaca interna
F. S4
G. anal levator muscle
H. a. iliaca externa
I. rectum
J. sphincter ani internus
K. sphincter ani externus
L. ischioanal fat

1. plexus hypogastricus superior
2. n. hypogastricus
3. truncus sympathicus
4. plexus pelvinus = plexus
    hypogastricus inferior
5. n. levator ani
6. nn. splanchnici pelvici
7. n. pudendus
8. nn. rectalis inferiores

Figure 13.2 Innervation of the rectum, sphincter, and anal levator muscle.

shoulder dystocia, persistent occipitoposterior position, and a perineal length less than 2.5 cm. In addition, induction of labor, prolonged labor and delivery, and a second stage longer than 1 hour are associated with third- and fourth-degree tears [LE A1/B].[3,4] All forms of operational deliveries are associated with an increased risk of sphincter injury, but forceps extraction clearly indicates the greatest

risk of sphincter injury [LE B]. Table 13.1 shows the risk factors for assisted deliveries as they were identified in an analysis of a 284 783 deliveries in a national obstetric database registry (Landelijke Verloskunde Registratie, LVR).

In contrast with a mediolateral episiotomy, a midline episiotomy is associated with an increased risk of sphincter injury [LE A1].[5] A mediolateral

Table 13.1 Risk of operational deliveries for the occurrence of sphincter injury [LE B][1]

	Performed in number of patients with sphincter injury/ performed in total number of women	OR (95% CI)
Forceps	348/7478	3.53 (3.11–4.02)
Vacuum	646/21 254	1.68 (1.52–1.86)
Fundus pressure (FP)	191/9176	1.83 (1.57–2.14)
Forceps with FP	27/522	4.62 (3.09–6.89)
Vacuum with FP	74/2661	1.78 (1.40–2.28)

Table 13.2 Classification of tears according to Sultan

Grade 1	Skin tear only
Grade 2	Skin and perineal tear with intact sphincter
Grade 3 Grade 3a Grade 3b Grade 3c	Tear to perineum and anal sphincter Tear <50% of EAS Tear >50% of EAS Tear in both the IAS and the EAS
Grade 4	Tear in perineum, anal sphincter, and anal mucosa

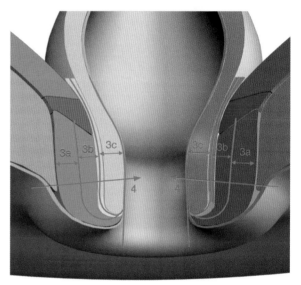

Figure 13.4 Classification of third- and fourth-degree tears.

1. symphysis
2. puborectal sling
3. axis of the rectal ampulla
4. axis of the anal canal
5. external anal sphincter

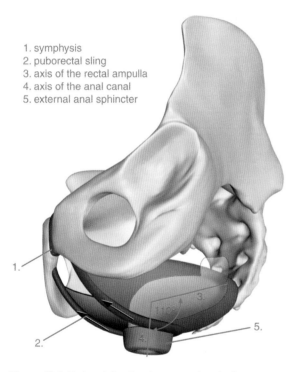

Figure 13.3 During defecation the anorectal angle changes through relaxation of the puborectal sling.

episiotomy can decrease the risk of sphincter injury (OR 0.21; 95% CI 0.19–0.23), but cannot prevent a sphincter injury in all cases [LE B].[5] The angle of the mediolateral episiotomy is important, because a greater angle of the episiotomy with respect to the midline is linked to a lower risk of sphincter injury (see also Figures 2.65–67) [LE B].[6]

Classification of Tears

In 2002, Sultan introduced a classification for perineal and sphincter tears. This classification has been adopted globally by international organizations as the standard classification (Table 13.2, Figure 13.4).[7]

In case of doubt of the classification of a third-degree tear, it is advised to choose the highest degree to avoid the risk of undertreatment.

A defect up to the anal mucosa behind the level of the sphincter, thus with an intact internal and external anal sphincter, is not classified as a fourth-degree tear, but must be described.

A rectal examination is essential for proper classification of the sphincter injury, not only to examine the anal mucosa, but also frequently stretching of the muscular fibers is needed to assess the sphincters

A
B

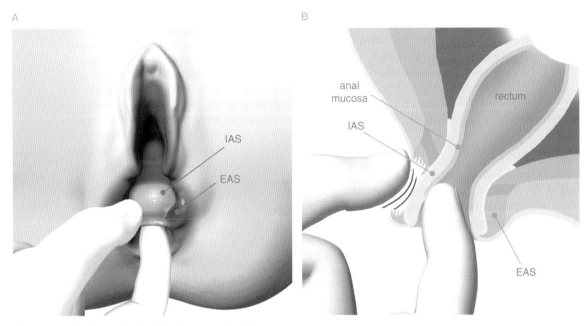

Figure 13.5 Rectal examination (A) and cross-section (B).

(Figure 13.5). In the anal examination, the index finger is in the anus and the thumb rests on the sphincter. The sphincter is palpated between the thumb and the index finger. In case of doubt, the patient may be asked to contract the anus. A defect can then be felt more clearly. A rectal examination must therefore precede any suturing.

Then, after the suturing, another rectal examination is performed to verify that there is good continuity again and to check whether the suturing caused any unintentional perforation in the mucous membrane. Reluctance to do a post-suturing rectal examination out of fear of damaging the sutures is not prudent. Obviously, this must be done with the necessary caution.

Technique

Background

There are two techniques to repair a sphincter defect: the end-to-end approximation of the sphincter and the overlapping technique, in which both sphincter halves are sutured on top of each other. In the literature there is no convincing evidence that one technique has a better outcome for the patient than the other technique [LE A1/2].[7–13] The most important aspect in the choice of technique is to choose the one

that is the most familiar to the surgeon. The disadvantage of the overlapping technique is that it cannot be used in grade 3a sphincter tears when the external sphincter is still largely intact. Surgeons using the overlapping technique in a grade 3b or higher sphincter tear must be trained and have practice in both methods, since in a grade 3a sphincter defect an end-to-end technique must always be used.

The internal and external anal sphincters each have their own function and must both be approximated in the suturing. It is therefore of utmost importance to identify the internal and external anal sphincters when closing the sphincter and to ensure the proper closure of both sphincters.

Some authors recommend closing the internal and external sphincters separately[12,14]; however, there is no supporting convincing evidence in the literature for this. To close the internal anal sphincter separately, both sphincter halves must be dissected. This can be technically difficult, with additional chances of complications and, in case of insufficient experience, even a risk of additional damage to the thin and delicate internal sphincter.

It is recommended to perform a sphincter repair under optimal conditions; this means, with good lighting and adequate pain management. These conditions are usually optimal in an operating room.

Until now, studies have not shown a difference in the outcome of fecal incontinence when a complete tear is repaired immediately after the delivery, compared to a repair done 8 to 12 hours after the delivery.[15] In such cases the disadvantage of waiting to repair the complete tear may be weighed against the advantage of asking a more experienced gynecologist to perform or supervise the operation.

Suturing Procedure

A grade 3a tear, in which the external anal sphincter is damaged by <50%, is closed with the end-to-end method. In a grade 3b tear or higher, either the end-to-end method or the overlapping technique may be used. In cases where the overlapping technique is chosen, the remaining fibers of the external sphincter that are still intact must be cut in order to be able to perform an overlap.

In higher stage sphincter defects, one half of the sphincter is often retracted into the muscle's fibrous capsule. On both sides, the internal and external anal sphincters are identified and grasped with Allis clamps. Besides Allis clamps, other atraumatic clamps can be used, such as Duval clamps.

Anal Mucosa

The anal mucosa is loosely sutured with the knots placed intraluminally (Figure 13.6). The most important argument for this is that the amount of foreign bodies in the tissue will be limited as much as possible and thereby provide the least chance of infection. The mucosa can also be sutured continuously. Locked sutures are preferred to prevent retraction of the mucous membrane.

Internal Anal Sphincter

The internal anal sphincter is sutured with side-by-side mattress sutures (Figure 13.7). The importance of using mattress sutures lies in the transverse traction orientation in a longitudinal muscle to prevent tearing.

External Anal Sphincter

It is important to view and approximate the entire length of the anal sphincter. This determines the length of the anal canal, which influences its resting tone and the risk of fecal incontinence [LF C].[16] If the entire length of the muscle is not approximated, the functional result will be inferior.

End-to-End Technique

The end-to-end technique for suturing the external anal sphincter is accomplished with *figure-of-eight* sutures or mattress sutures. With mattress sutures there is nevertheless a short overlap of the approximated muscle halves. Figure-of-eight sutures constitute real end-to-end suturing. Both methods have their pros and cons and the surgeon is free to decide on the method with which he or she is most familiar (Figure 13.8).

Detailed Description of End-to-End Technique: Figure-of-Eight

In the end-to-end technique, the figure-of-eight sutures are placed as follows (Figure 13.9):

- First, both sphincter halves are identified and atraumatic clamps are placed (Figure 13.9A).
- Suturing starts with the left half of the sphincter. The suture enters the top 1 cm from the edge and comes out at the bottom (Figure 13.9B). Then a switch is made to the right sphincter half. The suture enters the bottom 1 cm from the edge and comes out the top (Figure 13.9C). Next, another switch is made to the left sphincter half and there, 1 cm next to the previous stitch, again 1 cm from the edge, in at the top and out at the bottom (Figure 13.9D). Again a switch to the right sphincter half and the suture 1 cm next to the other stitch, 1 cm from the edge, in from the bottom and out the top (Figure 13.9E). This results

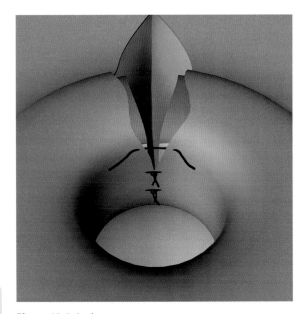

Figure 13.6 Anal mucosa.

A

B

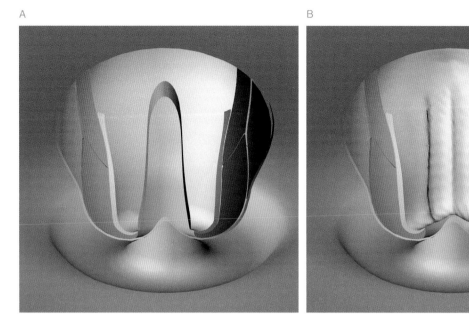

Figure 13.7A–B Internal anal sphincter.

A

B

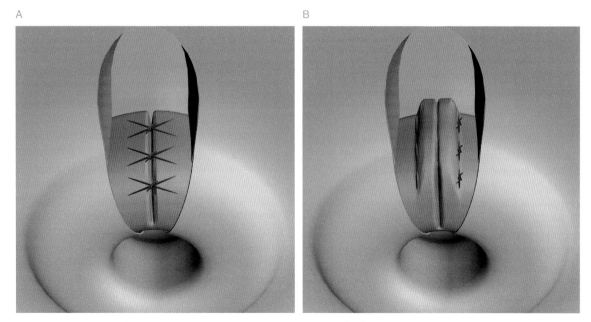

Figure 13.8 External anal sphincter in the end-to-end technique. (A) Figure-of-eight sutures. (B) Mattress sutures.

in sutures with two parallel lines at the bottom and a figure-of-eight at the top (Figure 13.9F).
- Two or three sutures are placed next to each other with a distance of 0.5 cm between them.

- After the sutures are placed, the clamps can be removed and the sutures can be tied.
- An overview of the situation after placing all of the sutures is illustrated in Figure 13.9G.

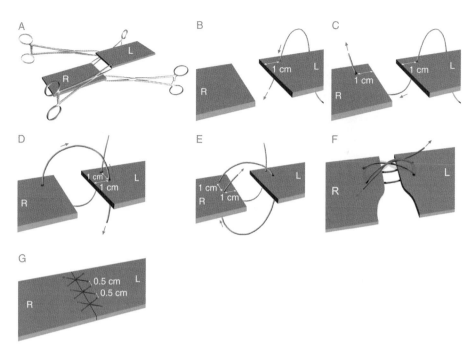

Figure 13.9A–G End-to-end technique, figure-of-eight suturing.

Detailed Description of End-to-End Technique: Mattress Sutures

In the end-to-end technique, mattress sutures are placed as follows (Figure 13.10):

- First, both sphincter halves are identified and atraumatic clamps are placed (Figure 13.10A).
- Suturing starts with the left half of the sphincter. The suture enters the top 1 cm from the edge and comes out at the bottom (Figure 13.10B). Then a switch is made to the right sphincter half. The suture enters the bottom 1 cm from the edge and comes out the top (Figure 13.10C). Next, the suture is inserted into the right sphincter half 0.5 cm next to the other stitch, 1 cm from the edge, in at the top and out at the bottom (Figure 13.10D). Again a switch to the left sphincter half and there 0.5 cm next to the previous stitch, again 1 cm from the edge, in from the bottom and out the top (Figure 13.10E).
- Two or three sutures are placed next to each other with a distance of 0.5 cm between them.
- After the sutures are placed, the clamps can be removed and the sutures can be tied.
- An overview of the situation after placing all of the sutures is illustrated in Figure 13.10F.

The Overlapping Technique

In the overlapping technique, the muscle halves that are grasped by the Allis clamps are placed over the top of each other, so that the sutures can be placed in the correct location. It is preferable to place three overlapping sutures next to each other (Figure 13.11).

Detailed Description of the Overlapping Technique

In the overlapping technique the sutures are placed as follows (Figure 13.12A–F and Animation 13.1):

- First, both sphincter halves are identified and atraumatic clamps are attached (Figure 13.12A).
- Suturing starts with the left half of the sphincter. The suture enters the top, 2 cm from the edge and comes out the bottom. Then a switch is made to the right sphincter half. The suture enters the top, 1 cm from the edge and comes out the bottom. After that, the suture enters the bottom of the right sphincter half and comes out the top in order to finish again in the left sphincter half, entering from the bottom and coming out the top (Figure 13.12B).
- Preferably, three stitches are made next to each other with a distance of 0.5 cm between them (Figure 13.12C).
- After the three sutures are placed, the clamps can be removed and the sutures can be tightened and tied, so that the two sphincter halves are pulled on top of each other (Figure 13.12D).
- Then, a second row is placed with support stitches. These go into the top 1 cm from the edge of the left

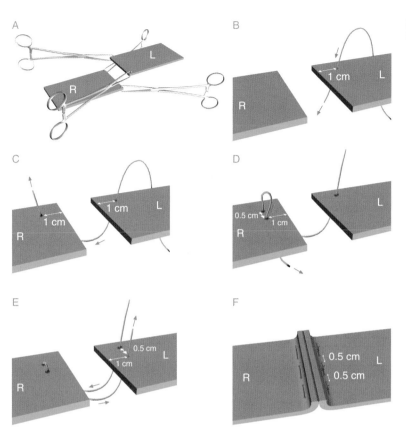

Figure 13.10A–F End-to-end technique, mattress sutures.

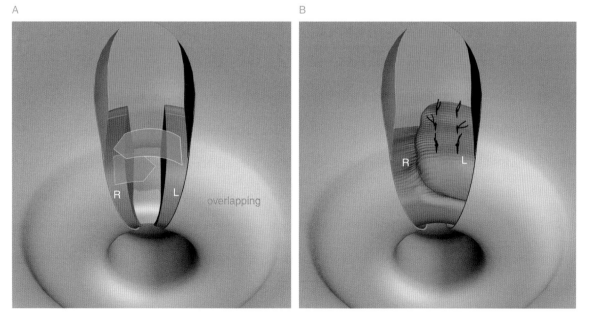

Figure 13.11 (A) Overview of the external anal sphincter in a grade 3b tear. (B) Overview of the location of the sutures after an overlap repair of a grade 3b tear.

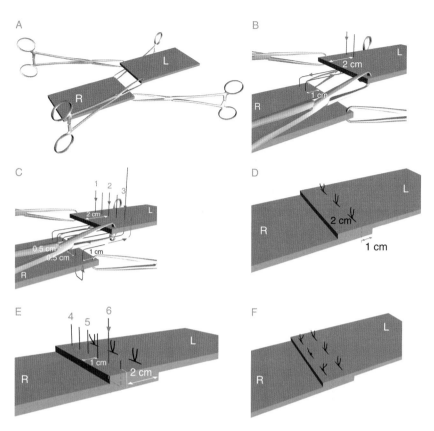

Figure 13.12A–F Detail of suturing with the overlapping technique.

sphincter half and come out the bottom. Then, 2 cm from the edge a firm transverse *bite* is taken into the right sphincter half, coming out the top. Then, the suture is finished in the left sphincter half, entering from below and coming out on top (Figure 13.12E).

- An overview of the situation after placing all of the sutures is illustrated in Figure 13.12F.

Perineum

When suturing the perineum it is important to build up the perineal body with loose or continuous sutures. The chance of a new sphincter injury is partially determined by the quality of the perineal body and the length of the perineum. To build up the perineal body, it is recommended, after suturing the sphincter, to place some additional support sutures in the bottom of the tear before approximating the bulbospongiosus muscle, the urethrovaginal muscle, and the transverse perineal muscle, as in a second-degree tear. The skin is sutured intracutaneously.

Suturing Material

The anal mucosa is sutured with atraumatic polyglactin 910, polyglycolic acid, or a comparably absorbable material with a thickness of 3–0. The internal and the external anal sphincters are sutured with polydioxanone (PDS) 3–0 or other comparable monofilament, slowly dissolvable material. An atraumatic and monofilament suture is preferred in view of infections. The sphincter must be sutured with dissolvable material since non-dissolvable sutures can lead to abscess formation. The tensile strength and reabsorption time must be sufficiently long for proper healing of the sphincter. Sharp ends of sutures can cause irritation and must therefore be cut short and must be covered with a good protective layer. The perineum and the skin must be sutured with polyglactin 910, polyglycolic acid, or comparable rapidly absorbable material with a thickness of 2–0 or 3–0.

Antibiotics

According to the surgical wound classification (according to Mayhall), a third-degree tear is considered to be a "contaminated wound" and a fourth-degree tear is a "dirty wound" because of the contamination with fecal matter.[17] Treatment with antibiotics is advised in both cases. An infection causes a risk of wound problems and a chance of developing incontinence or fistula formation; therefore, it is not prudent to withhold treatment with antibiotics [LE A1].[17] If the total tear is repaired immediately after childbirth, a single pre-operative dose of antibiotics will be sufficient. If the repair time of the tear is more than 3 hours, a repeated dose of antibiotics should be considered. Prophylaxis for more than 24 hours is not advisable and causes unnecessary disturbance of the microbial flora [LE A1].[17] Antibiotics must be administered immediately after the sphincter injury is diagnosed. Therefore, the antibiotics must be administered in the delivery room and not wait until getting to the operating room.

Postoperative Phase

Postoperative Management

- *Laxatives:* it is advised to prescribe laxatives for several weeks [LE D].[12] Lactulose can lead to intestinal gas formation, which may cause flatulence and false defecation pressure. In that case, macrogol/electrolytes or magnesium hydroxide is preferred. If defecation does not occur, there is a risk of bolus formation, with the possible result of severe anal dilatation. Where defecation does not occur, enemas are recommended.
- *Pain relief:* paracetamol and NSAIDs are the medicines of first choice when pain relief is needed. Preparations with codeine must be avoided, as they may cause constipation.
- *Pelvic floor exercises:* the advice is to start pelvic floor physiotherapy or pelvic floor exercises after a few weeks [LE D].[13]

Follow-Up and Consequences of Sphincter Injuries

Follow-Up

The follow-up must be longer than only one postpartum check-up. If a patient has residual symptoms of fecal incontinence, it is important to refer her to a pelvic floor physiotherapist, provide dietary measures, perform additional diagnostic testing by means of ultrasound imaging and ultimately refer the patient to a colorectal surgeon or urogynecologist.

Complications: Postpartum and Late Consequences

Recent studies show that after 12 months of follow-up, 60–80% of the patients are asymptomatic [LE A2].[12]

Frequent complaints after a sphincter injury are: perineal pain, dyspareunia, wound dehiscence, rectovaginal fistulas, and most importantly, incontinence for flatulence and feces and fecal *urgency.*[12,18,19] There are many women suffering from a persistent sphincter defect despite primary recovery, who initially do not have any symptoms [LE C].[20–22] Young women can compensate quite well with the residual sphincter fibers and the puborectal sling. Nevertheless, these women have an insecure future since the anal sphincter function deteriorates with age due to prolonged conduction times of the pudendal nerve and fibrosis ring of the internal and external anal sphincter. A large section of women with a sphincter defect only develop symptoms at a later age.

Management of Subsequent Pregnancies

The literature provides little data for providing *evidence-based* guidelines for managing subsequent pregnancies after prior sphincter injury.[12,13]

Ninety-five percent of the women with a sphincter injury do not experience a new sphincter injury during a subsequent pregnancy [LE C].[23] The risk of having a (transitory) deterioration of fecal symptoms after a subsequent pregnancy varies in the studies from 17% to 24% [LE C].[12,13] This risk is not only caused by further damage of the sphincter, but can also arise due to further neurogenic compromise because of engagement of the fetal head during pregnancy and delivery. Especially women who after their first childbirth had a transitory period of fecal incontinence run an increased risk of worsening symptoms after a subsequent childbirth [LE C].[24]

A number of recommendations can be formulated for a subsequent pregnancy [LE D][12,13]:

- In patients *without residual symptoms* there are insufficient reasons for advising against a vaginal delivery after a sphincter injury. Counseling on the risk of developing symptoms should be offered. If an episiotomy is indicated, a mediolateral episiotomy with a sufficiently large angle of 45° to 60° from the vertical midline must be made. There is insufficient evidence that a routine episiotomy can prevent a recurrence of sphincter injury and therefore should only be performed on the indication of risk factors.

- Women who continue to have *(temporary) residual symptoms* after a sphincter injury and women with mild residual symptoms should be counseled that a subsequent vaginal delivery has a risk of compromised sphincter function. Upon proper counseling a choice should be made for a vaginal delivery or an elective cesarean section.
- In *serious persistent symptoms* of fecal incontinence and a demonstrable sphincter defect there is an indication of secondary reconstructive surgery. If women still have a clear desire to have children, it may be contemplated to avoid the risk of a cesarean section by first delivering vaginally and only then do a reconstruction. The risk that further damage in a subsequent delivery will influence the result after a secondary sphincter reconstruction appears to be minimal on theoretical grounds.
- *After reconstructive surgery* of a sphincter, a cesarean section is indicated.

Important Points and Recommendations

- Training in diagnosing, classifying, and repairing sphincter injuries is of great importance. Repairing an injury is only done after precise diagnosis [LE B].
- All forms of operative deliveries are associated with an increased risk of sphincter injury, in which forceps extraction clearly indicates the greatest risk of sphincter injury. Considering the major avoidable risk of a sphincter injury, forceps extraction should be performed with reservation [LE B].
- The overlapping technique is just as effective as the end-to-end technique. It is therefore recommended to choose the technique which is the most familiar to the surgeon.
- Of all patients with a sphincter injury, 60–80% are asymptomatic after 12 months [LE A2]. Of all patients with a sphincter injury, 95% have no recurrent sphincter injury during the next childbirth [LE C].
- Recommendations for the next pregnancy are [LE D]:
  - *no residual symptoms:* no contraindication for vaginal delivery, counseling regarding the risk of recurrent symptoms, episiotomy on indication of risk factors;
  - *residual symptoms (temporary):* counseling on the risk of a compromised sphincter function after a subsequent delivery, consultation between the woman and the gynecologist about vaginal delivery versus elective cesarean section;
  - *serious residual symptoms:* if an indication for reconstructive surgery, first vaginal delivery, then reconstruction;
  - *after reconstructive surgery:* elective cesarean section.

References

1 Leeuw JW de, Struijk PC, Vierhout ME, et al. Risk factors for third degree perineal ruptures during delivery. BJOG. 2001;**108**(4):383–7.

2 Andrews V, Sultan AH, Thakar R, et al. Occult anal sphincter injuries – myth or reality? BJOG. 2006;**113**:195–200.

3 Eason E, Labrecque M, Wells G, et al. Preventing perineal trauma during childbirth: a systematic review. Obstet Gynecol. 2000;**95**(3):464–71.

4 Sultan AH, Kamm MA, Hudson CN, et al. Third degree obstetric anal sphincter tears: risk factors and clinical outcome of primary repair. BMJ. 1994;**308**:887–91.

5 Carroli G, Belizan J. Episiotomy for vaginal birth (Cochrane Review). The Cochrane Library Issue 3, 2004. Chichester, UK: John Wiley & Sons, Ltd.

6 Eogan M, Daly L, O'Connell PR, et al. Does the angle of episiotomy affect the incidence of anal sphincter injury? BJOG. 2006;**113**:190–4.

7 Fernando R, Sultan AH, Kettle C, et al. Methods of repair for obstetric anal sphincter injury. Cochrane Database Syst Rev. 2008;**3**:CD002866.

8 Williams A, Adams EJ, Tincello DG, et al. How to repair an anal sphincter injury after vaginal delivery: results of a randomized controlled trial. BJOG. 2006;**113**(2):201–7.

9 Farrell SA, Gilmour D, Turnbull GK, et al. Overlapping compared with end-to-end repair of third- and fourth-degree obstetric anal sphincter tears: a randomized controlled trial. Obstet Gynecol. 2010;**116**(1):16–24.

10 Fernando R, Sultan AH, Kettle C, Thakar R, Radley S. Methods of repair for obstetric anal sphincter injury. Cochrane Database Syst Rev. 2013;**12**:CD002866. DOI: 10.1002/14651858.CD002866.pub3.

11 Rygh AB, Korner H. The overlap technique versus end-to-end approximation technique for primary repair of obstetric anal sphincter rupture: a randomized controlled study. Acta Obstet Gynecol Scand. 2010;**89**(10):1256–62.

12 Fernando RJ, Williams AA, Adams EJ. The management of third- and fourth-degree perineal tears. RCOG Green-top Guideline 2007;**29**.

13 Richtlijn NVOG. Totaal Ruptuur. 2013. http://richtlij nendatabase.nl/richtlijn/totaalruptuur/risicofactoren_ en_preventie_van_totaalruptuur.html

14 Lindqvist PG, Jernetz M. A modified surgical approach to women with obstetric anal sphincter tears by separate suturing of external and internal anal sphincter. A modified approach to obstetric anal sphincter injury. BMC Pregnancy Childbirth. 2010;**10**:51.

15 Nordenstam J, Mellgren A, Altman D, López A, Zetterström J. Immediate or delayed repair of obstetric anal sphincter tears – a randomized controlled trial. BJOG. 2008;**115**:857–65.

16 Hooi GR, Lieber ML, Church JM. Postoperative anal canal length predicts outcome in patients having sphincter repair for fecal incontinence. Dis Colon Rectum. 1999;**42**(3):313–18.

17 van Kasteren MEE, Gijssens IC, Kullberg BJ, et al. Optimaliseren van het antibioticabeleid in Nederland. V. SWAB-richtlijnen voor perioperatieve antibiotische profylaxe. Ned Tijdschr Geneeskd. 2000;**144**(43): 2049–55.

18 Fernando R, Sultan AH, Kettle C, et al. Repair techniques for obstetric anal sphincter injuries: a randomized controlled trial. Obstet Gynecol. 2006;**107**:1261–8.

19 Sultan AH, Thakar R, Fenner DE. Perineal and anal sphincter trauma. London: Springer, 2007.

20 Pinta TM, Kylanpaa ML, Salmi TK, et al. Primary sphincter repair: are the results of the operation good enough? Dis Colon Rectum. 2004;**47**(1):18–23.

21 Mackenzie N, Parry L, Tasker M, et al. Anal function following third degree tears. Colorectal Dis. 2004;**6**(2):92–6.

22 Goffeng AR, Andersch B, Andersson M, et al. Objective methods cannot predict anal incontinence after primary repair of extensive anal tears. Acta Obstet Gynecol Scand. 1998;**77**(4):439–43.

23 Harkin R, Fitzpatrick M, O'Connell PR, et al. Anal sphincter disruption at vaginal delivery: is recurrence predictable? Eur J Obstet Gynecol Reprod Biol. 2003;**109**(2):149–52.

24 Bek KM, Laurberg S. Risk of anal incontinence from subsequent vaginal deliveries after a complete obstetric anal sphincter tear. Br J Obstet Gynaecol. 1992;**99**: 724–6.

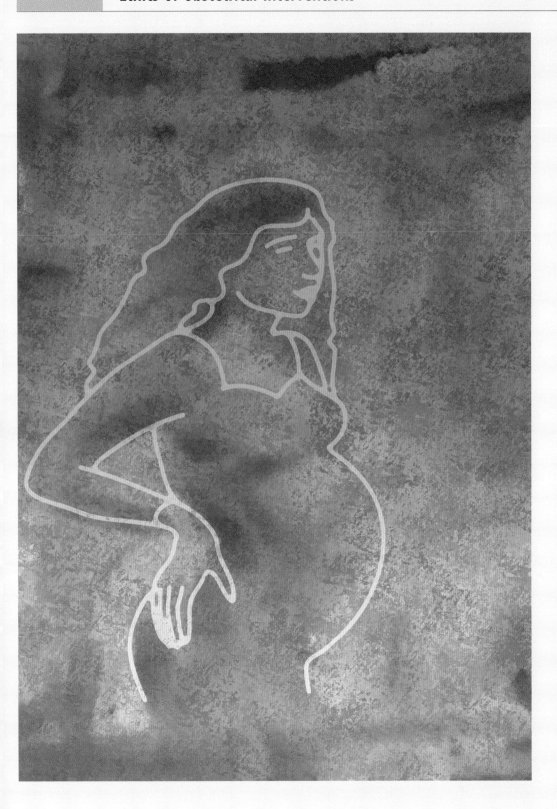

Ethical Dimensions of Obstetrical Interventions

F.A. Chervenak, A. Grunebaum, and L.B. McCullough

Introduction

Ethics is an essential dimension of obstetrical intervention.[1-3] In this chapter, we therefore develop a framework for clinical judgment and decision-making about the ethical dimensions of obstetrical interventions. We emphasize a preventive ethics approach that appreciates the potential for ethical conflict and adopts ethically justified strategies to prevent those conflicts from occurring by use of the informed consent process. Preventive ethics helps to build and sustain a strong physician–patient relationship.

We begin by defining ethics, medical ethics, and the fundamental ethical principles of medical ethics, beneficence, and respect for autonomy. The central ethical challenge for obstetrical interventions is an adequate informed consent process. We therefore show how these two ethical principles should shape the informed consent process between the obstetrician and the pregnant woman, identifying the appropriate roles for each.

Key Concepts

Medical Ethics

Ethics is the disciplined study of morality that aims to provide practical guidance in our lives. Medical ethics is the disciplined study of morality in medicine and provides practical guidance to physicians by identifying their obligations to patients as well as the obligations of patients.[4] It is important not to confuse medical ethics with the many sources of morality in modern pluralistic societies. These include, but are not limited to, law, history, the world's religions, ethnic and cultural traditions, families, the traditions and practices of medicine (including medical education and training), and personal experience. Medical ethics

since the eighteenth century European and American Enlightenments has been secular.[5] It makes no reference to God or revealed tradition, but to results of argument-based reasoning. At the same time, secular medical ethics is not intrinsically hostile to religious beliefs. Therefore, ethical principles and virtues should be understood to apply to all physicians, regardless of their personal religious and spiritual beliefs.[6] Secular medical ethics has the distinct advantage of being transcultural and transnational.

The traditions and practices of medicine constitute an obvious source of morality for physicians. These provide an important reference point for medical ethics because they are based on the obligation to protect and promote the health-related interests of the patient. This obligation tells physicians what morality in medicine ought to be, but in very general, abstract terms. Providing a practical, clinically applicable account of this general ethical obligation is the central task of medical ethics, using ethical principles.[4]

The Ethical Principle of Beneficence

The ethical principle of beneficence in its general meaning and application requires one to act in a way that is expected reliably to produce the greater balance of benefits over harms in the lives of others.[6] To put this principle into clinical practice requires a reliable account of the benefits and harms relevant to the care of the patient, and of how those goods and harms should be reasonably balanced against each other when not all of them can be achieved in a particular clinical situation, such as a request for an elective cesarean delivery.[7] In medicine, the principle of beneficence requires the physician to act in a way that is reliably expected to produce the greater balance of clinical benefits over harms for the patient.[4]

Obstetric Interventions, ed. P. Joep Dörr, Vincent M. Khouw, Frank A. Chervenak, Amos Grunebaum, Yves Jacquemyn, and Jan G. Nijhuis. Published by Cambridge University Press. © Cambridge University Press 2017.

Beneficence-based clinical judgment has an ancient pedigree, with its first expression found in the Hippocratic Oath and accompanying texts.[8] It makes an important claim: to interpret reliably the health-related interests of the patient from medicine's perspective. This perspective is provided by the commitment to evidence-based reasoning in the deliberative practice of medicine. As rigorously evidence-based,[9] beneficence-based judgment is not the function of the individual clinical perspective of any particular physician and therefore should not be based merely on the clinical impression or intuition of an individual physician. On the basis of this rigorous clinical perspective, focused on the best available evidence, beneficence-based clinical judgment identifies the clinical benefits that can be achieved for the patient in clinical practice based on the competencies of medicine. The benefits that medicine is competent to seek for patients are the prevention and management of disease, injury, disability, and unnecessary pain and suffering, and the prevention of premature or unnecessary death. Pain and suffering become unnecessary when they do not result in achieving the other goods of medical care, e.g., allowing a woman to labor without effective analgesia.[4]

Nonmaleficence means that the physician should prevent causing harm and expresses the limits of beneficence. Nonmaleficence is better known as *"primum non nocere"* or "first do no harm." This commonly invoked dogma is really a Latinized misinterpretation of the Hippocratic texts, which emphasized beneficence while avoiding harm when approaching the limits of medicine.[4] Nonmaleficence should be incorporated into beneficence-based clinical judgment: when the physician approaches the limits of beneficence-based clinical judgment, i.e., when the evidence for expected benefit diminishes and the risks of clinical harm increase, then the physician should proceed with great caution. The physician should be especially concerned to prevent serious, far-reaching, and irreversible clinical harm to the patient.

The Ethical Principle of Respect for Autonomy

In contrast to the principle of beneficence, there has been increasing emphasis in medical ethics on the principle of respect for autonomy.[6] This principle requires the physicians to empower the decision-making role of the pregnant woman about the management of her pregnancy.

Beneficence and Respect for Autonomy in the Informed Consent Process for Obstetrical Interventions

The ethical principles of beneficence and respect for autonomy both shape the informed consent process. As to beneficence, it is important to note that there is an inherent risk of paternalism in beneficence-based clinical judgment. By this we mean that beneficence-based clinical judgment, if it is *mistakenly* considered to be the sole source of moral responsibility and therefore moral authority in medical care, invites the unwary physician to conclude that beneficence-based judgments can be imposed on the pregnant woman in violation of her autonomy. Paternalism can be experienced as a dehumanizing response to the patient and, therefore, should be avoided in the practice of obstetrics.

The preventive ethics response to this inherent paternalism is for the physician to explain the diagnostic, therapeutic, and prognostic reasoning that leads to his or her clinical judgment about what is in the interest of the patient so that the patient can assess that judgment for herself and provide consent. The practical steps for doing so are the following: The physician should disclose and explain to the patient the major factors of this reasoning process, including matters of uncertainty. In neither medical law nor medical ethics does this require that the patient be provided with a complete medical education.[10] The physician should then explain how and why other clinicians might reasonably differ from his or her clinical judgment. The physician should then present a well-reasoned response to this critique. The outcome of this process is that beneficence-based clinical judgments take on a rigor that they sometimes lack, and the process of their formulation includes explaining them to the patient. It should be apparent that beneficence-based clinical judgment can result in the identification of a continuum of obstetrical interventions that protect and promote the patient's health-related interests, when these alternatives are supported in evidence-based clinical judgment. Beneficence-based clinical judgment provides an important preventive ethics antidote to paternalism by increasing the likelihood that one or more of these medically reasonable, evidence-based alternatives will be acceptable to the patient. All beneficence-based alternatives must be identified and explained to all patients, regardless of how the physician is paid, especially those that are well established in evidence-based obstetrical interventions.

This informed consent process is also a response to the reality that pregnant women increasingly bring to their medical care their own perspectives on what is in their interest. The principle of respect for autonomy translates this fact into autonomy-based clinical judgment. Because each patient's perspective on her interests is a function of her values and beliefs, it is impossible to specify the benefits and harms of autonomy-based clinical judgment in advance. Indeed, it would be inappropriate for the physician to do so, because the definition of her benefits and harms and their balancing are the prerogative of the patient. Not surprisingly, autonomy-based clinical judgment is strongly antipaternalistic in nature.[4]

The practical steps that the pregnant woman needs to complete in the informed consent process are the following: pay attention to information that she is provided with about the progress of her labor and beneficence-based intrapartum management; absorb and retain this information; appreciate that this information does indeed apply to her; evaluate beneficence-based alternatives on the basis of her own values and beliefs; and express a value-based preference. The obstetrician needs to complete complementary steps: recognize the capacity of each pregnant woman to deal with clinical information (and not to underestimate that capacity); provide information (disclose and explain all medically reasonable alternatives, i.e., those supported in beneficence-based clinical judgment); recognize the validity of the values and beliefs of the patient; not interfere with and, when necessary, assist the patient in her evaluation and ranking of diagnostic and therapeutic alternatives for managing her condition; and elicit and implement the patient's value-based preference.[4,11]

The ethical obligations of physicians in the informed consent process and the practical steps for fulfilling these obligations were developed first in medical ethics and practice. These ethical obligations were subsequently codified into law. In the United States this process occurred in the common law, i.e., the law written by courts in deciding civil litigation, starting early in the twentieth century. In 1914, *Schloendorff v. The Society of The New York Hospital*

established the concept of simple consent, i.e., whether the patient says "yes" or "no" to surgical management of a "fibroid tumor."[10,12] This decision is frequently quoted: "Every human being of adult years and sound mind has the right to determine what shall be done with his body, and a surgeon who performs an operation without his patient's consent commits an assault for which he is liable in damages."[12] The legal requirement of consent further evolved to include disclosure of information sufficient to enable patients to make informed decisions about whether to say "yes" or "no" to medical intervention.[10] These legal developments should be interpreted as giving the force of law to best ethical practices. There is an important lesson to be learned from this history: best ethical practices in obstetrics should be fostered by obstetricians, to lead and appropriately shape the development of law and health policy.

How should the obstetrician decide on the scope of information to be provided to the pregnant woman, to ensure giving her enough information without overwhelming her with information? The reasonable person standard provides guidance, with its clinical ethical concept of "material" information: what any patient in the patient's condition needs to know and the lay person of average sophistication should not be expected to know. Patients need to know what the physician thinks is clinically salient, i.e., the physician's beneficence-based clinical judgment about obstetrical interventions such as the use of forceps versus cesarean delivery. This reasonable person should be adopted in obstetric practice. On this standard, the obstetrician should disclose to the pregnant woman information about her current condition and the medically reasonable alternatives to diagnose and manage the patient's condition, along with the clinical benefits and risks of each such alternative. When evidence-based reasoning identifies only one such alternative or when such reasoning identifies an alternative as clinically superior, it should be recommended. Making beneficence-based recommendations enhances, and does not interfere with, patient autonomy.

Conclusion

While this book emphasizes techniques of obstetrical interventions, it is apparent that the clinical application of these techniques should incorporate the ethical dimensions that we have discussed in this chapter. Specifically, obstetricians should routinely engage their pregnant patients in a decision-making process, starting with evidence-based reasoning and then shaped by both beneficence and respect for autonomy in the practical steps that we have described. In the United States and other countries throughout the world the professional liability crisis has, unfortunately, influenced physicians' behaviors in decision-making with patients.[13] While risk-reduction strategies to improve patient safety and thereby reduce professional liability are fully ethically justified,[14] the performance of unnecessary cesarean deliveries through distortion of the informed consent process is unethical and should be eschewed, as a matter of professional integrity, by obstetricians throughout the world.[13,15,16]

References

1 American College of Obstetricians and Gynecologists. Ethics in Obstetrics and Gynecology. 2nd edn. Washington, DC: American College of Obstetricians and Gynecologists; 2004.

2 Association of Professors of Gynecology and Obstetrics. Exploring Medical-legal Issues in Obstetrics and Gynecology. Washington, DC: APGO Medical Education Foundation; 1994.

3 FIGO Committee for the Study of Ethical Aspects of Human Reproduction. Recommendations of Ethical Issues in Obstetrics and Gynecology. London: International Federation of Gynecology and Obstetrics; 1997.

4 McCullough LB, Chervenak FA. Ethics in Obstetrics and Gynecology. New York, NY: Oxford University Press; 1994.

5 Engelhardt HT Jr. The Foundations of Bioethics, 2nd edn. New York, NY: Oxford University Press; 1995.

6 Beauchamp TL, Childress JF. Principles of Biomedical Ethics. 5th edn. New York, NY: Oxford University Press; 2001.

7 Chervenak FA, McCullough LB. An ethically justified algorithm for offering, recommending, and performing cesarean delivery and its application in managed care practice. Obstet Gynecol. 1996;**87**:302–5.

8 Hippocrates. Oath of Hippocrates. In: Temkin O, Temkin CL, eds. Ancient Medicine: Selected Papers of Ludwig Edelstein. Baltimore, MD: Johns Hopkins University Press; 1976:6.

9 McCullough LB, Coverdale JH, Chervenak FA. Argument-based medical ethics: a formal tool for critically appraising the normative medical ethics literature. Am J Obstet Gynecol. 2004;**191**:1097–1102.

10 Faden RR, Beauchamp TL. A History and Theory of Informed Consent. New York, NY: Oxford University Press; 1986.

11 Wear S. Informed Consent: Patient Autonomy and Clinician Beneficence within Health Care. 2nd edn. Washington, DC: Georgetown University Press; 1998.

12 Schloendorff v. The Society of The New York Hospital, 211 N.Y. 125, 126, 105 N.E. 92, 93; 1914.

13 Chervenak JL, McCullough LB, Chervenak FA. A new approach to professional liability reform: placing obligations of stakeholders ahead of their interests. Am J Obstet Gynecol. 2010;**203**:203.e1–7.

14 Grunebaum A, Chervenak F, Skupski D. Effect of a comprehensive obstetric patient safety program on compensation payments and sentinel events. Am J Obstet Gynecol. 2011;**204**:97–105.

15 Chervenak FA, McCullough LB. Neglected ethical dimensions of the professional liability crisis. Am J Obstet Gynecol. 2004;**190**:1198–200.

16 Chervenak FA, McCullough LB. Planned home birth: the professional responsibility response. Am J Obstet Gynecol. 2013;**208**:31–8.

Index

Page numbers in bold are definitions/main points.